BIOPHARMACEUTICAL SEQUENTIAL STATISTICAL APPLICATIONS

STATISTICS: Textbooks and Monographs

A Series Edited by

1. The Generalized Jackknife Statistic, *H. L. Gray and W. R. Schucany*
2. Multivariate Analysis, *Anant M. Kshirsagar*
3. Statistics and Society, *Walter T. Federer*
4. Multivariate Analysis: A Selected and Abstracted Bibliography, 1957–1972, *Kocherlakota Subrahmaniam and Kathleen Subrahmaniam*
5. Design of Experiments: A Realistic Approach, *Virgil L. Anderson and Robert A. McLean*
6. Statistical and Mathematical Aspects of Pollution Problems, *John W. Pratt*
7. Introduction to Probability and Statistics (in two parts), Part I: Probability; Part II: Statistics, *Narayan C. Giri*
8. Statistical Theory of the Analysis of Experimental Designs, *J. Ogawa*
9. Statistical Techniques in Simulation (in two parts), *Jack P. C. Kleijnen*
10. Data Quality Control and Editing, *Joseph I. Naus*
11. Cost of Living Index Numbers: Practice, Precision, and Theory, *Kali S. Banerjee*
12. Weighing Designs: For Chemistry, Medicine, Economics, Operations Research, Statistics, *Kali S. Banerjee*
13. The Search for Oil: Some Statistical Methods and Techniques, *edited by D. B. Owen*
14. Sample Size Choice: Charts for Experiments with Linear Models, *Robert E. Odeh and Martin Fox*

15. Statistical Methods for Engineers and Scientists, *Robert M. Bethea, Benjamin S. Duran, and Thomas L. Boullion*
16. Statistical Quality Control Methods, *Irving W. Burr*
17. On the History of Statistics and Probability, *edited by D. B. Owen*
18. Econometrics, *Peter Schmidt*
19. Sufficient Statistics: Selected Contributions, *Vasant S. Huzurbazar (edited by Anant M. Kshirsagar)*
20. Handbook of Statistical Distributions, *Jagdish K. Patel, C. H. Kapadia, and D. B. Owen*
21. Case Studies in Sample Design, *A. C. Rosander*
22. Pocket Book of Statistical Tables, *compiled by R. E. Odeh, D. B. Owen, Z. W. Birnbaum, and L. Fisher*
23. The Information in Contingency Tables, *D. V. Gokhale and Solomon Kullback*
24. Statistical Analysis of Reliability and Life-Testing Models: Theory and Methods, *Lee J. Bain*
25. Elementary Statistical Quality Control, *Irving W. Burr*
26. An Introduction to Probability and Statistics Using BASIC, *Richard A. Groeneveld*
27. Basic Applied Statistics, *B. L. Raktoe and J. J. Hubert*
28. A Primer in Probability, *Kathleen Subrahmaniam*
29. Random Processes: A First Look, *R. Syski*
30. Regression Methods: A Tool for Data Analysis, *Rudolf J. Freund and Paul D. Minton*
31. Randomization Tests, *Eugene S. Edgington*
32. Tables for Normal Tolerance Limits, Sampling Plans and Screening, *Robert E. Odeh and D. B. Owen*
33. Statistical Computing, *William J. Kennedy, Jr., and James E. Gentle*
34. Regression Analysis and Its Application: A Data-Oriented Approach, *Richard F. Gunst and Robert L. Mason*
35. Scientific Strategies to Save Your Life, *I. D. J. Bross*
36. Statistics in the Pharmaceutical Industry, *edited by C. Ralph Buncher and Jia-Yeong Tsay*
37. Sampling from a Finite Population, *J. Hajek*
38. Statistical Modeling Techniques, *S. S. Shapiro*
39. Statistical Theory and Inference in Research, *T. A. Bancroft and C.-P. Han*
40. Handbook of the Normal Distribution, *Jagdish K. Patel and Campbell B. Read*
41. Recent Advances in Regression Methods, *Hrishikesh D. Vinod and Aman Ullah*
42. Acceptance Sampling in Quality Control, *Edward G. Schilling*
43. The Randomized Clinical Trial and Therapeutic Decisions, *edited by Niels Tygstrup, John M Lachin, and Erik Juhl*
44. Regression Analysis of Survival Data in Cancer Chemotherapy, *Walter H. Carter, Jr., Galen L. Wampler, and Donald M. Stablein*
45. A Course in Linear Models, *Anant M. Kshirsagar*
46. Clinical Trials: Issues and Approaches, *edited by Stanley H. Shapiro and Thomas H. Louis*
47. Statistical Analysis of DNA Sequence Data, *edited by B. S. Weir*
48. Nonlinear Regression Modeling: A Unified Practical Approach, *David A. Ratkowsky*

49. Attribute Sampling Plans, Tables of Tests and Confidence Limits for Proportions, *Robert E. Odeh and D. B. Owen*
50. Experimental Design, Statistical Models, and Genetic Statistics, *edited by Klaus Hinkelmann*
51. Statistical Methods for Cancer Studies, *edited by Richard G. Cornell*
52. Practical Statistical Sampling for Auditors, *Arthur J. Wilburn*
53. Statistical Methods for Cancer Studies, *edited by Edward J. Wegman and James G. Smith*
54. Self-Organizing Methods in Modeling: GMDH Type Algorithms, *edited by Stanley J. Farlow*
55. Applied Factorial and Fractional Designs, *Robert A. McLean and Virgil L. Anderson*
56. Design of Experiments: Ranking and Selection, *edited by Thomas J. Santner and Ajit C. Tamhane*
57. Statistical Methods for Engineers and Scientists: Second Edition, Revised and Expanded, *Robert M. Bethea, Benjamin S. Duran, and Thomas L. Boullion*
58. Ensemble Modeling: Inference from Small-Scale Properties to Large-Scale Systems, *Alan E. Gelfand and Crayton C. Walker*
59. Computer Modeling for Business and Industry, *Bruce L. Bowerman and Richard T. O'Connell*
60. Bayesian Analysis of Linear Models, *Lyle D. Broemeling*
61. Methodological Issues for Health Care Surveys, *Brenda Cox and Steven Cohen*
62. Applied Regression Analysis and Experimental Design, *Richard J. Brook and Gregory C. Arnold*
63. Statpal: A Statistical Package for Microcomputers—PC-DOS Version for the IBM PC and Compatibles, *Bruce J. Chalmer and David G. Whitmore*
64. Statpal: A Statistical Package for Microcomputers—Apple Version for the II, II+, and IIe, *David G. Whitmore and Bruce J. Chalmer*
65. Nonparametric Statistical Inference: Second Edition, Revised and Expanded, *Jean Dickinson Gibbons*
66. Design and Analysis of Experiments, *Roger G. Petersen*
67. Statistical Methods for Pharmaceutical Research Planning, *Sten W. Bergman and John C. Gittins*
68. Goodness-of-Fit Techniques, *edited by Ralph B. D'Agostino and Michael A. Stephens*
69. Statistical Methods in Discrimination Litigation, *edited by D. H. Kaye and Mikel Aickin*
70. Truncated and Censored Samples from Normal Populations, *Helmut Schneider*
71. Robust Inference, *M. L. Tiku, W. Y. Tan, and N. Balakrishnan*
72. Statistical Image Processing and Graphics, *edited by Edward J. Wegman and Douglas J. DePriest*
73. Assignment Methods in Combinatorial Data Analysis, *Lawrence J. Hubert*
74. Econometrics and Structural Change, *Lyle D. Broemeling and Hiroki Tsurumi*
75. Multivariate Interpretation of Clinical Laboratory Data, *Adelin Albert and Eugene K. Harris*
76. Statistical Tools for Simulation Practitioners, *Jack P. C. Kleijnen*

77. Randomization Tests: Second Edition, *Eugene S. Edgington*
78. A Folio of Distributions: A Collection of Theoretical Quantile-Quantile Plots, *Edward B. Fowlkes*
79. Applied Categorical Data Analysis, *Daniel H. Freeman, Jr.*
80. Seemingly Unrelated Regression Equations Models: Estimation and Inference, *Virendra K. Srivastava and David E. A. Giles*
81. Response Surfaces: Designs and Analyses, *Andre I. Khuri and John A. Cornell*
82. Nonlinear Parameter Estimation: An Integrated System in BASIC, *John C. Nash and Mary Walker-Smith*
83. Cancer Modeling, *edited by James R. Thompson and Barry W. Brown*
84. Mixture Models: Inference and Applications to Clustering, *Geoffrey J. McLachlan and Kaye E. Basford*
85. Randomized Response: Theory and Techniques, *Arijit Chaudhuri and Rahul Mukerjee*
86. Biopharmaceutical Statistics for Drug Development, *edited by Karl E. Peace*
87. Parts per Million Values for Estimating Quality Levels, *Robert E. Odeh and D. B. Owen*
88. Lognormal Distributions: Theory and Applications, *edited by Edwin L. Crow and Kunio Shimizu*
89. Properties of Estimators for the Gamma Distribution, *K. O. Bowman and L. R. Shenton*
90. Spline Smoothing and Nonparametric Regression, *Randall L. Eubank*
91. Linear Least Squares Computations, *R. W. Farebrother*
92. Exploring Statistics, *Damaraju Raghavarao*
93. Applied Time Series Analysis for Business and Economic Forecasting, *Sufi M. Nazem*
94. Bayesian Analysis of Time Series and Dynamic Models, *edited by James C. Spall*
95. The Inverse Gaussian Distribution: Theory, Methodology, and Applications, *Raj S. Chhikara and J. Leroy Folks*
96. Parameter Estimation in Reliability and Life Span Models, *A. Clifford Cohen and Betty Jones Whitten*
97. Pooled Cross-Sectional and Time Series Data Analysis, *Terry E. Dielman*
98. Random Processes: A First Look, Second Edition, Revised and Expanded, *R. Syski*
99. Generalized Poisson Distributions: Properties and Applications, *P. C. Consul*
100. Nonlinear L_p-Norm Estimation, *Rene Gonin and Arthur H. Money*
101. Model Discrimination for Nonlinear Regression Models, *Dale S. Borowiak*
102. Applied Regression Analysis in Econometrics, *Howard E. Doran*
103. Continued Fractions in Statistical Applications, *K. O. Bowman and L. R. Shenton*
104. Statistical Methodology in the Pharmaceutical Sciences, *Donald A. Berry*
105. Experimental Design in Biotechnology, *Perry D. Haaland*
106. Statistical Issues in Drug Research and Development, *edited by Karl E. Peace*
107. Handbook of Nonlinear Regression Models, *David A. Ratkowsky*
108. Robust Regression: Analysis and Applications, *edited by Kenneth D. Lawrence and Jeffrey L. Arthur*
109. Statistical Design and Analysis of Industrial Experiments, *edited by Subir Ghosh*

112. Data Quality Control: Theory and Pragmatics, *edited by Gunar E. Liepins and V. R. R. Uppuluri*
113. Engineering Quality by Design: Interpreting the Taguchi Approach, *Thomas B. Barker*
114. Survivorship Analysis for Clinical Studies, *Eugene K. Harris and Adelin Albert*
115. Statistical Analysis of Reliability and Life-Testing Models: Second Edition, *Lee J. Bain and Max Engelhardt*
116. Stochastic Models of Carcinogenesis, *Wai-Yuan Tan*
117. Statistics and Society: Data Collection and Interpretation: Second Edition, Revised and Expanded, *Walter T. Federer*
118. Handbook of Sequential Analysis, *B. K. Ghosh and P. K. Sen*
119. Truncated and Censored Samples: Theory and Applications, *A. Clifford Cohen*
120. Survey Sampling Principles, *E. K. Foreman*
121. Applied Engineering Statistics, *Robert M. Bethea and R. Russell Rhinehart*
122. Sample Size Choice: Charts for Experiments with Linear Models: Second Edition, *Robert E. Odeh and Martin Fox*
123. Handbook of the Logistic Distribution, *edited by N. Balakrishnan*
124. Fundamentals of Biostatistical Inference, *Chap T. Le*
125. Correspondence Analysis Handbook, *J.-P. Benzécri*
126. Quadratic Forms in Random Variables: Theory and Applications, *A. M. Mathai and Serge B. Provost*
127. Confidence Intervals on Variance Components, *by Richard K. Burdick and Frank A. Graybill*
128. Biopharmaceutical Sequential Statistical Applications, *edited by Karl E. Peace*
129. Item Response Theory: Parameter Estimation Techniques, *by Frank B. Baker*

Additional Volumes in Preparation

Nonparametric Statistical Inference: Third Edition, Revised and Expanded, *by Jean Dickinson Gibbons and Subhabrata Chakraborti*

Design and Analysis of Bioavailability and Bioequivalence Studies, *by Shein-Chung Chow and Jen-Pei Liu*

Survey Sampling: Theory and Methods, *by Arijit Chaudhuri and Horst Stenger*

Bivariate Discrete Distribution, *by Subrahmaniam Kocherlakota and Kathleen Kocherlakota*

BIOPHARMACEUTICAL SEQUENTIAL STATISTICAL APPLICATIONS

edited by

Karl E. Peace
Biopharmaceutical Research Consultants, Inc.
Ann Arbor, Michigan

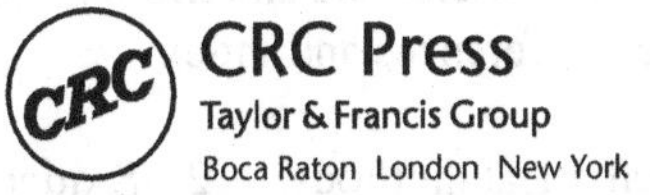

CRC Press is an imprint of the
Taylor & Francis Group, an **informa** business

First published 1992 by Marcel Dekker, Inc.

Published 2020 by CRC Press
CRC Press
Taylor & Francis Group
6000 Broken Sound Parkway NW, Suite 300
Boca Raton, FL 33487-2742

First issued in paperback 2020

ISBN 13: 978-0-367-57998-2 (pbk)
ISBN 13: 978-0-8247-8628-1 (hbk)

Visit the Taylor & Francis Web site at
http://www.taylorandfrancis.com

and the CRC Press Web site at
http://www.crcpress.com

Library of Congress Cataloging-in-Publication Data

Biopharmaceutical sequential statistical applications / edited by Karl E. Peace.
p. cm. – (Statistics, textbooks and monographs ; v. 128)
Includes bibliographical references and index.
ISBN 0-8247-8628-9
1. Drugs --Testing--Statistical methods. 2. Sequential analysis. I. Peace, Karl E. II. Series.
[DNLM: 1. Biopharmaceutics. 2. Clinical Trials. 3. Drug Evaluation. 4. Statistics. QV 771 B6153]
RM307.27.B55 1992
615'.1901'072--dc20
DNLM/DLC

92-4530
CIP

Preface

Successful drug, biological, and medical device development for human use requires aggressive, highly dedicated, competent, and diversified discovery, basic research program teams, clinical development teams, and associated research programs and clinical development plans. These programs and plans must reflect good science and adequately address requirements of regulatory agencies for approval to market.

The pharmaceutical industry is highly competitive. There are enormous pressures and incentives to make the regulatory dossier available for registrational filing as early as possible. Although speed is of the essence, speed in the absence of quality is likely to require a longer development time. Many have heard the saying "Never enough time to do it right, always enough time to do it over." Sequential statistical procedures, when incorporated into quality research and development programs, represent one way of possibly making the regulatory dossier available more rapidly.

Incorporating sequential procedures into pharmaceutical research and development programs is not to be taken lightly, nor is it without risks. Good planning, execution, monitoring, data collection and management, statistical analysis, communication and report writing skills, and resources are required.

However, each clinical development program, particularly Phase III and other large-scale clinical trials, should be assessed as to the feasibility of incorporating sequential or interim procedures. Not only may it be possible to terminate some trials (and therefore complete a clinical program earlier) on the basis of efficacy, it may be ethically imperative in some trials to be able to terminate earlier on the basis of safety or lack of efficacy.

This book presents several applications of statistical sequential procedures. Many of the applications have formed a part of New Drug Applications (NDAs) that have been approved by the Food and Drug Administration (FDA). Most of the applications are presented as case studies. *Biopharmaceutical Sequential Statistical Applications* is intended to reflect both theoretical and applied aspects of sequential statistical procedures used in the biopharmaceutical areas. A variety of sequential methods are presented, with real applications in both the preclinical and clinical areas of pharmaceutical research and development.

This book has seven parts. The first part presents the methodologic aspects of sequential procedures. The second part reflects applications to drug screening preclinical programs. The third through seventh parts reflect applications in the clinical development of drugs. Applications in anticancer clinical drug development are presented in the third part. Applications in antiviral clinical drug development are presented in the fourth part. Part five presents applications in cardiovascular clinical drug development. Applications in gastrointestinal clinical drug development appear in part six. Finally, part seven presents a variety of applications in other areas of clinical research.

The seven parts represent a total of 22 chapters, which are self-contained. The first three chapters reflect methods and are somewhat more theoretical; the remaining chapters focus attention to practical aspects of applying sequential procedures to real applications. The authors provide a background or introduction to the application or disease area, details of the protocol, details of monitoring and data collection, details of the sequential statistical analysis plan and statistical analyses, conclusions, discussion, and complete references.

Biopharmaceutical Sequential Statistical Applications is a resource for statisticians, scientists, and clinicians who desire or need to know methodological aspects of statistical, sequential procedures as they are applied in the regulated environments of pharmaceutical research and development. This book could serve as a desk or library reference, or as a textbook for graduate students in biostatistics or other targeted seminars. It will be particularly useful to preclinical scientists engaged in drug screening, namely, pharmacologists, pathologists, and toxicologists; those engaged in clinical research and development, particularly clinicians and data monitoring personnel; regulatory affairs personnel who want to know about how interim analysis may impact submissions;

and statisticians providing support to preclinical screening and clinical development programs.

I wish to express deep and sincere thanks to the 39 authors of the chapters for their remarkable and excellent contributions. Their collective efforts should have a profound impact on the future utilization and application of biopharmaceutical, sequential, statistical procedures—particularly to the preclinical screening and clinical development areas of pharmaceutical research. Special thanks go to Marcel Dekker, Inc., for interest in this project, to Dr. J. P. Hsu for reading the manuscripts, and to the secretarial staff at Biopharmaceutical Research Consultants, Inc., 4600 Stein Road, Ann Arbor, MI 48105.

Karl E. Peace

Contents

Contributors

Donald A. Berry* School of Statistics, University of Minnesota, Minneapolis, Minnesota

George J. Bosl Department of Medicine, Memorial Sloan-Kettering Cancer Center, New York, New York

Richard G. Cornell Department of Biostatistics, University of Michigan, Ann Arbor, Michigan

David D. Cuthbertson Department of Biostatistics, University of Michigan, Ann Arbor, Michigan

Robert L. Davis Clinical Biostatistics, Merck Sharp & Dohme Research Laboratories, West Point, Pennsylvania

Federico Dies Clinical Investigation and Regulatory Affairs, Lilly Research Laboratories, Eli Lilly and Company, Indianapolis, Indiana

---

Current affiliation:

*Institute of Statistics and Decision Sciences, Comprehensive Cancer Center, Duke University, Durham, North Carolina

Charles Du Mond Institute for Research Data Management, Syntex Research, Palo Alto, California

Gregory G. Enas Department of Statistical and Mathematical Sciences, Eli Lilly and Company, Indianapolis, Indiana

Nathan H. Enas Department of Statistical and Mathematical Sciences, Eli Lilly and Company, Indianapolis, Indiana

Paul I. Feder Statistics and Data Analysis Systems, Battelle, Columbus, Ohio

Nancy L. Geller Biostatistics Research Branch, National Heart, Lung, and Blood Institute, National Institutes of Health, Bethesda, Maryland

Albert J. Getson Clinical Biostatistics, Merck Sharp & Dohme Research Laboratories, West Point, Pennsylvania

Samuel V. Givens Department of Biostatistics, Hoffmann-La Roche, Inc., Nutley, New Jersey

Clare Gnecco* Department of Biostatistics, Memorial Sloan-Kettering Cancer Center, New York, New York

Celedon R. Gonzales Lilly Research Laboratories, Eli Lilly and Company, Indianapolis, Indiana

Harry Haber Department of Biometrics, Warner-Lambert/Parke-Davis Pharmaceutical Research Division, Ann Arbor, Michigan

David W. Hobson Medical Research and Evaluation Facility, Battelle, Columbus, Ohio

Irving K. Hwang Clinical Biostatistics and Research Data Systems, Merck Sharp & Dohme Research Laboratories, Rahway, New Jersey

R. L. Joiner† Applied Statistics and Computer Applications Section, Battelle, Columbus, Ohio

Kyungmann Kim Department of Biostatistics, Harvard School of Public Health, and Dana-Farber Cancer Institute, Boston, Massachusetts

Current affiliations:
*Statistical Evaluation and Research Branch, Food and Drug Administration, Rockville, Maryland
†TSI Redfield Laboratories, Redfield, Arkansas

Amy H. Lin Department of Biostatistics, Hoffmann-La Roche, Inc., Nutley, New Jersey

Katherine H. Lipschutz Clinical Biostatistics, Merck Sharp & Dohme Research Laboratories, West Point, Pennsylvania

M. Claire Matthews Statistics and Data Analysis Systems, Battelle, Columbus, Ohio

Paula K. Norwood Department of Medical Biostatistics and Data Operations, R. W. Johnson Pharmaceutical Research Institute, Raritan, New Jersey

Carl T. Olson Medical Research and Evaluation Facility, Battelle, Columbus, Ohio

Karl E. Peace Biopharmaceutical Research Consultants, Inc., Ann Arbor, Michigan

Ronald Pedersen Department of Clinical Biostatistics, Wyeth-Ayerst Research, Radnor, Pennsylvania

Kathleen J. Propert Department of Biostatistics, Harvard School of Public Health, Boston, Massachusetts

Frank W. Rockhold U.S. Medical Affairs and Clinical Development, SmithKline Beecham Pharmaceuticals, King of Prussia, Pennsylvania

Bruce E. Rodda Biostatistics and Data Management, Bristol-Myers Squibb Company, Princeton, New Jersey

Daniel J. Schaid Cancer Center Statistics, Mayo Clinic, Rochester, Minnesota

Anthony C. Segreti Department of Clinical Statistics, Burroughs Wellcome Company, Research Triangle Park, North Carolina

Weichung Joseph Shih Clinical Biostatistics and Research Data Systems, Merck Sharp & Dohme Research Laboratories, Rahway, New Jersey

Steven M. Snapinn Clinical Biostatistics and Research Data Systems, Merck Sharp & Dohme Research Laboratories, West Point, Pennsylvania

Robert R. Starbuck Department of Clinical Biostatistics and Data Management, Wyeth-Ayerst Research, Radnor, Pennsylvania

Dei-In Tang Statistical Science and Epidemiology Division, Nathan S. Kline Institute for Psychiatric Research, Orangeburg, New York

Balasamy Thiyagarajan Clinical Biostatistics and Research Data Systems, Merck Sharp & Dohme Research Laboratories, West Point, Pennsylvania

Karen L. Walton-Bowen Clinical Biostatistics and Research Data Systems, Merck Sharp & Dohme Research Laboratories, West Point, Pennsylvania

Samuel Wieand Cancer Center Statistics, Mayo Clinic, Rochester, Minnesota

BIOPHARMACEUTICAL SEQUENTIAL STATISTICAL APPLICATIONS

I

SEQUENTIAL METHODS

1

Overview of the Development of Sequential Procedures

Irving K. Hwang

Merck Sharp & Dohme Research Laboratories, Rahway, New Jersey

I. INTRODUCTION

Since Sir Austin Bradford Hill in 1946 introduced the controlled clinical trial for the Streptomycin in Tuberculosis Trials Committee of the Medical Research Council (1948), the use of double-blind, randomized, and controlled clinical trials has emerged as a principal method for the evaluation of new drugs or therapeutic procedures in medicine. Ethical and economic considerations are prominent in all clinical trials in new drug research and development. With the exception of phase I and early phase II studies, most clinical trials are multicenter studies, in which patient entry is usually sequential and staggered. There is a strong ethical or economic obligation for the sponsor or research group to review or analyze the interim data periodically for evidence of efficacy and safety over the course of the trial. As compelling evidence emerges, either favoring or disfavoring the new therapy, it may become ethically or economically necessary to terminate the trial before schedule. Although periodic evaluation of interim data is a frequent and necessary practice in drug development, particular statistical problems of multiple testing and bias do appear. Classical clinical trial designs do not formally provide the option for early termination. Rather, classical designs consider only fixed-sample-size trials. When data from a fixed-sample-size trial are analyzed repeatedly, the true type I (α, false positive) and type II (β, false negative) error probabilities associated with the testing of hypotheses will be inflated above the prespecified levels (Armitage et al., 1969; McPherson and Armitage, 1971; McPherson, 1974; Abt, 1981). For example, when we choose the conventional $\alpha = 0.05$ level for the type I error probability, the corresponding two-sided standard normal critical value will be $z = 1.96$. If this critical value were naively used for each repeated test, the true type I error probability would be inflated as follows: It will be 0.05 for testing once; 0.08, twice; 0.11, three times; 0.14, five times; 0.19, ten times; and to 0.25, twenty times, which is fivefold the true value of $\alpha = 0.05$ [see Table 2 in Armitage et al. (1969)]. To control the undesirable escalation of the true error probabilities, sequential methods were developed.

A brief overview of the development of sequential methods over the past 40 years is presented. In Section II we provide a general review of these sequential methods along with discussions on their advantages and disadvantages. These methods include the classical open and closed sequential designs, response adaptive and Bayesian approaches, group sequential methods, and pseudosequential and semi-Bayesian approaches. Technical details of these methods are not given, but extensive references are provided. The development of sequential methods has been reviewed by DeMets and Lan (1984), and more recently, by Davis and Hwang (1992) and the PMA Ad Hoc Committee on Interim Analysis (1991).

II. DEVELOPMENT OF SEQUENTIAL METHODS

A. Classical Open and Closed Sequential Designs

To control type I and type II error probabilities, Wald (1947) introduced the *sequential probability ratio test* (SPRT) to test a simple null hypothesis H_0: $\theta = \theta_0$, against a simple alternative hypothesis $H_1: \theta = \theta_1$. The SPRT is often referred to as an *open sequential design*, which needs continuous evaluation after each new observation. The procedure forms the basis for classical sequential designs, where the type I and type II error probabilities are approximately equal to α and β, respectively. It possesses certain optimal properties (Wald and Wolfowitz, 1948; Lai, 1973; Simons, 1976) that minimize the expected sample size at θ_0 and θ_1 among all tests with the same or smaller error probabilities. However, there are three major drawbacks to the SPRT that severely restrict its applications: (1) the continuation region is open and it provides no upper bound on the number of observations; (2) the expected sample size is minimized only at values of θ_0 and θ_1; and (3) it impractically requires continuous analysis of the data after each new observation.

To minimize the number of observations to test H_0 against H_1, Armitage (1957) and Anderson (1960) proposed *closed* or *restricted sequential designs*. The triangular test introduced by Anderson is a special case of the modified SPRT, which requires analysis after every outcome. The sequential designs developed by Armitage require pairing the data, one observation from each of the two groups. The patient pairs are usually formed on the basis of entry time, which are not necessarily matched on biological or medical grounds. Later, Armitage (1975) proposed *repeated significant tests* (RSTs) for paired data, based on the earlier work of Armitage et al. (1969). Since the RST boundaries are nearly identical to the closed sequential boundaries, the optimal properties are also similar. Independently, Samuel-Cahn (1974a, b, c) studied the behavior of RST in cases of uniform and normal distributions. She demonstrated that the asymptotic results remain valid when the variance is unknown under normality and in the general case of a one-parameter exponential family. Although the closed sequential design and the RST are superior to the open sequential design, their use has been limited due to the requirement for patient pairing or continuous evaluation after each new observation.

Both the open and closed sequential designs assume that patient response is immediate; these sequential methods are generally not useful for time-to-event data in mortality trials with long-term patient follow-up. Nevertheless, Breslow (1969), Breslow and Haug (1972), Koziol and Petkau (1978), Jones and Whitehead (1979), Whitehead and Jones (1979), Nagelkerke and Hart (1980), Joe et al. (1981), Whitehead and Stratton (1983), and Whitehead (1983) addressed the applications of classical sequential designs to survival data. Again, the limitations of these designs in general are patient pairing or continuous testing of data after each outcome and the need to specify an alternative in constructing stopping boundaries.

B. Response Adaptive and Bayesian Approaches

Methods were also proposed to adjust the treatment allocation sequentially based on patient response (Noel et al., 1975; Simon, 1977). The *play-the-winner rule* developed by Robbins (1952) and Zelen (1969) is one of the simpler models. Similar to their idea, Bolognese (1983) suggested the *up-and-down designs* for an early phase II dose-finding trial such that the dose range of a new test drug can be estimated. These methods all require extensive patient monitoring; the optimality and stopping rules, if they exist, are not well defined.

A wealth of literature in Bayesian framework is also available in the development of sequential methodology. The *decision theoretic approach*, which minimizes the posterior expected loss, was formulated by Anscombe (1963) and Colton (1963) for sequential medical trials. Mehta (1981) extended this approach to sequential comparison of two exponential distributions with censored data. The optimal criterion is to minimize the posterior expected regret of stopping. Cornfield (1966a, b) proposed another approach, termed *relative betting odds* (RBOs). Although the RBO approach was used by Cornfield and later explored by Lachin (1981), it has not been used extensively. Recently, Berry (1985, 1987, 1989) criticized the arbitrariness of α and β in the hypothesis testing (Neyman–Pearson) formulation and failure of frequentists to exploit a priori information. He repeatedly argued that the virtue of the Bayesian approach lies in the fact that subsequent Bayesian inferences are not affected by frequent or even continuous evaluations. However, the need to prespecify and adhere to a prior distribution on the parameters remains one of the major barriers for the adaptation of a Bayesian approach to clinical trials. Using previous trial information to develop a priori is not as straightforward as it may seem; not to mention the ever-changing patient population characteristics and medical practices. In advocating the use of the fixed-sample p-value without adjusting for sequential tests as a *pragmatic compromise,* Dupont (1983) argued that the primary use of p-values, which are most familiar and almost universally accepted in medicine, is as measures of *inferential strength.* However, Brown (1983) called it a *deliberate misusage* for not providing any necessary adjustments.

C. Group Sequential Methods

1. Ad Hoc Rules

A few ad hoc rules, which are not based on a precise theoretical model, were proposed by Haybittle (1971) and subsequently by Peto et al. (1976). The typical ad hoc rule suggests the use of a two-sided critical value of $z = 3.0$ at each interim analysis, but retains the conventional $z = 1.96$ at the final analysis. Instead, the Aspirin Myocardial Infarction Study Research Group (1980) used $z = 2.6$ as a constant boundary throughout. These ad hoc rules may be simple to use for interim analyses, but they do not precisely guarantee any prespecified type I and type II error probabilities.

2. Pocock and O'Brien–Fleming Boundaries

Instead of pairing patients, Pocock (1977) adapted Armitage's RST to develop *group sequential methods* (GSMs), which drastically changed the design and analysis of sequential clinical trials. The GSM performs repeated significance tests at longer, equally spaced intervals on equally sized groups of patients, so that the difficulty of continuous assessment of the response of each pair of patients is overcome. Pocock obtained exact results for discrete group sequential boundaries for a normal response with known variance through numerical integration using numerical quadrature for a multivariate normal distribution

(Armitage et al., 1969; Milton, 1972). Pocock demonstrated, via Monte Carlo simulations, that normal results are readily adapted to other types of response data (e.g., binomial and exponential). Independently, O'Brien and Fleming (1979) introduced different discrete group sequential boundaries for comparing two treatments when the response is both dichotomous and immediate. Whereas Pocock boundaries remain constant throughout the repeated significance tests (e.g., for $\alpha = 0.05$ and a total of $N = 3$ analyses, the two-sided boundary is 2.289 throughout), O'Brien–Fleming boundaries decrease over time (e.g., for $\alpha = 0.05$ and $N = 3$, the corresponding boundary is 3.471, 2.455, and 2.004 for the first, second, and third analysis, respectively). Although the theoretical derivations are similar for these two types of boundaries (Lan and Wittes, 1988), the stopping rules are different, resulting in quite different operating characteristics. For example, the critical value of 2.004 for the third analysis of O'Brien–Fleming boundary gives an adjusted α level of 0.045, which is only slightly smaller than 0.05, the prespecified signficance level. The penalty paid in terms of the final α for performing interim analyses is relatively small, and therefore, the use of O'Brien–Fleming-like boundaries has been popular in practice.

3. Other Developments

Subsequently, DeMets and Ware (1980, 1982), Whitehead and Stratton (1983), and Bristol (1988) developed one-sided as well as asymmetric group sequential boundaries. Pocock (1982) and McPherson (1982) examined the number of interim analyses, and Pocock (1982) suggested performing no more than five interim analyses. Gould and Pecore (1983) considered group sequential designs allowing acceptance of the null hypothesis and incorporating cost. Whitehead (1983) and Whitehead and Stratton (1983) discussed the common problems of *overshooting* and *overrunning* in group sequential trials. Whitehead and Stratton provided a comparison of group sequential designs based on RST with those based on the double triangular test. Whitehead (1990) further discussed the overrunning and underrunning issues. A number of authors also addressed the designs of two-stage group sequential boundaries [e.g., Elashoff and Reedy (1984), Chi et al. (1986), Case et al. (1987), Wieand and Therneau (1988), and Thall et al. (1988)]. Wang and Tsiatis (1987) proposed a general class of group sequential boundaries that yields approximately optimal boundaries for minimizing the expected sample size. Jennison (1987) discussed efficient group sequential tests with variable sample size. Armitage et al. (1985), Geary (1988), Wei et al. (1990), and a few other authors investigated sequential tests in the settings of repeated measures. Instead of using repeated significance tests, Jennison (1982) and Jennison and Turnbull (1984, 1989) proposed stopping rules using group sequential confidence intervals. Since early stopping rules in clinical trials can lead to bias in point estimation of the true treatment effect, Siegmund (1978, 1985), Tsiatis et al. (1984), Chang and O'Brien (1985), Kim and DeMets (1987b), Rosner and Tsiatis (1988), Chang (1989), Kim (1990), and Facey and Whitehead (1990) approached the estimation problems using confidence intervals following sequential tests. Peace (1987) investigated the power issues in trials with repeated tests. Geller and Pocock (1987, 1988) discussed a number of group sequential designs and stopping rules and suggested a few guidelines for practitioners for conduct of interim analysis. Hughes and Pocock (1988) examined stopping rules and estimation problems. Pocock and Hughes (1989) discussed practical problems in interim analyses, including unplanned analyses and estimation. Enas et al. (1989), Davis and Hwang (1992), and the PMA Ad Hoc Committee on Interim Analysis (1991) addressed various interim analysis issues in the pharmaceutical industry. In sequential analysis of multiple endpoints, Tang et al. (1989) combined the solutions to the multiple endpoint (O'Brien, 1984; Pocock et al., 1987) and multiple testing problems by using the generalized least squares procedure of O'Brien. Compared to univariate methods for a single endpoint, the proposed multivariate method for multiple endpoints demonstrated quite favorable results in terms of sample size. Gould (1991) and Gould and Shih (1991) proposed procedures for interim analysis that do not affect the type I error rate for binomial data and normally distributed data, respectively. The advantages of these procedures are that not only can sample size be reestimated without unblinding the interim data, but the type I error rate is not affected. However, without knowing the observed treatment effect at the time of interim analysis, the sample size may be increased unnecessarily. In advocating Bayesian over group sequential approach, Freedman and Spiegelhalter (1989) identified four problems with group sequential methods for monitoring clinical trials. Whitehead (1991) countered the problems of Freedman and Spiegelhalter and raised problems that appeared to be inherent in their own Bayesian approach.

4. Applications to Survival Data

Many authors illustrated that group sequential methods are also applicable to time-to-event or survival response, which may require staggered patient entry and long-term follow-up. Tsiatis (1981a, b, 1982), Slud and Wei (1982), Harrington et al. (1982), Sellke and Siegmund (1983), Slud (1984), and Hwang (1988) studied the asymptotic group sequential distribution of either the logrank statistic (Mantel, 1966; Peto and Peto, 1972; Cox, 1972), the modified Wilcoxon statistic (Prentice, 1978), or the general class of linear rank statistics (Chatterjee and Sen, 1973; Tarone and Ware, 1977; Prentice, 1978; Prentice and Marek, 1979; Harrington and Fleming, 1982; Tsiatis, 1982). Gail et al. (1982) and DeMets and Gail (1985) investigated, via simulations, the use of both Pocock and O'Brien–Fleming boundaries with the logrank test, both when the analyses are scheduled at equal numbers of deaths and at equal intervals of calendar times.

5. The α Spending (Use) Function Approach

Group sequential methods such as Pocock (1977) and O'Brien and Fleming (1979) were developed based on the *partial sum process,* which requires that (1) the maximum number of interim analyses be prespecified, and (2) the sequence of response variables that form the partial-sum process be independent and identically distributed. The second condition requires that the interim analyses be equally spaced in terms of the information time of the trial. More specifically, analyses must be conducted at times which are spaced so that the amount of information accruing to each analysis is equal. The total information of a clinical trial is represented by either the total number of patients, the total number of endpoint events, or surrogates such as patient-weeks or patient-years. The information time (ranging between 0 and 1) is the process time rescaled in terms of the total information of the trial. During the course of a trial, various factors may influence the frequency and timing of interim analyses. If the frequency or timing of the analyses is substantially altered from equally spaced information times, the above-described group sequential boundaries would be inapplicable (Lan and DeMets, 1989a). Slud and Wei (1982) suggested the construction of group sequential boundaries by choosing a steadily increasing sequence of error probabilities α_i, $i = 1, 2, \ldots, N,$ such that the sum of these probabilities is equal to the prespecified significance level α. Although the design of Slud and Wei does not require analyses at equally spaced information times, the number and timing of analyses still need to be prespecified.

The work by Lan and DeMets (1983) and Kim and DeMets (1987) avoids these problems through the use of an α *spending (use) function*, which allows the trialist to define in advance the way in which the overall α is to be spent over the information time. This approach provides the flexibility of not having to prespecify the number and timing of interim analyses. Interim analyses may often be scheduled at specific calendar times, while theoretically they should occur in terms of information times. [See Lan and DeMets (1989b) for a discussion of calendar time versus information time.] When the α spending function approach is employed, one only need prespecify the overall α allowed and the spending rate of using it. The group sequential boundary constructed by the α spending function is determined by past and current, not by future information or the total number of analyses. Hwang (1988) and Hwang et al. (1990) extended the α spending function approach to a general one-parameter family of α spending functions called the γ-*family*. This family generalizes the α spending functions of Lan and DeMets (1983) and Kim and DeMets (1987).

The boundaries constructed by this family have optimal properties, in terms of minimizing the expected sample size, similar to those of the well-known boundaries.

Therefore, one can use a preselected α spending function to construct a customized group sequential boundary for analyses at arbitrarily (or unequally) spaced information times. The α spending function approach is also applicable to cases involving repeated measures and unplanned interim analyses if the rate of α spending is prespecified. Kim (1989) considered three point estimators following group sequential tests using the α spending function approach. The procedure of Kim can easily be adapted to the sequential logrank test for survival data. Flexibility appears to be the main amenity of the α spending function approach, and recently, it has gained more use in many clinical trials.

D. Pseudosequential and Semi-Bayesian Approaches

An approach that has been developed parallel to group sequential methods is that of the *pseudosequential* or *curtailing procedures*. Whereas the classical sequential and group sequential methods focus on data already available, the curtailing procedures focus on both existing and future data. Lan et al. (1982, 1984) and Halperin et al. (1982) proposed the *stochastic curtailing* approach, which considers early termination of a trial when the probability of a trend being reversed is extremely small. Using stochastic curtailing, conditional probabilities given the interim data (under either the null or alternative hypothesis) are calculated to project future trial outcome at the scheduled end. The procedure can be useful in justifying early termination of a fixed-sample-size trial and as a means for evaluating the performance of a trial when formal interim analyses were not planned in advance. Stochastic curtailing of a nonsequential trial is extremely conservative in terms of early stopping, and it is generally advisable not to use this procedure for early stopping until at least two-thirds of the total information of the trial is available. In an extension of stochastic curtailing, Herson (1979), Choi et al. (1985), Spiegelhalter et al. (1985), Andersen (1987), and Choi and Pepple (1989) proposed the calculation of *predictive probabilities* with respect to current belief about the unknown parameters. The major difference between the curtailing and predictive probability procedures lies in the assumptions made regarding the distribution of future, not-yet-observed data. To reject (or not to reject) the null hypothesis, the former assumes that future data follow the same distribution [or different distributions per Lan (personal communication, 1990)] under the null and alterative hypotheses, and it calculates the conditional probabilities given the interim data accumulated thus far to project future outcome. On the other hand, the latter assumes that the distribution of future data is a mixture based on estimates derived from the observed data as well as from a priori assumption, and it calculates the predictive power by averaging the conditional probabilities. The predictive probability approach is considered *semi-Bayesian.* Neither the stochastic curtailing nor the predictive probability approach preserves exact overall type I and II error probabilities. Recently, Snapinn (1991) described a conditional probability procedure that attempts to maintain the overall α and β by balancing the probabilities of false early rejection and acceptance.

III. DISCUSSION

The development of sequential methodology has had a major impact on the design and analysis of controlled clinical trials. This is especially evident in large clinical trials with extensive patient follow-up or trials that are of pivotal or confirmatory nature in the pharmaceutical industry. For ethical, economic, or administrative reasons, interim analyses are often conducted on data accrued in clinical trials for evidence of efficacy and safety. Interim analysis may introduce bias and inflate true type I and II error probabilities. Many papers in the literature have addressed these issues, and in particular, the Food and Drug Administration (FDA) has raised serious concerns about improper planning and conduct of interim analysis (FDA, 1988). However, developments during the past 15 years (e.g., group sequential methods, stochastic curtailing, and predictive power approach) have brought better insights and provided logical avenues of handling the statistical problems in sequential analysis of clinical trials.

Whereas sequential analysis of data in an ongoing trial is a crucial element of good clinical practice and management, it is difficult to establish a particular procedure or a definitive decision rule for ongoing data monitoring and interim analysis. Nevertheless, regardless of the sequential methods or decision rules chosen, they should be planned and executed in a coherent way; the primary goal should always be to minimize bias and control error probabilities, and ultimately, to maintain the scientific and ethical integrity of the trial. This has been well stated by Canner (1981): "Decision-making in clinical trials is complicated and often protracted. . . . No single statistical decision rule or procedure can take place of well-reasoned consideration at all aspects of the data by a group of concerned, competent and experienced persons with a wide range of scientific backgrounds and points of view."

REFERENCES

Abt, K. (1981). Problems of repeated significance testing. *Controlled Clin. Trials 1*: 377.

Andersen, P. K. (1987). Conditional power calculation as an aid in the decision whether to continue a clinical trial. *Controlled Clin. Trials 8*: 67.

Anderson, T. W. (1960). A modification of the sequential probability ratio test to reduce sample size. *Ann. Math. Stat. 31*: 165.

Anscombe, F. J. (1963). Sequential medical trials. *J. Am. Stat. Assoc. 58*: 365.

Armitage, P. (1957). Restricted sequential procedures. *Biometrika 44*: 9.

Armitage, P. (1975). *Sequential Medical Trials*, 2nd ed., Blackwell, Oxford.

Armitage, P., McPherson, C. K., and Rowe, B. C. (1969). Repeated signficance tests on accumulating data. *J. R. Stat. Soc. A 132*: 235.

Armitage, P., Stratton, I. M., and Worthington, H. V. (1985). Repeated significance tests for clinical trials with a fixed number of patients and variable follow-up. *Biometrics 41*: 353.

Aspirin Myocardial Infarction Study Research Group (1980). A randomized controlled trial of aspirin in persons recovered from myocardial infarction. *J. Am. Med. Assoc. 243*: 661.

Berry, D. A. (1985). Interim analyses in clinical trials: classical vs. Bayesian approaches. *Stat. Med. 4*: 521.

Berry, D. A. (1987). Interim analysis in clinial trials: the role of the likelihood principle. *Am. Stat. 41*: 117.

Berry, D. A. (1989). Monitoring accumulating data in a clinical trial. *Biometrics 45*: 1197.

Bolognese, J. B. (1983). A Monte Carlo study of three up-and-down designs for dose-ranging. *Controlled Clin. Trials 4*: 187.

Breslow, N. E. (1969). On large sample sequential analysis with application to survivalship data. *J. Appl. Probab. 6*: 261.

Breslow, N., and Haug, C. (1972). Sequential comparison of exponential survival curves. *J. Am. Stat. Assoc. 67*: 691.

Bristol, D. R. (1988). A one-sided interim analysis with binary outcomes. *Controlled Clin. Trials 9*: 206.

Brown, B. W., Jr., (1983). Comments on Dupont manuscript: Sequential stopping rules and sequentially adjusted *p* values: does one require the other? *Controlled Clin. Trials 4*: 11.

Canner, P. L. (1981). Practical aspects of decision-making in clinical trials: the Coronary Drug Project as a case study. *Controlled Clin. Trials 1*: 363.

Case, L. D., Morgan, T. M., and Davis, C. E. (1987). Optimal restricted two-stage designs. *Controlled Clin. Trials 8*: 146.

Chang, M. N. (1989). Confidence intervals for a normal mean following a group sequential test. *Biometrics 45*: 247.

Chang, M. N., and O'Brien, P. C. (1985). Confidence intervals following group sequential tests. *Controlled Clin. Trials 7*: 18.

Chatterjee, S. K., and Sen, P. K. (1973). Nonparametric testing under progressive censorship. *Calcutta Stat. Assoc. Bull. 22*: 13.

Chi, P. Y., Bristol, D. R., and Castellana, J. U. (1986). A clinical trial with an interim analysis. *Stat. Med. 5*: 387.

Choi, S. C., and Pepple, P. A. (1989). Monitoring clinical trials based on predictive probability of significance. *Biometrics 45*: 317.

Choi, S. C., Smith, P. J., and Becker, D. P. (1985). Early decision in clinical trials when treatment differences are small. *Controlled Clin. Trials 6*: 280.

Colton, T. (1963). A model for selecting one of two medical treatments. *J. Am. Stat. Assoc. 58*: 388.

Cornfield, J. (1966a). Sequential trials, sequential analysis and the likelihood principle. *Am. Stat. 20*: 18.

Cornfield, J. (1966b). A Bayesian test of some classical hypothesis—with applications to sequential clinical trials. *J. Am. Stat. Assoc. 61*: 577.

Cox, D. R. (1972). Regression models and life tables (with discussion). *J. R. Stat. Soc. B 34*: 187.

Davis, R. L., and Hwang, I. K. (1992). Interim analysis in clinical trials. In *Statistics in the Pharmaceutical Industry,* 2nd ed. (C. R. Buncher and J. Y. Tsay, eds.), Marcel Dekker, New York.

DeMets, D. L., and Gail, M. H. (1985). Use of logrank tests and group sequential methods at fixed calendar times. *Biometrics 41*: 1039.

DeMets, D. L., and Lan, K. K. G. (1984). An overview of sequential methods and their application in clinical trials. *Commun. Stat. Theory Methods 13*: 2315.

DeMets, D. L., and Ware, J. H. (1980). Group sequential methods for clinical trials with a one-sided hypothesis. *Biometrika 67*: 651.

DeMets, D. L., and Ware, J. H. (1982). Asymmetric group sequential boundaries for monitoring clinical trials. *Biometrika 69*: 661.

Doll, R. (1982). Clinical trials: retrospect and prospect. *Stat. Med. 1*: 337

Dupont, W. D. (1983). Sequential stopping rules and sequentially adjusted *p* values: does one require the other? *Controlled Clin. Trials 4*: 3.

Elashoff, J. D., and Reedy, T. J. (1984). Two-stage clinical trial stopping rules. *Biometrics 40*: 791.

Enas, G. G., Dorseif, B. E., Sampson, C. B., Rockhold, R. W., and Wuu, J. (1989). Monitoring versus interim analysis of clinical trials: a perspective from the pharmaceutical industry. *Controlled Clin. Trials 10*: 57.

Facey, K. M., and Whitehead, J. (1990). An improved approximation for calculation of confidence intervals after a sequential clinical trial. *Stat. Med. 9*: 1277.

FDA (1988). *Guideline for the Format and Content of the Clinical and Statistical Sections of an Application*, Center for Drug Evaluation and Research, Food and Drug Administration, Washington, D. C., p. 64.

Freedman, L. S., and Spiegelhalter, D. J. (1989). Comparison of Bayesian with group sequential methods for monitoring clinical trials. *Controlled Clin. Trials 10*: 357.

Gail, M. H., DeMets, D. L., and Slud, E. V. (1982). Simulation studies on increments of the two-sample logrank score tests for survival time data with application to group sequential boundaries. *Survival Analysis,* IMS Monograph Series, Institute of Mathematical Statistics, Hayward, Calif., p. 287.

Geary, D. N. (1988). Sequential testing in clinical trials with repeated measurements. *Biometrika 75*: 311.

Geller, N. L., and Pocock, S. J. (1987). Interim analysis in randomized clinical trials: ramifications and guidelines for practitioners. *Biometrics 43*:213.

Geller, N. L., and Pocock, S. J. (1988). Design and analysis of clinical trials with group sequential stopping rules. In *Biopharmaceutical Statistics for Drug Develop-*

ment (K. E. Peace, ed.), Marcel Dekker, New York, p. 489.

Gould, A. L. (1991). Interim analyses for monitoring clinical trials that do not affect the type I error rate. To appear in Stat. Med.

Gould, A. L., and Pecore, V. J. (1982). Group sequential methods for clinical trials allowing early acceptance of H_0 and incorporating costs. *Biometrika 69*: 75.

Gould, A. L., and Shih, W. J. (1991). Sample size reestimation without unblinding for normally distributed outcomes with unknown variance. Submitted to *Commun. Stat. Theory Methods.*

Halperin, M., Lan, K. K. G., Ware, J. H., Johnson, N. J., and DeMets, D. L. (1982). An aid to data monitoring in clinical trials. *Controlled Clin. Trials 3*: 311.

Harrington, D. P., and Fleming, T. R. (1982). A class of rank test procedures for censored survival data. *Biometrika 69*: 553.

Harrington, D. P., Fleming, T. R., and Green, S. J. (1982). Procedures for serial testing in censored survival data. *Survival Analysis,* IMS Monograph Series, Institute of Mathematical Statistics, Hayward, Calif., p. 269.

Haybittle, J. L. (1971). Repeated assessment of results in clinical trials of cancer treatment. *Br. J. Radiol. 44*: 793.

Herson, J. (1979). Predictive probability early termination plans for phase II clinical trials. *Biometrics 35*: 775.

Hughes, M. D., and Pocock, S. J. (1988). Stopping rules and estimation problems in clinical trials. *Stat. Med. 7*: 1231.

Hwang, I. K. (1988). Group sequential signficance tests for clinical trials, Ph.D. dissertation, Department of Statistics, The Wharton School, University of Pennsylvania.

Hwang, I. K., Shih, W. J., and de Cani, J. S. (1990). Group sequential designs using a family of type I error probability spending functions. *Stat. Med. 9*: 1439.

Jennison, C. (1982). Sequential methods for medical experiments. Ph.D. dissertation, Department of Industrial Engineering and Operations Research, Cornell University.

Jennison, C. (1987). Efficient group sequential tests with unpredictable group sizes. *Biometrika 74*: 155.

Jennison, C., and Turnbull, B. W. (1984). Repeated confidence intervals for group sequential trials. *Controlled Clin. Trials 5*: 33.

Jennison, C., and Turnbull, B. W. (1989). Interim analyses: the repeated confidence interval approach (with discussion). *J. R. Stat. Soc. B. 51*: 305.

Joe, H., Koziol, J. A., and Petkau, A. J. (1981). Comparison of procedures for testing for equality of survival distributions. *Biometrics 37*: 327.

Jones, D., and Whitehead, J. (1979). Sequential forms of the logrank and modified Wilcoxon tests for censored data. *Biometrika 66*: 105.

Kim, K. (1989). Point estimation following group sequential tests. *Biometrics 45*: 613.

Kim, K., and DeMets, D. L. (1987a). Design and analysis of group sequential tests based on the type I error spending rate function. *Biometrika 74*: 149.

Kim, K., and DeMets, D. L. (1987b). Confidence intervals following group sequential tests in clinical trials. *Biometrics 43*: 857.

Koziol, J. A., and Petkau, A. J. (1978). Sequential testing of the equality of two survival curves using modified Savage statistics. *Biometrika 65*: 615.

Lachin, J. M. (1981). Sequential clinical trials for normal variates using interval composite hypotheses. *Biometrics 37*: 87.

Lai, T. L. (1973). Optimal stopping and sequential tests which minimize the maximum expected sample size. *Ann. Stat. 1*: 659.

Lan, K. K. G., and DeMets, D. L. (1983). Discrete sequential boundaries for clinical trials. *Biometrika 70*: 659.

Lan, K. K. G., and DeMets, D. L. (1989a). Changing frequency of interim analysis in sequential monitoring. *Biometrics 45*: 1017.

Lan, K. K. G., and DeMets, D. L. (1989b). Group sequential procedures: calendar versus information time. *Stat. Med. 8*: 1191.

Lan, K. K. G., and Wittes, J. (1988). The *B*-value: a tool for monitoring data. *Biometrics 44*: 579.

Lan, K. K. G., DeMets, D. L., and Halperin, M. (1984). More flexible sequential and non-sequential design in long-term clinical trials. *Commun. Stat. Theory Methods 13*: 2339.

Lan, K. K. G., Simon, R., and Halperin, M. (1982). Stochastically curtailed tests in long-term clinical trials. *Commun. Stat. Sequential Anal. 1*: 207.

Mantel, N. (1966). Evaluation of survival data and two new rank order statistics arising in its consideration. *Cancer Chemother. Rep. 50*: 163.

McPherson, C. K. (1974). Statistics: the problem of examining accumulating data more than once. *N. Engl. J. Med. 290*: 501.

McPherson, C. K. (1982). On choosing the number of interim analyses in clinical trials. *Stat. Med. 1*: 25.

McPherson, C. K., and Armitage, P. (1971). Repeated significance tests on accumulating data when the null hypothesis is not true. *J. R. Stat. Soc. A 134*: 15.

Mehta, C. R. (1981). Sequential comparison of two exponential distributions with censored survival data. *Biometrika 68*: 669.

Nagelkerke, N. J. D., and Hart, A. A. M. (1980). The sequential comparison of survival curves. *Biometrika 67*: 247.

Noel, D. G., Sobel, M., and Weiss, G. H. (1975). A survey of adaptive sampling for clinical trials. In *Perspectives in Biometrics* (R. M. Elashoff, ed.), Academic Press, New York.

O'Brien, P. C. (1984). Procedures for comparing samples with multiple endpoints. *Biometrics 40*: 1079.

O'Brien, P. C., and Fleming, T. R. (1979). A multiple testing procedure for clinical trials. *Biometrics 35*: 549.

Peace, K. E. (1987). *P*-values and power computation in multiple-look trials. *J. Chronic Dis. 40*: 23.

Peto, R., and Peto, J. (1972). Asymptotically efficient rank invariant test procedures. *J. R. Stat. Soc. A 135*: 185.

PMA Ad Hoc Committee on Interim Analysis (1991). Interim analysis in the pharmaceutical industry. To appear in *Controlled Clin. Trials.*

Pocock, S. J. (1977). Group sequential methods in the design and analysis of clinical trials. *Biometrika 64*: 191.

Pocock, S. J. (1982). Interim analysis for randomized clinical trials: the group sequential approach. *Biometrics 38*: 153.

Pocock, S. J., and Hughes, M. D. (1989). Practical problems in interim analyses, with particular regard to estimation. *Controlled Clin. Trials 10*: 209S.

Pocock, S. J., Geller, N. L., and Tsiatis, A. A. (1987). The analysis of multiple endpoints in clinical trials. *Biometrics 43*: 487.

Prentice, R. L. (1978). Linear rank tests with right-censored data. *Biometrika 65*: 167.

Prentice, R. L., and Marek, P. (1979). A qualitative discrepancy between censored data rank tests. *Biometrics 35*: 861.

Robbins, H. (1952). Some aspects of the sequential design of experiments. *Bull. Am. Math. Soc. 58*: 527.

Rosner, G. L., and Tsiatis, A. A. (1988). Exact confidence intervals following a sequential trial: a comparison of methods. *Biometrics 75*: 723.

Samuel-Cahn, E. (1974a). Two kinds of repeated significance tests, and their application for the uniform distribution. *Commun. Stat. 3*: 419.

Samuel-Cahn, E. (1974b). Repeated significance test II, for hypotheses about the normal distribution. *Commun. Stat. 3*: 711.

Samuel-Cahn, E. (1974c). Repeated significance tests I and II. *Commun. Stat. 3*: 735.

Sellke, T., and Siegmund, D. (1983). Sequential analysis of the proportional hazards model. *Biometrika 70*: 315.

Siegmund, D. (1978). Estimation following sequential tests. *Biometrika 65*: 341.

Siegmund, D. (1985). *Sequential Analysis: Tests and Confidence Intervals*, Springer-Verlag, New York.

Simon, R. (1977). Adaptive treatment assignment methods and clinical trials. *Biometrics 33*: 743.

Simons, G. (1976). An improved statement of optimality for sequential probability ratio tests. *Ann. Stat. 4*: 1240.

Slud, E. V. (1984). Sequential linear rank tests for two-sample censored survival data. *Ann. Stat. 12*: 551.

Slud, E., and Wei, L. J. (1982). Two-sample repeated significance tests based on the modified Wilcoxon statistic. *J. Am. Stat. Assoc. 77*: 862.

Snapinn, S. M. (1991). Monitoring clinical trials with a conditional probability stopping rule. To appear in *Stat. Med.*

Spiegelhalter, D. J., Freedman, L. S., and Blackburn, P. R. (1986). Monitoring clinical trials: conditional or predictive power? *Controlled Clin. Trials 7*: 8.

Tang, D. I., Gnecco, C., and Geller, N. L. (1989). Design of group sequential clinical trials with multiple endpoints. *J. Am. Stat. Assoc. 84*: 776.

Tarone, R. E., and Ware, J. (1977). On distribution-free tests for equality of survival distributions. *Biometrika 64*: 156.

Thall, P. F., Simon, R., Ellenberg, S. S., and Shrager, R. (1988). Optimal design for clinical trials with binary response. *Stat. Med. 7*: 571.

Tsiatis, A. A. (1981a). A large sample study of Cox's regression model. *Ann. Stat. 9*: 93.

Tsiatis, A. A. (1981b). The asymptotic joint distribution of the efficient scores test for the proportional hazards model calculated over time. *Biometrika 68*: 311.

Tsiatis, A. A. (1982). Repeated significance testing for a general class of statistics used in censored survival analysis. *J. Am. Stat. Assoc. 77*: 855.

Tsiatis, A. A., Rosner, G. L., and Mehta, C. R. (1984). Exact confidence intervals following a group sequential test. *Biometrics 40*: 797.

Wald, A. (1947). *Sequential Analysis*, Wiley, New York.

Wald, A., and Wolfowitz, J. (1948). Optimal character of the sequential probability ratio test. *Ann. Math. Stat. 19*: 326.

Wang, S. K., and Tsiatis, A. A. (1987). Approximately optimal one-parameter boundaries for group sequential trials. *Biometrics 43*: 193.

Wei, L. J., Su, J. Q., and Lachin, J. M. (1990). Interim analysis with repeated measurements in a sequential clinical trial. *Biometrika 77*: 359.

Whitehead, J. (1983). *The Design and Analysis of Sequential Clinical Trials*, Ellis Horwood, Chichester, West Sussex, England.

Whitehead, J. (1990). Overrunning and underrunning in sequential clinical trials. Submitted to *Controlled Clin. Trials.*

Whitehead, J. (1991). Letter to editor on 'Comparison of Bayesian with group sequential methods for monitoring clinical trials?' Freedman and Spiegelhalter, 1989). *Controlled Clin. Trials 12*: 340.

Whitehead, J., and Jones, D. (1979). The analysis of sequential clinical trials. *Biometrika 66*: 443.

Whitehead, J., and Stratton, I. (1983). Group sequential clinical trials with triangular continuation regions. *Biometrics 39*: 227.

Wieand, S., and Therneau, T. (1987). A two-stage design for randomized trials with binary outcomes. *Controlled Clin. Trials 8*: 20.

Zelen, M. (1969). Play-the-winner rule and the controlled clinical trial. *J. Am. Stat. Assoc. 64*: 131.

2

Practical Approaches to the Design and Conduct of Interim Analyses

Frank W. Rockhold

SmithKline Beecham Pharmaceuticals, King of Prussia, Pennsylvania

Gregory G. Enas

Eli Lilly and Company, Indianapolis, Indiana

I. INTRODUCTION

Sequential statistical methods are receiving more prominent positions in the design and conduct of clinical drug development programs within the pharmaceutical industry than they were 10 years ago. This recent attention to interim analysis may be attributed to many factors, including the following. First, much of the early work in sequential methods, as pioneered by Wald (1947), Armitage (1975), and others, has now been tailored so as to be more compatible with the realities and logistical problems of clinical trial conduct. Second, the need to develop new drugs for life-threatening or severely debilitating diseases is more pronounced than ever. Development must take place in the shortest time possible without compromising the inferences drawn from the studies involved. Investigators are realizing that interim analysis techniques can aid this rapid drug development process immensely. Third, the decisions that the pharmaceutical industry company must make are requiring better information more quickly. Whether it be for making a decision to build a new manufacturing facility for a promising new treatment or to abandon a lost cause, industry is catching on to the need for decision making based on rigorous interim analyses instead of by the "seat of the pants."

Last, but not least, continual assessment of the benefit-to-risk ratio is of critical importance to the patient, investigator, sponsor, and regulatory agency alike. Sequential methods are now available that can help make better decisions regarding the benefit-to-risk ratio in a timely fashion. For example, a study was recently completed that compared to a placebo an experimental drug designed to prevent heart failure. The medical monitor observed during the course of the study that of the first five patients who died all died during the infusion period of the drug. All the investigators from the multicenter trial reviewed the data and concurred that the trial should continue.

After 60 patients had been studied, the death rate in the drug group was 13/31 (41.9%), compared to 7/29 (24.1%) in the placebo group. An interim anlaysis for efficacy when 100 patients had been studied had been planned in the protocol. This observed death rate concerned the monitor, and an unplanned interim analysis of the safety data was carried out. Using an O'Brien–Fleming adjustment, under the assumption that 100 patients had been studied (even though 60 patients had actually been studied), the p-value comparing the mortality rates was not statistically significant. The study was stopped anyway. The final safety picture would be compromised even if the planned number of patients were to be enrolled and no mortality was observed in the additional patients.

The sequence of events described above is a good example of a circumspect monitor, with the other investigators doing their jobs properly. Decisions were made based on accumulating evidence. The decisions were weighted by the prior experience of the investigators. The more data available, the less prior experience became a factor in the final decision.

In the past, interim statistical analyses of safety data were usually carried out only after a series of untoward events had been observed. Planning for interim analyses of safety or efficacy data was rarely done. It is now true that in many studies, plans are laid out in the protocol for interim analyses to be performed during the course of the trial.

The need to make decisions from data accumulated in ongoing studies has provided the impetus to apply methods which for the most part have been developed for clinical trials outside the pharmaceutical industry. It has proved to be no minor task to implement sequential methods in an industrial context. The purpose of this chapter is to outline some of the formidable challenges that present themselves when conducting a clinical drug development program and to give some practical ways in which these challenges can be addressed.

II. MONITORING VERSUS INTERIM ANALYSIS

What does or does not constitute an interim analysis is often confused with the ongoing task of monitoring a clinical trial. The process of monitoring a clinical trial has been defined as "scrutinizing the logistics of a clinical trial so that the intended plan of the trial protocol is realized." On the other hand, interim analysis has been defined as "the process of scientific inference and decision making throughout the course of a clinical trial. This includes the process of estimation and hypothesis testing before the scheduled end of a trial." (Enas et al., 1989).

Monitoring is overseeing the ongoing conduct of a study. Activities associated with monitoring include checking of protocol compliance and individual patient safety. Both investigator and patient compliance with the protocol have to be assessed on an ongoing basis. Investigator compliance assessments should include checks for (1) timeliness of patient enrollment, (2) timeliness of data submission to sponsor, (3) data quality, and (4) proper inclusion/exclusion of patients. Patients must comply as well with the protocol, although the task to ensure this falls largely on the investigators. With respect to the actual logistics of carrying out a trial, the sponsor oversees the investigators and the investigators oversee the patients.

However, when it comes to patient safety, both the sponsor and the individual investigators have important roles. The investigators have the responsibility to discontinue any patients in a study who have serious adverse events that they believe are treatment related. The sponsor is in a position to assess any overall trends in discontinuations and/or other safety indicators by pooling pertinent information from all study centers. The need to terminate the study early if patient safety is in jeopardy may require that an actual interim statistical analysis be performed.

Regulatory agencies have to be informed of any serious adverse event. Form FDA-1639 (Drug Experience Report) is used in the United States to report these events to the Food and Drug Administration (FDA). Our own experience indicates a variance of opinion within the FDA as to whether or not a patient must be unblinded to treatment if such an event takes place. We personally believe that unblinding should take place only if knowledge of such treatment is necessary for decisions about subsequent treatment of the patient. If a patient is unblinded at the study center, the patient is discontinued from the study immediately. Our own experience within the industry tells us that unblinding of the sponsor always takes place when form 1639 is filed. However, unnecessary unblinding may possibly impair the credibility of a study even if the study site is still blinded. These and other dangers of unblinding are areas for future discussion. For now it is sufficient to say that this practice and its impact on patients and studies should be assessed.

Monitoring, then, is an ongoing process. Inspection, "cleaning," and validation of data should be performed in a blinded manner. Descriptive summary statistics can be produced for the study population as a single group, not categorized into treatment groups. These processes can be aided using standard computer-generated reports which can be run easily and as often as necessary. For example, if age and gender are important descriptions of an intended study population, a report showing the proportion of the patients randomized that are male and the proportion of those randomized that are over 65 years old can be generated as often as necessary. This would help the monitors ensure that the planned study populations were in fact those being studied.

In summary, monitoring activities are concerned primarily with the patients in the trial and are performed as often as necessary so that proper study conduct is maintained. On the other hand, many decisions made during the course of a clinical trial affect not only the patients currently in the study but future patients as well. The uncertainty surrounding such inferences made before the scheduled end of a study may need to be quantified using interim analysis techniques.

III. REASONS FOR INTERIM ANALYSES

There are five primary reasons for performing analyses before a study is completed: (1) trends in aggregate safety data, (2) abandoning lost causes, (3) generation of new hypotheses, (4) resource and production decisions, and (5) overwhelming efficacy in life-threatening conditions. We discuss these below.

A. Trends in Aggregate Safety Data

An increased frequency of extremely serious adverse events in one group compared to another may warrant study discontinuation. An increased frequency of moderately serious adverse events may not warrant discontinuation but may warrant some type of countermeasure such as stricter characterization of pharmacodynamics (e.g., Holter monitoring) or taking more laboratory measurements.

B. Abandoning Lost Causes

If an experimental compound does not have the intended effect, this should be detected as early as possible in the study so that patients are not exposed to nonbeneficial treatments and sponsor resources can be reallocated to more promising projects.

C. Generation of New Hypotheses

Preliminary data might suggest that future studies should be conducted to confirm or refute possibly unexpected findings in the present study. Protocol amendments might also be in order, given early results. It might be determined early in the study that some important prognostic variables were not balanced between the treatment groups, or the baseline characteristics of the sample were suggestive of concomitant disorders that should be investigated.

D. Resource and Production Decisions

Decisions to begin expensive and resource-intensive endeavors such as manufacturing scaleup need to be based on data. Excessive waiting in making such decisions might result in very costly delays to both patients and the sponsor. Resource allocation decisions and project prioritization need to be made as the trial progresses, based on the current database.

E. Overwhelming Efficacy in Life-Threatening Conditions

If a very large, beneficial effect was observed in a trial involving cancer, AIDS, or other life-threatening illness, there might be justification to stop the trial early when it became apparent that the benefit of treatment clearly outweighed the risks of treatment. In other situations, though, reasons for trial termination will not be so clear cut. In less life-threatening conditions the benefit/risk ratio is less well defined. Studies in these conditions should generally be carried to completion in order to carefully evaluate the benefit/risk ratio. Another situation, in which large consistent treatment differences over time warrant study termination, occurs when sample sizes are based on what turns out to be an overly conservative estimate of variability. These cases are apparently rare, however.

IV. LOGISTICAL ISSUES IN THE INTERIM ANALYSIS PROCESS

Many of the issues surrounding the decision to conduct an interim analysis of a randomized clinical trial (RCT) are very pragmatic in nature. The numerous statistical issues involved in the performance of interim analyses are discussed elsewhere in this book. A number of philosophical issues revolving around data monitoring and interim analyses have been outlined and discussed in the first part of this chapter. The remainder of the chapter deals with the logistical issues involved in actually carrying out the analyses. The objective is to orient the reader to the fact that the "interim analysis" is a *comprehensive process* requiring time, resources, and logistical coordination and not just a "statistical analysis." The salient issues involved in this exercise will also be outlined.

Although many logistical issues involved in the performance of interim analyses are similar to those for the clinical trial as a whole, the problems are amplified in the setting of the interim evaluation. In addition, some additional issues are unique to the interim look itself. The primary cause and common thread of many of the issues unique to interim analyses in an RCT is time. This is discussed now, followed by a discussion of issues related to resource allocation, data retrieval, data management, risk management, and dissemination of results.

A. Timing and Speed of Analyses

One of the primary considerations in the planning of the timing and execution of interim analyses in an RCT is the safety and well-being of the patients currently enrolled and soon to be enrolled in the trial. This applies to both the safety and efficacy aspects of the treatment under study. For the most part, the decision risks inherent in the interim analysis process affect patients in future trials or in the marketplace. The logistical issues discussed here relate to the duration of the analysis and speed of accrual of the patients into the trial. If the decision relates to a significant efficacy or safety issue, it is of importance to arrive at an answer quickly if it is necessary to terminate the trial.

In addition, and perhaps more important, patients continue to be enrolled while the analysis is being conducted. This *enrollment lag time* presents a logistical challenge that encompasses ethical, regulatory, and statistical aspects. If accrual is expected to be rapid and response immediate, only a very few looks may be feasible. Since it is practically impossible to conduct the analysis before the next patient is enrolled, this problem will be ever present. The only other option is to suspend enrollment while the analysis is being conducted. Anyone who is involved in RCT implementation would cringe at the thought of this action, due to the difficulty in "re-priming the pump." Initiation and maintenance of the RCT is a resource-intensive exercise, and if the decision is made to continue the trial, the risk in cost and time of restarting may be substantial and momentum will be lost. This must, of course, be balanced against the ethical concern of continuing to enroll while the *interim analysis process* is carried out. The ultimately conservative approach would be to suspend treatment while the analysis proceeds. This is in reality too ethically and logistically complex to consider. Thus the patients who are enrolled during the interim analysis process fall into a special category. A critical time frame includes the time from the moment the last patients to be included in the analysis is enrolled until they complete enough of the protocol to be used in the interim evaluation. Thus for a chronic or subacute condition, 1 to 12 weeks may elapse while treatment of the last-included patients progresses. Added to this is the time required to perform the analysis. During this time, patients continue to be enrolled. The potential contribution of this information to the interim decision process is unknown. The issue becomes particularly acute if the decision is to terminate trial enrollment. This problem will be exacerbated if the analysis must be reviewed by an outside data monitoring committee and scheduling becomes a problem. In addition, if the analysis takes place too early in the trial, the data base may lack "maturity." Each investigator in a trial has a learning curve to climb, and early results may not look like later results. It is important that each investigator reach "steady state" before an analysis is conducted, if possible.

B. Resources

The number and frequency of analyses raise very real resource constraint issues. The effort that goes into data collection, processing, and analysis on an interim basis is almost as great as that used in the final analysis. The amount of resources required is very much affected by the number of variables needed in the interim analysis. The amount of information necessary to arrive at a decision must be balanced with the effort expended to obtain it. To be sure, one should be wary of this factor at the final analysis as well. Indeed, if one can arrive at a sensible decision point with a restricted data base in the interim, one wonders why that could not be accomplished at the end of the trial as well. Additionally, if the interim analysis is completed just prior to the end of the trial when all the available information can be reviewed, one wonders why the analysis would be performed at all. One of the objectives (albeit minor) of conducting interim analyses is to save on time and resources. It is thus imperative that one determine that this will be the case for the benefits of the interim look to be fully realized.

C. Data Retrieval

One of the significant costs of doing the interim analysis is the increased pressure on the field monitoring staff to keep files current and to ensure that source document reviews are kept up to date. Scheduling of monitoring visits also becomes a logistical issue for data collection, due to compressed timing. From a trial monitoring point of view, however, up-to-date monitoring results in the ability to assess protocol compliance of the investigators and performance of the field monitoring staff in a timely manner. This should allow the detection of problems occurring consistently across centers earlier than normal in the trial. Once again, it is always of importance to do this in a RCT, but the goal of performing an interim analysis forces timely adherence to the process.

Nonetheless, there are a number of activities that would not be performed until the end of the trial, such as checking drug accountability, checking pharmacy records, drug assignments, and patient follow-up. The presence of an interim analysis causes these processes to be monitored on an interim basis, which generates additional workload. This is done so that in the event the decision is made to terminate enrollment and proceed with a submission or publication, the data will be as high in quality as though the trial had gone to completion.

D. Data Management

As with the trial monitoring staff, the data management area is required to compress its timing of events. Although in the monitoring area there are certain advantages to developing and testing systems in a manner contemporaneous with the trial to detect problems early, it does force tight scheduling of resources.

One of the biggest determinants of the workload and logistics of data processing is the decision on the quality of the data to be used in the analysis. This decision as to whether to use "clean" or "dirty" data again has logistical as well as clinical and regulatory implications. One is caught in the conundrum that if clean data are always required to arrive at a decision in a completed trial, why are "dirty" data adequate for an interim analysis? This decision will depend on many factors, not the least of which relates to the nature and complexity of the variables(s) being analyzed and what ethical issues, if any, are being considered as part of the analysis process.

Interim analysis of unvalidated data is reasonable in some situations. It would be assumed, of course, that the majority of the data are correct as collected and that there are no systematic biases in the incorrect fields. Systematic biases that are associated with the hypothesis being investigated can substantially compromise the validity of the inferences. If no such biases exist, missing and/or aberrant data may be considered as being randomly distributed, and although possibly increasing estimated variability (and decreasing power), the hypothesis-testing procedures would not be invalidated.

Interim analyses should be performed on data that have at least been screened by use of simple diagnostic procedures such as descriptive statistics. There is rarely a need to validate an entire paient record before an analysis can be performed on a particular variable. To expedite complete monitoring of the RCT process as well as assessing the overall compliance with the protocol, data-entry screens, edit checks, audit trails, and computer programs should be tested before study data arrive at the data center. Computer programs may be used to spot suspected erroneous data values.

E. Interim Analysis Risk Management

Although the potential gains to be realized from a clinical, regulatory, and commercial standpoint seem all too clear to those involved in the industry, it must be documented that there are definable risks associated with interim analyses. Some of these, such as the potential for biases in the data and additional data coming in while the analysis is going on have been outlined above. Since one of the major objectives secondary to making a decision on the hypothesis of interest is to estimate treatment differences, the practitioner must be conscious of the pitfalls. Under the best of circumstances, it has been shown that repeated looks at the data can lead to a bias in the estimation of treatment differences in an RCT (Jennison and Turnbull, 1984).

The subset analyzed in the interim analysis has associated with it all of the potential pitfalls that the complete patient sample in the final analysis has—and then some. Although most practitioners would choose to rely on the "intent-to-treat" or all-patients subset, some questions may require the "evaluable" patient subset as defined in the protocol. Balance on protocol-defined prognostic variables should also be checked when performing an interim analysis, especially early in the trial, when imbalance is more sensitive to the smaller sample size. Information from study sites should be approximately proportional to those expected at trial's end. It is commonly believed that the best results in the trials occur early from the best-enrolling investigators.

Another factor that needs to be monitored closely is the maintenance of the treatment code blind. If the trial is to be monitored in a blinded fashion, the person responsible for the generation of the randomization sequence should not be associated with the actual conduct of the study. For purposes of reporting to regulatory authorities, only serious adverse events should warrant unblinding of any individual patient in the study. Any patient so unblinded should immediately be discontinued from the study, although the person's data should be used in the analysis. The treatment groups should be unblinded only at a group level for interim analyses.

F. Dissemination of the Results of the Analysis

Dissemination of unblinded group results should be restricted before the study is completed. In many cases, especially when the possibility of early stopping is great, it is best if only persons not directly involved in the trial view interim results. This group of people is commonly called a *data monitoring board*. In general, persons directly involved with the study sites (e.g., clinical research associates, medical monitors, etc.) may have access to interim results only if strict procedures are followed to prevent disclosure of results to study site personnel. The people who discuss the clinical trial with the various investigators should see only the pooled results across treatment groups. This would prevent premature and/or inadvertent disclosure to those who are actually evaluating patients. Results on interesting but equivocal findings should be held confidential to avoid acting on insignificant results. People not directly associated with the study sites may need to see unblinded group results in order to make internal decisions.

In most trials the people reviewing the data include the medical monitor and other clinical research scientists. These persons should exercise total restraint on any disclosure to the investigator or other study site personnel of the interim analysis results. Only when the decision is made to terminate the trial early should individual investigators and data-handling personnel be informed of the results. This would ensure that the study sites remain blinded throughout the study. Patients with life-threatening diseases, for example, should be told in the informed consent that interim analyses will be conducted and that the study will be stopped early if warranted.

V. CONCLUSION

Interim analyses and their interpretations must be done carefully and judiciously. In this chapter we have outlined various factors that must be considered when undertaking interim analyses. Although the logistical constraints are formidable, they are not insurmountable. The rules for interim analyses should be defined in the protocol. The statistical risks involved with making such decisions can be estimated using the statistical methods discussed throughout this book. The philosophical, logistical, regulatory, and clinical risks were outlined briefly in this chapter.

The return on investment made to monitor a study properly and to perform interim analyses in a careful, scientific manner can be measured not only in terms of the most efficient use of time and resources in bringing a new therapy to clinical practice but in the benefit to current and future patients. We have demonstrated that the decision to perform an interim analysis should not be made on the basis of the natural tendency toward "intellectual curiosity," but for sound scientific, regulatory, commercial, or medical reasons.

REFERENCES

Armitage, P., (1975) *Sequential Medical Trials*, 2nd ed., Wiley, New York.

Enas, G. G., Dornseif, B. E., Sampson, C. B., Rockhold, F. W., and Wuu, J. (1989). Monitoring versus interim analysis of clinical trials: a perspective from the pharmaceutical industry. *Controlled Clin. Trials 10*: 57–70.

Jennison, C., and Turnbull, B. W., (1984). Repeated confidence intervals for group sequential clinical trials. *Controlled Clin. Trials 5*: 33–45.

Wald, A. (1947). *Sequential Analysis*, Wiley, New York.

3

Group Sequential Designs for Trials with Multiple Endpoints

Nancy L. Geller

National Heart, Lung, and Blood Institute, National Institutes of Health, Bethesda, Maryland

Clare Gnecco*

Memorial Sloan-Kettering Cancer Center, New York, New York

Dei-In Tang

Nathan S. Kline Institute for Psychiatric Research, Orangeburg, New York

I. INTRODUCTION

The first two sections of this chapter describe methodology for a certain multiplicity problem in clinical trials. Group sequential designs allow multiple significance testing, yet maintain a preassigned overall significance level and allow a trial to be stopped before all data are collected. In randomized clinical trials, a second multiplicity problem often arises: that of multiple endpoints.

A single endpoint is not natural in many clinical trials. O'Brien (1984) discussed a randomized trial of standard versus experimental treatment for diabetes in which improvement in nerve function was measured by 34 correlated variables. The problem of one-sided hypothesis testing for multiple endpoints was first addressed in a very theoretical way in the 1960s and received renewed and more practical attention in the context of clinical trials in the mid 1980s. The papers of Kudo (1963) and Perlman (1969) gave discussions of likelihood ratio tests for one-sided alternatives with different conditions on the covariance structures, but the required *p*-values were computationally infeasi-

*Current affiliation: Food and Drug Administration, Rockville, Maryland

ble. O'Brien (1984) surveyed the methods used in clinical trials and provided new practical statistics designed to detect one-sided alternatives. The generalized least squares (GLS) procedure he proposed was further explored by Pocock et al. (1987) for two-armed clinical trials to illustrate its applicability to continuous, dichotomous, or censored endpoints.

These two multiplicity problems, repeated significance testing of data as they accumulate and multiple endpoints, usually occur together in clinical trials. Early stopping when one treatment is vastly superior to the other is as desirable in trials with multiple endpoints as in trials with a single endpoint. It is our purpose to review how the separate solutions to the multiple endpoint and repeated significance-testing problems have been combined for two-armed clinical trials to yield a more realistic trial design. Using O'Brien's statistics, we discuss methods for the design of two-armed clinical trials that allow for interim analyses *and* consider all endpoints simultaneously. Our development is similar to that of Pocock et al. (1987) and Tang et al. (1989a), but slightly more general. As it turns out, any of the methods in the group sequential literature will still be of use, with only minimal change in the definition of certain parameters. Compared to univariate methods based on any single endpoint, the multivariate methods described here can be quite favorable as far as sample size is concerned. We also discuss when a multiple-endpoint approach is appropriate, describing several examples.

Another multiple-endpoint statistic, which is not included here, was discussed by Tang et al. (1989b). The group sequential use of that and other multiple-endpoint statistics was discussed by Tang et al. (1991).

II. METHODS

It is clear that any group sequential method for multiple endpoints must be based on a method for single-stage, fixed-sample-size analysis of multiple endpoints. Several of these are described here, with their group sequential implementation.

A. Bonferroni Correction

A simple way to deal with multiple endpoints is the Bonferroni correction, discussed by Pocock et al. (1987). This approach is attractive because no joint distribution theory is required. Pocock et al. (1987) showed that under multivariate normality, the Bonferroni correction is only slightly conservative when the pairwise correlation between endpoints is less than 0.5. Thus in a multiple-endpoint trial, one might divide the overall significance level by the number of endpoints and set nominal significance levels for each endpoint based on the resulting group sequential boundaries.

Pocock et al. (1987) noted that the Bonferroni approach has greatest power for the alternative hypothesis for which only one of the endpoints had a nonzero treatment difference and the endpoint having the difference is unspecified. When multiple endpoints each showed moderate treatment differences in the same direction, the approach lacked power and so might not detect certain differences.

Alternative approaches making better use of overall clinical trial information, such as the covariance structure, would be useful. The approaches that follow assume multivariate normality. Under this assumption, for two-sided alternatives, Hotelling's T^2 test or a χ^2 test are the classical tests. However, in clinical trials, the alternative hypothesis is one-sided, and the use of this more restricted alternative hypothesis will result in significant improvements in power (Robertson et al., 1988).

B. O'Brien's Statistics

We consider testing the hypothesis that two treatments have the same efficacy, as measured by k ($\geqslant 2$) endpoints. Let μ_i, $i = 1, 2$, denote the mean vector of the first and second treatment effects, respectively. O'Brien (1984) proposed tests of the null hypothesis

$$H_0: \quad \mu_1 = \mu_2 \tag{1}$$

against the alternative hypothesis

$$H_A: \quad \mu_1 - \mu_2 = \delta\lambda \tag{2}$$

where δ is a $(k \times 1)$ column vector of specified treatment differences and λ is a scalar. Here, as in Tang et al. (1989a), δ can be any prespecified vector with nonnegative components. The null hypothesis is then $\lambda = 0$ and (without loss of generality) the one-sided alternative of interest is $\lambda > 0$.

For a sample of n observations per arm, O'Brien's GLS statistic is

$$\frac{(n/2)^{1/2}\delta'\Sigma^{-1}Y}{(\delta'\Sigma^{-1}\delta)^{1/2}} \tag{3}$$

where Y denotes the vector of mean treatment differences based on the n observations per arm, δ' denotes the transpose of δ, and $2\Sigma/n$ is the covariance matrix of the Y vector. The statistic (3) is a linear combination of the mean treatment differences for each endpoint, with the linear coefficients a function of the vector δ and the covariance matrix Σ. If Y has a multivariate normal distribution and Σ is known, O'Brien's GLS statistic also is normally distributed. When Y is asymptotically normal and Σ is estimated consistently, (3) is asymptotically normal (Pocock et al., 1987).

The choice of the δ in O'Brien's GLS statistic reflects the investigator's belief about the direction in which the alternative lies. However, Pocock et al. (1987) pointed out that the weight vector, $\Sigma^{-1}\delta$, for combining individual endpoints in O'Brien's GLS statistic may have some negative components, which they considered "untenable from a practical point of view."

Any δ for which $\Sigma^{-1}\delta$ has only nonnegative components would avoid the problem of negative weights. When the variances of the endpoints are equal, one choice is $\delta = \Sigma J$, where $J = (1, 1, \ldots, 1)^T$, which corresponds to the ordinary least squares (OLS) statistic, also discussed by O'Brien (1984). The OLS statistic for multiple endpoints is thus a function of the unweighted average of the normalized treatment differences for the individual endpoints.

C. Use of O'Brien's Statistics in Group Sequential Trials

Tang et al. (1989a) showed how O'Brien's GLS statistic could be used in group sequential trials. Because the OLS statistic also is a linear combination of asymptotically normally distributed test statistics, the same development based on standard univariate group sequential theory applies, with a small modification in the multiplier used to set the sample size. Specifically, for two-armed clinical trials, any of the sequences of nominal signficance levels for group sequential trials is applicable to either of O'Brien's statistics. Furthermore, the sample size needed to detect the specific alternative $\lambda = \lambda_0$ in equation (2) can be determined using existing tables, such as Table 2 of Geller and Pocock (1987), with $\lambda_0^{-2}(\delta'\Sigma^{-1}\delta)^{-1}$ substituting for σ^2/δ^2 when using O'Brien's GLS statistic and with $\lambda_0^{-2}(J'\Sigma J)^{-1}$ substituting for σ^2/δ^2 when using O'Brien's OLS statistic.

Finally, Tang et al. (1989a) proved that an analysis of multiple endpoints against the alternative (2) using O'Brien's GLS statistic will always be more powerful than an analysis of any single endpoint using any one of the (asymptotically) normal test statistics comprising O'Brien's GLS statistic.

III. DISCUSSION

It is worth considering examples of situations where the methodology described should be employed as well as examples where a single-endpoint design would be superior. Certain clinical trials do not have one natural endpoint. One example is an antiviral trial for a chronic episodic disease such as genital herpes, where the goals of treatment include ending an episode, increasing the length of time from one episode to the next, and symptomatic relief. Time to pain relief, time to relief from itching, time to crusting or healing of lesions, and duration of the episode are all endpoints of interest. Several of these might be taken as primary multiple endpoints in a clinical trial. Trials of lung function or immune modulators also often consider a number of changes in several parameters, and these, too, might be appropriately regarded as primary multiple endpoints. Another area in which these methods may well be appropriate is psychological studies, in which multi-item rating scales are commonplace.

In cancer therapy trials, a short-term endpoint, "response," is usually defined and long-term outcomes, such as disease-free interval and overall survival, are also of interest. It is arguable that these should not be combined because one is short term (evaluable within several months of starting treatment) and the others take a longer time to be evaluated. The question of which of these endpoints would be primary would depend on the goal of treatment. Of course, each specific trial has its own special features, and this may make selection of a single endpoint either important or impossible.

In adopting the multiple-endpoint approach to clinical trial design described here, the statistician should not forget that the sample-size savings can be considerable. This implies that the power to detect differences in the individual endpoints will be compromised if the multiple-endpoint approach is taken in design. Thus if results on single endpoints will be demanded at the end of the trial, the sample size should be set so that estimates for individual endpoints will be sufficiently precise.

Some further examples of clinical trials to which these methods have been applied are given in Tang et al. (1989a, b) and Tang et al. (1991).

REFERENCES

Geller, N. L., and Pocock, S. J. (1987). Interim analyses in randomized clinical trials: ramifications and guidelines for practitioners. *Biometrics 43*: 213–224.

Geller, N. L., and Pocock, S. J. (1988). Design and analysis of clinical trials with group sequential stopping rules. In *Biopharmaceutical Statistics for Drug Development*, Karl E. Peace, (ed.), Marcel Dekker, New York, pp. 489–508.

Kudo, A. (1963). A multivariate analogue of the one-sided test. *Biometrika 50*: 403–418.

O'Brien, P. C. (1984). Procedures for comparing samples with multiple endpoints. *Biometrics 40*: 1079–1087.

Perlman, M. D. (1969). One-sided testing problems in multivariate analysis. *Ann. Math. Stat. 40*: 549–567.

Pocock, S. J., Geller, N. L., and Tsiatis, A. A. (1987). The analysis of multiple endpoints in clinical trials. *Biometrics 43*: 487–498.

Robertson, T., Wright, F. T., and Dykstra, R. L. (1988). *Order Restricted Statistical Inference*, Wiley, New York.

Tang, D.-I., Geller, N. L., and Pocock, S. J. (1991). On the design and analysis of randomized clinical trials with multiple endpoints. *Biometrics* (in press).

Tang, D.-I., Gnecco, C., and Geller, N. L. (1989a). Design of group sequential clinical trials with multiple endpoints. *J. Am. Stat. Assoc. 84*: 776–779.

Tang, D.-I., Gnecco, C., and Geller, N. L. (1989b). An approximate likelihood ratio test for a normal mean vector with nonnegative components with application to clinical trials. *Biometrika 76*: 577–583.

II

APPLICATIONS IN DRUG SCREENING

4

Statistical Design Considerations for Stagewise, Adaptive Dose Allocation in Dose-Response Studies

Paul I. Feder, David W. Hobson, Carl T. Olson, R. L. Joiner,* and M. Claire Matthews

Battelle, Columbus, Ohio

I. INTRODUCTION

Dose-response experiments are very frequently carried out as parts of drug and chemical development and evaluation programs in many areas of toxicology, pharmacology, and the biomedical sciences. In this chapter we discuss an approach to the experimental design of such studies when the responses are dichotomous (i.e., success or failure, yes or no, 0 or 1, etc.). The results from such quantal response studies are used to estimate dose-response distributions that specify the relation between dose and effect. For example, in the case of a drug development application, the dose-response distribution might represent the probability of obtaining an efficacious response (e.g., alleviation of disease symptoms) as a function of drug dose. Usually, but not always, the probability of efficacious response increases in a monotonic fashion as the administered drug dose increases.

A principal design objective of many dose-response studies is the estimation of particular dose-response distribution percentiles. The ED_{100p} is defined as that dose at which $100p$ percent of the subjects respond positively (e.g., 50% respond positively at the ED_{50} dose, 95% respond positively at the ED_{95} dose, etc.).

* Current affiliation: TSI Redfield Laboratories, Redfield, Arkansas

The statistical design problem is to estimate specified aspects of the dose-response distribution, such as the ED_{50}, the ED_{95}, or the slope, as precisely as feasible using small-to-moderate numbers of experimental subjects. The sensitivity of an experimental design depends very heavily on the specific dose levels that are selected for inclusion in the design, as well as on the sample size. Ideally, the design doses should bracket each of the dose-response percentiles to be estimated; they should be spread widely enough to permit estimation of the shape of the dose-response distribution, if this is also an objective. Estimation of extreme percentiles requires asymmetric dose allocations, due to unequal variability of response.

At first glance it appears that to achieve these aims, it is necessary to know the dose-response distribution prior to the experiment. In that event, however, the experiment itself would be unnecessary! To circumvent this apparent paradox, a stagewise, adaptive dose allocation strategy has been adopted. An initial (a priori) dose-response relation is hypothesized based on historical data, on results of pilot experiments, on results of literature values, or on toxicological judgment. The first-stage dose allocation is based on this initial hypothesis. The first-stage experimental results are combined with the a priori information to update the hypothesized dose-response distribution. The second-stage dose allocation is based on this updated dose-response distribution. The entire process is iterated until the appropriate number of stages has been completed.

In this chapter we discuss the stagewise, adaptive experimental design approach in detail, covering the assumptions made, the theory and methods used, and the specialized algorithms and associated computer programs that are used to implement the methods. The procedures are illustrated by example.

In Section II we discuss the objectives, assumptions, methods, and theory underlying the stagewise, adaptive design approach. The individual aspects of the design procedure are discussed in some detail and are illustrated by example. A case study of the effectiveness of the stagewise, adaptive dose allocation strategy in a particular application is presented in detail in Section III. The case study illustrates how the components of the process interface. In Section IV we describe briefly the application of the methodology in the design stages of a number of other programs. In some of the programs, the flexibility of the adaptive approach permitted beneficial midstudy design modifications to be made, in response to early stage results that differed substantially from what had been anticipated prior to the study. In Section V we review the methods and the assumptions underlying them, as well as a number of areas for possible extension. The specific methods discussed in this chapter pertain to dichotomous responses, to relatively simple dose-response models, and to an estimation of specialized aspects of those relations. The general logic and design approaches, however, are applicable to more general types of responses, models, and studies, and to alternative design objectives.

A number of papers have been published in the statistical literature pertaining to aspects of and strategies for stagewise experimental designs for dose-response experiments. Dixon (1965) and others consider sequential up–down experimental strategies for estimating specified percentiles of a dose-response distribution. Dixon's original procedure pertained to estimation of the LD_{50} value using one observation at a time, at a series of prespecified and equally spaced dose levels. Following each death, the dose would be decreased to the next lower level in the series; following each survival the dose would be raised to the next higher level in the series. The aim of this procedure is for the test doses to converge rapidly to the vicinity of the LD_{50}. Wetherill et al. (1966) generalized this procedure to estimate percentiles other than the fiftieth. Hsi (1969) generalized the procedure to incorporate the use of multiple tests at each stage.

The objectives of the up–down procedure differ from those of the design strategies considered in this chapter and are less flexible. The principal aim of the procedure is to concentrate testing near the LD_{50} value. This concentration of tests near the LD_{50} value results in relatively imprecise estimation of the distribution slope. The up–down method generally involves just one observation at a time, and even its extension to multiple observations per stage concentrates all the testing at a single dose per stage.

Lai and Robbins (1978, 1979) consider adaptive stochastic approximation design schemes for estimating the level θ at which a response function, $M(x)$, is equal to some desired value. Their goal, like that of the up–down method, is for the test doses to converge to θ as rapidly as possible and remain there. Such a goal would be appropriate if θ represents the dosage of a drug that results in an optimal drug level in the blood. This goal, however, precludes precise determination of other points on the response distribution or precise estimation of the overall shape of the distribution, such as its (local) slope. Their method also involves using just one dose level per stage.

Tsutakawa (1980) evaluates the performance of experimental designs for estimating a percentage point of a two-parameter logistic dose-response distribution. He takes a Bayesian approach and formulates the design problem by selecting a design to minimize the expected posterior variance of the percentage point of interest. Tsutakawa's approach thus takes into account the amount of uncertainty that is present in the estimates of the dose-response distribution parameters. He reports that "although the Bayesian approach . . .can be simply fomulated. . . . Exact solutions require an impractical amount of computation. . . ." He thus restricts attention to a simplified class of designs that consist of k replicates at each of m equally spaced dose levels. Tsutakawa reports that for a relatively concentrated prior distribution, the design efficiency does not vary greatly with the number of dose levels used. For a diffuse (i.e., relatively uninformative) prior distribution, however, the designs involving greater numbers of dose levels are more efficient than those designs with fewer dose levels. Although Tsutakawa's design evaluations pertain to single-stage studies, they can easily be extended to multistage procedures.

McLeish and Tosh (1983) consider a sequential method for estimating an extreme percentile of a dose-response distribution. Their method is most applicable when the expected response (e.g., lethality) level is low. The aim of their method is to gain more information about the extreme distribution percentile while controlling the total number of deaths rather than the total sample size. This is analogous to the use, in the one sample problem, of negative binomial sampling rather than binomial sampling. McLeish and Tosh suggest specifying a series of equally spaced doses. An observation is made at the first (lowest) dose, and dose levels are incremented sequentially until a response (e.g., death) is obtained. The observed random variable is N, the number of dose increments until the first response. The procedure is repeated a specified number of times, each time starting at the first (lowest) dose. The starting points and increments are functions of the percentage point to be estimated.

Abdelbasit and Plackett (1983) evaluate the characteristics of alternative experimental designs for estimating the parameters of logistic dose-response distributions. They utilize the D-optimality precision criterion, which is a global criterion, not directly related to the estimation precision for distribution percentiles. They consider stagewise designs in a small number of stages, which update the initial parameter estimates after each stage. Abdelbasit and Plackett are concerned primarily with the robustness of the designs, as the initial parameter estimates differ from the true parameters.

Abdelbasit and Plackett restrict attention to two- and three-dose designs, with equal sample sizes per dose. They choose the dose levels at those distribution percentiles that result in D-optimality. They report that two-dose designs are more efficient than three-dose designs *if* the initial parameter specifications are correct. The three-dose designs are, however, more robust than the two-dose designs to departures of the initial parameter estimates from the true parameters. A too narrowly spread out design is less robust to the effects of poor initial parameter estimates than is a widely spread out design.

Abdelbasit and Plackett also compare the relative efficiencies of single-stage designs and multistage designs having the same total numbers of observations. The initial parameter estimates are updated following each stage. They report that the multistage designs are more efficient relative to the single-stage designs for poor initial parameter estimates than for good initial estimates. A succession of stages permits improvement in the initial estimates when such improvement is needed but is wasteful when little improvement is required. The relative efficiency of multistage designs increases with the total sample size, N, because the initial parameter estimates converge to the true parameters more and more rapidly. Thus for large N, multistage designs are preferable to single-stage designs since they are somewhat more efficient for poor initial parameter estimates, yet are nearly as efficient for good initial estimates.

These results, in conjunction with those of Tsutakawa, suggest that multistage designs with multiple dose levels per stage are to be recommended when the initial parameter estimates are incorrectly or imprecisely determined. This is the situation against which the stagewise, adaptive experimental design procedures discussed in this chapter are intended to protect.

II. STAGEWISE, ADAPTIVE DESIGN APPROACH: THEORY AND METHODS

In this section we discuss the assumptions, methods, and theory underlying the stagewise, adaptive design approach. In Section A we discuss the objectives of the design process and the assumptions made. In Section B we briefly review the steps in the stagewise, adaptive design process. Various aspects of the design procedure and associated displays are described in greater detail in Sections C to F. Section G describes a SAS computer procedure that has been developed to implement these ideas.

A. Assumptions and Objectives

A treatment or exposure regimen is administered to experimental subjects at a series of graded doses. It is desired to design and carry out an experimental program to study the relation between the treatment dose and the response level. A number of assumptions are made here concerning the responses, the dose-response relations, and the experimental populations. These assumptions result in technical simplifications; the basic ideas and methods, however, are applicable in a much more general framework.

It is assumed that the response is dichotomous (i.e., response, nonresponse). It is assumed that the dose-response relation can be described by a probit model in the (common) logarithm of dose, at least in the central portion (e.g., between the 10th and 90th percentiles). Let d denote the drug dose and $x = \log_{10}(d)$. Let $P(d)$ denote the probability of a response at dose d. Then

$$P(d) = \Phi(\beta_0 - 5 + \beta_1 x) \tag{1}$$

$\Phi(\cdot)$ denotes the standard normal cumulative distribution function and β_0 and β_1 are unknown parameters to be estimated from the data. In the subsequent discussion $\Phi^{-1}(\cdot)$ represents the inverse normal (i.e., probit) function and $\hat{\beta}_0$ and $\hat{\beta}_1$ are maximum likelihood estimates of β_0 and β_1.

This model assumes that the probability of response increases monotonically from 0 when $d = 0$, to 1 as d increases without limit. It does not incorporate provisions for background response, for upper bounds on response probability strictly less than 1, or for the effects of covariates. This model is applicable in many situations. For example, if response is acute lethality (e.g., within 48 hours) following dose *d* of a toxicant, this model asserts that there would be no acute lethality in the absence of toxicant and that there would be essentially complete lethality with a sufficiently high challenge dose.

In other situations the model might need to be extended. For example, if response represents recovery from an illness after receiving dose *d* of a particular drug treatment, some subjects might recover even in the absence of drug, while others might not recover no mattrer how high a drug dose they received.

The model does not account for covariate effects such as age, body weight, or initial level of a particular enzyme. The model also assumes absence of drift or other stage-to-stage variation in the response characteristics of the population over the course of the experiment. Possible modifications in design strategy to detect and adjust for stage-to-stage drift or variation are suggested briefly in Section V. They are not, however, considered elsewhere in the chapter.

The design objectives are to estimate those aspects of the dose-response relation that are of interest, with relatively high precision based on the available resources. The procedures are also designed for flexibility. The stagewise, adaptive dose allocation process permits information obtained in previous stages to influence the dose selection in current and future stages. This enables the experimenters to modify the experimental procedures or dose allocations in midstudy if the a priori or early stage assumptions concerning treatment efficacy are contradicted by the experimental results observed in the early stages.

No formal optimization criteria and algorithms are built into the design approach. Often, several formal design objectives may compete with one another and with other, more formal objectives. For example, "optimal" designs for estimating the ED_{50} value would differ from "optimal" designs for estimating the ED_{95}, which in turn would differ from "optimal" designs for estimating the slope.

Rather than generate a single design for each objective, the approach taken is to generate multiple "target" designs and to evaluate their sensitivity relative to each experimental objective. Generally, a design that is best for one objective (e.g., the ED_{95}) may be relatively inefficient for other objectives. Thus the aim is to arrive at a compromise design, which is nearly as sensitive as the "best" with respect to each of the objectives. Sensitivity analyses are carried out to evaluate the performance of each design over a range of underlying dose-response distributions. Thus "robustness" to departures from assumptions is also taken into account when selecting a target design.

Toxicological judgment and logistical considerations have essential roles in the experimental planning process. Generally, for a specified total sample size, considerations of design sensitivity and design flexibility suggest utilizing the largest number of stages and the smallest sample size per stage (one per treatment, if possible) that are feasible. Conversely, considerations of program logistics and elapsed time often suggest utilizing the smallest number of stages and the largest sample size per stage that are feasible. Toxicological input is needed to arrive at a compromise between these two extremes. For some programs a constant sample size per stage evens out the scheduling and workload. For other programs it is desired to start cautiously, with just one subject per treatment per stage, and then gradually increase the sample size per stage as information is accumulated concerning the underlying dose-response relations. For yet other programs, sample sizes for some treatment regimens are tapered down in the later stages and are reallocated to more promising treatment regimens. The strategy for each experimental program needs to be decided jointly by statistical and toxicological personnel in light of the statistical and logistical goals for the program.

Another area of design flexibility pertains to early termination of the study. If the attained midstudy results are substantially inferior to the a priori expectations, the study may be stopped. Aspects of the study could be modified and the study resumed. An example where this proved to be beneficial is discussed in Section IV. If the midstudy results provide conclusive statistical evidence that some treatment regimens are far superior to others, the study may be stopped, or at least the inferior treatment regimens deleted. Toxicological input is also incorporated into such decisions.

B. Design Process During the Experiment

This section reviews the steps involved in the stagewise, adaptive design process. The components of this process are summarized below. They are schematically displayed in Figure 1 and are discussed in greater detail in the subsequent sections.

1. Determine the a priori (stage 0) dose-response distribution based on historical data, literature values, or toxicological judgment.
2. Choose the first-stage dose allocation to approximate the target design, based on the a priori dose-response distribution.
3. Carry out stage 1 testing.
4. Estimate the current distribution percentiles based on the updated dose-response distribution assessment.
5. Choose doses for the next stage to approximate the target design as closely as possible, over and above the past and current dose allocations.
6. Evaluate the sensitivities of alternative dose allocations for the next stage, over and above the current data.
7. Choose the next-stage dose allocation.
8. Carry out next-stage testing.
9. Iterate.

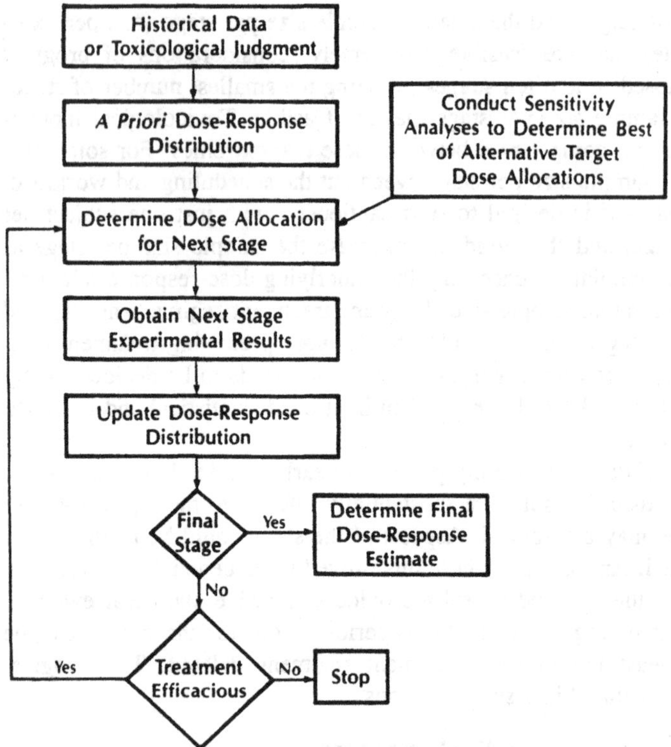

Figure 1 Design process during the experiment.

C. Design Strategy Prior to the Experiment: Target Designs

It can be shown that under model (1) the estimation sensitivity of any design depends solely on the numbers of subjects allocated to the various dose-response distribution percentiles. More precisely, let x_p denote the logarithm of the pth percentile of the distribution in (1):

$$x_p = \frac{\Phi^{-1}(p) - (\beta_0 - 5)}{\beta_1} \tag{2}$$

Then

$$\text{std err}[(\hat{\beta}_0 - 5) + \hat{\beta}_1 x_p] = f(\text{design percentile allocation}) \tag{3}$$

Let $\hat{x}_p$ denote the estimated pth percentile

$$\hat{x}_p = \frac{\Phi^{-1}(p) - (\hat{\beta}_0 - 5)}{\hat{\beta}_1} \tag{4}$$

Then

$$\text{std err}(\hat{x}_p) = \frac{1}{\beta_1} f(\text{design percentile allocation}) \tag{5}$$

Equation (5) indicates that the standard error of the estimated pth percentile is inversely proportional to the dose-response distribution slope, but otherwise depends only on the percentile allocation in the design. Thus, to evaluate the relation between sensitivity of percentile estimation and allocation of experimental subjects to dose-response distribution percentiles, it can be assumed without loss of generality that $\beta_0 - 5 = 0$ and $\beta_1 = 1$. The resulting standard errors appropriate for the standardized distribution need only be divided by the true slope, β_1, to obtain the standard errors appropriate for the same percentile allocation in the actual dose-response distribution.

The foregoing implies that the relative sensitivities of alternative dose allocations can be evaluated *before* any data have been collected. This permits "target designs" to be selected before the start of the experiment. Their sensitivities for estimating distribution percentiles of interest as well as the distribution slope can be compared based on the a priori estimates of the dose-response distributions. Doses are selected for the first stage based on the a priori most sensitive target design. Following each experimental stage, the estimates of the underlying dose-response distributions are updated. Doses are selected for the next stage to best approximate the currently most sensitive target design, over and above the previous dose allocations, based on the updated dose-response distributions. At each stage the relative sensitivities of the alternative target designs depend only on the percentile dose allocations. This process is iterated until the completion of all the stages or until the endpoints of interest are determined with the desired levels of precision.

The a priori evaluation of alternative target designs is illustrated by a study in the planning stage. The response is 48-hour lethality following exposure to graded doses of a toxicant and treatment with a single, standard regimen. The primary objective is to estimate the 50th percentile of the underlying dose-response distribution. Secondary objectives are to estimate the 90th percentile and the slope. Table 1 displays alternative target designs for the study. Each design corresponds to the allocation of 100 subjects to the doses indicated, which are based on specified percentiles of the a priori dose-response distribution. For example, design GD2 corresponds to the essentially equal allocation of the 100 subjects to the 10th, 20th, . . . , 90th percentiles of the a priori dose-response distribution. These a priori dose-response percentiles are based

Table 1 Specifications of Alternative Target Designs, Proposed Doses, and Numbers of Subjects per Dose

Design ID.	Dose 1	No. subj.	Dose 2	No. subj.	Dose 3	No. subj.	Dose 4	No. subj.	Dose 5	No. subj.	Dose 6	No. subj.	Dose 7	No. subj.	Dose 8	No. subj.	Dose 9	No. subj.
GD 1	7.7	25.00	11.1	25.00	15.2	25.00	21.9	25.00										
GD 2	5.9	11.11	7.7	11.11	9.4	11.11	11.1	11.11	13.0	11.12	15.2	11.11	18	11.11	21.9	11.11	28.7	11.11
GD 3	5.9	20.00	9.4	20.00	13.0	20.00	18.0	20.00	28.7	20.00								
GD 4	7.7	33.33	13.0	33.34	21.9	33.33												
GD 5	7.7	30.00	13.0	40.00	21.9	30.00												
GD 6	9.4	33.33	13.0	33.34	18.0	33.33												
GD 7	5.9	25.00	11.1	25.00	15.2	25.00	28.7	25.00										
GD 8	5.9	10.00	7.7	20.00	11.1	20.00	15.2	20.00	21.9	20.00	28.7	10.00						
GD 9	5.9	33.33	13.0	33.34	28.7	33.33												
GD10	5.9	10.00	7.7	25.00	13.0	30.00	21.9	25.00	28.7	10.00								

on the results of a similar study that was carried out a number of years ago. Note that the *relative* sensitivities of the designs would remain the same if we scaled the sample sizes for each dose in each design up or down by the same scale factor (e.g., by dividing by 10). Since the sample sizes are used for planning purposes only, they do not necessarily have to be whole numbers. Note also that the design sensitivities depend on the specified doses only through the underlying dose-response percentiles.

D. A Priori Dose-Response Distributions and Past Data

The a priori assumptions about the dose-response distributions applicable to the forthcoming study are based on the results of previous studies, on information in the literature, or on toxicological judgment. These assumptions are expressed by specifying the a priori parameters (β_0 and β_1) of the dose-response distribution as well as a variance–covariance matrix indicating the uncertainty in these parameters. Table 2 displays the parameters of the a priori dose-response distribution for the example being considered in this section. These parameters are based on the results of a similar study that was carried out several years ago.

In general, the source(s) of the a priori information and the assumptions about its strength, weakness, and relevance to the current program are identified by toxicological experts and are subject to toxicological judgment and review. The aim is to utilize information as similar to the current study as possible. The most informative situation would be to have historical data based on a previous study conducted with the same animal model, the same responses recorded (e.g., at the same time intervals), the same toxicant challenge regimen, and the same therapy regimen. Less informative situations might involve studies with different animal models, different exposure regimens (route, length, or dose), or different therapy regimens (route, length, or dose). In the absence of a priori information or toxicological opinion concerning the nature of the present dose-response relations, a preliminary up–down study (Dixon, 1965; Hsi, 1969) might be carried out to provide some indication of the central regions and the general steepness of the dose-response distributions.

Table 2 Parameters Specifying the A Priori Probit Dose-Response Distribution and a Variance–Covariance Matrix Indicating the Uncertainty in These Parameters

BO	B1	VO	CO1	VI
0.843	3.732	0.338	−0.299	0.274

It is sometimes possible to use historical data based on other animal models or other exposure or therapy regimens to obtain partial a priori information. It is known, for example, that while an ED_{50} dose may vary widely across species or across therapy regimens, the slopes of the dose-response distributions tend to be much more consistent. For example, an a priori dose-response distribution for rats might be obtained from one for mice by assuming the same slope and by extrapolating the ED_{50} dose (on a body weight basis) from one species to another based on the ratio of the body surface areas. Alternatively, one might obtain an a priori estimate of the ED_{50} in rats based on a small preliminary up–down experiment in rats by assuming the same dose-response distribution slope as that for mice and using the limited rat data to estimate the center of the distribution.

After each stage of experimentation the a priori distribution is updated based on the results from all the previous stages in the current experiment. The historical results could be discounted relative to the current results by treating each historical observation as w observations (where $0 \leqslant w \leqslant 1$) and each current observation as one observation. This is most easily accomplished by inflating the a priori variances and covariances by the factor $1/w$ before combining them with the current data. The choice $w = 0$ totally disregards the historical data.

Prior to the first stage there are no current data. This is indicated by specifying a single "dummy dose" at which 0 animals and 0 responses were observed. Such an a priori specification is illustrated in Table 3. The stagewise, adaptive design procedure incorporates these current data into the evaluations of the target designs in a manner discussed in the next subsection.

E. Expected Information from the Target Designs

After one or more experimental stages have been completed, there are two components of information associated with each dose allocation in the subsequent stages: (1) the attained or "local" information, based on the results observed in the previous stages, and (2) the expected or "Fisher" information, based on the anticipated results to be obtained in subsequent stages. The total information is the sum of these two components.

Table 3 Experimental Results from Previous Stages[a]

Stage	Dose	X	NN	Y
1	20	1.30103	0	0

[a] Prior to the first stage, the numbers of animals (NN) and the numbers of responses (Y) are each zero.

1. Attained (Local) Information

The data from the previous stages can be summarized as (n_1, d_1, y_1), $(n_2, d_2, y_2), \ldots, (n_k, d_k, y_k)$. These data result from placing n_i subjects on test at dose d_i and observing y_i responses, $i = 1, 2, \ldots, k$. Each triple is binomially distributed with response probability $P(d)$ satisfying the probit model, as specified in equation (1). Let $\Phi(\cdot)$ and $\phi(\cdot)$ denote the standard normal cumulative distribution function and the standard normal probability density function, respectively. Let $L(\beta_0,\beta_1)$ denote the likelihood function associated with these data. The local information is given by the negative of the second derivative matrix of the (natural) log-likelihood function:

$$I(\beta_0,\beta_1 \mid y_1, \ldots, y_k) = -\begin{bmatrix} \dfrac{\partial^2 \ln L}{\partial\beta_0\,\partial\beta_0} & \dfrac{\partial^2 \ln L}{\partial\beta_0\,\partial\beta_1} \\ \dfrac{\partial^2 \ln L}{\partial\beta_0\,\partial\beta_1} & \dfrac{\partial^2 \ln L}{\partial\beta_1\,\partial\beta_1} \end{bmatrix} \tag{6}$$

It can be shown by straightforward calculations that

$$I(\beta_0,\beta_1 \mid y_1, \ldots, y_k) = \sum \left[\left(\frac{y_i}{\Phi_i^2} + \frac{n_i - y_i}{(1-\Phi_i)^2} \right) \phi_i^2 + \left(\frac{y_i}{\Phi_i} - \frac{n_i - y_i}{1-\Phi_i} \right) A_i \phi_i \right] \begin{pmatrix} 1 & x_i \\ x_i & x_i^2 \end{pmatrix} \tag{7}$$

where $x_i = \log_{10}(d_i)$, $A_i = \beta_0 - 5 + \beta_1 x_i$, $\Phi_i = \Phi(A_i)$, and $\phi_i = \phi(A_i)$. Note that the local information depends on the unknown parameters β_0, β_1 through the A_i's.

2. Expected (Fisher) Information

The attained information from the previous stages is common to all the candidate dose allocations for future stages. The expected information, however, differs for each of these candidate dose allocations. Suppose that a particular candidate dose allocation for one or more future stages places m_j subjects on test at dose d_j, $j = 1, 2, \ldots, H$. The expected information is given by the expectation (with respect to the true, underlying dose-response distribution) of the negative of the second derivative matrix of the (natural) log likelihood function. The expectation of the information matrix in equation (7), after changing notation from i to j, from n_i to m_j, and from k to H, is

$$J(\beta_0,\beta_1) = \sum_{j=1}^{H} \frac{m_j \phi_j^2}{\Phi_j(1-\Phi_j)} \begin{pmatrix} 1 & x_j \\ x_j & x_j^2 \end{pmatrix} \tag{8}$$

where x_j, A_j, Φ_j, and ϕ_j are defined in direct analogy to the local information.

The expected information depends on the unknown parameters β_0, β_1 through the A_j's.

3. Total Information and Anticipated Precision

The total information for a specified dose allocation is the sum of the attained local information from the previous stages and the expected Fisher information from the future stages:

$$T(\beta_0,\beta_1 \mid y_1, \ldots, y_k) = I(\beta_0,\beta_1 \mid y_1, \ldots, y_k) + J(\beta_0,\beta_1) \equiv \begin{bmatrix} t_{00} & t_{01} \\ t_{01} & t_{11} \end{bmatrix} \tag{9}$$

where the 2×2 matrices $I(\cdot)$ and $J(\cdot)$ are defined in equations (7) and (8), respectively.

For a particular dose allocation the variance–covariance matrix of the slope and intercept estimates, $\hat{\beta}_0$ and $\hat{\beta}_1$, is the inverse of T:

$$\text{var}(\hat{\beta}_0,\hat{\beta}_1) = T^{-1}\frac{1}{t_{00}t_{11} - t_{01}^2}\begin{bmatrix} t_{11} & -t_{01} \\ -t_{01} & t_{00} \end{bmatrix} \equiv \begin{bmatrix} v_2 & c_{01} \\ c_{01} & v_1 \end{bmatrix} \tag{10}$$

The estimated asymptotic standard errors of quantities of interest based on the dose-response model are functions of this variance–covariance matrix. The standard error of the slope estimate $\hat{\beta}_1$ is

$$\text{std err}(\hat{\beta}_1) = [(0,1)T^{-1}(0,1)']^{1/2} = v_1^{1/2} \tag{11}$$

The standard error of the estimated probit of response probability at logarithmic dose x is

$$\text{std err}(\hat{\beta}_0 - 5 + \hat{\beta}_1 x) = [(1,x)T^{-1}(1,x)']^{1/2} \tag{12}$$

Let x_{100p} denote the logarithm of the $100p$ percentile of the dose-response distribution:

$$x_{100p} = \frac{\Phi^{-1}(p) - \beta_0 + 5}{\beta_1} \tag{13}$$

The estimated $100p$ percentile, $\hat{x}_{100p}$, is obtained by substituting $\hat{\beta}_0$, $\hat{\beta}_1$ for β_0, β_1 in equation (13). The standard error of the estimated $100p$ percentile is

$$\text{std err}(\hat{x}_{100p}) = \frac{1}{\beta_1}[(1,x_{100p})T^{-1}(1,x_{100p})']^{1/2} \tag{14}$$

The standard errors in equations (11) to (14) involve the parameters of the (unknown) underlying dose-response distribution. These are specified via the a priori dose-response distribution, which is discussed in Section II. C and illustrated in Table 2.

The a priori distribution is updated following each stage, as additional current data are obtained. In updating the a priori distribution, the historical data may be discounted relative to the current data or deleted, as discussed in Section II.C.

F. Sensitivity Analysis

Detailed sensitivity analyses are carried out for each target design to assess its performance under a variety of distributions that might be likely to occur. The central distribution in the sensitivity analysis is based on the specified parameters of the a priori distribution, such as that shown in Table 2. Each target design is evaluated at the central distribution as well as at perturbations about the central distribution. The aim is to determine how well the target designs perform over a class of distributions rather than at just the single a priori distribution. The sensitivity analysis thus accounts for robustness of the target designs to departures from assumptions.

The parameters of the distributions that enter into the sensitivity analysis are perturbed over a range determined by the specified variance–covariance matrix of the a priori distribution, such as that shown in Table 2. This tacitly assumes that the dose-response distribution underlying the results to be obtained in the current test program is statistically compatible with the a priori distribution. The confidence imparted in the a priori distribution is thus reflected in the size of the variance–covariance. This matrix can be scaled up or down by multiplication by a constant factor, as discussed in Section II. C. The methods used to select the distributions that enter into the sensitivity analysis are discussed in the Appendix to this chapter.

The results of the sensitivity calculations are expressed in terms of predicted standard errors of distribution (logarithmic) percentiles of interest as well as the predicted standard error of the slope. Table 4 displays the detailed sensitivity results for design GD1. This design is specified in Table 1 and consists of equal division of 100 subjects among the 20th, 40th, 60th, and 80th percentiles of the a priori dose-response distribution. The middle line in the table (underlined) corresponds to the central distribution. The remaining 48 lines correspond to perturbations about this central distribution. Standard errors of the estimates of (logarithmic) percentiles of interest (50th, 80th, 90th in Table 4) as well as standard errors of the slope are calculated for each of these distributions. The right-hand column (labeled "factor") corresponds to the probability associated with each distribution. The calculation of these probabilities is discussed in the Appendix.

The results of the sensitivity analyses for each target design are summarized in Tables 5 and 6. Table 5 displays weighted averages of the standard errors,

Table 4 Detailed Sensitivity Analysis Results for Design GD1[a]

	Design ID	BO	B1	PCT1	PCT2	PCT3	SEPCT1	SEPCT2	SEPCT3	SEB1	Factor
1	GD1	1.55686	2.91972	50	80	90	0.0475553	0.105432	0.144400	0.811355	0.007225
2	GD1	1.20344	3.24360	50	80	90	0.0425211	0.087692	0.119305	0.825290	0.012325
3	GD1	0.94630	3.47924	50	80	90	0.0395914	0.077833	0.105347	0.836581	0.014450
4	GD1	0.87048	3.73200	50	80	90	0.0369559	0.069308	0.093270	0.849757	0.017000
5	GD1	0.37462	4.00312	50	80	90	0.0345812	0.061943	0.082831	0.885239	0.014450
6	GD1	0.05727	4.29394	50	80	90	0.0324384	0.055585	0.073817	0.883449	0.012325
7	GD1	0.46251	4.77025	50	80	90	0.0296066	0.047653	0.062573	0.917088	0.007225
8	GD1	1.83080	2.91972	50	80	90	0.0458485	0.099725	0.138222	0.807840	0.012325
9	GD1	1.27738	3.24360	50	80	90	0.0413883	0.083288	0.114485	0.821842	0.021025
10	GD1	1.02024	3.47924	50	80	90	0.0387140	0.074149	0.101283	0.832958	0.024850
11	GD1	0.74442	3.73200	50	80	90	0.0362952	0.086245	0.089881	0.848208	0.029000
12	GD1	0.44858	4.00312	50	80	90	0.0340894	0.059413	0.079987	0.861758	0.024650
13	GD1	0.13121	4.29394	50	80	90	0.0320774	0.053511	0.071482	0.880045	0.021025
14	GD1	0.38857	4.77025	50	80	90	0.0293862	0.046141	0.060826	0.913844	0.012325
15	GD1	1.88010	2.91972	50	80	90	0.0451534	0.096097	0.134306	0.806163	0.014450
16	GD1	1.32667	3.24360	50	80	90	0.0409168	0.080498	0.111440	0.820226	0.024650
17	GD1	1.06953	3.47824	50	80	90	0.0383808	0.071824	0.098721	0.831596	0.028900
18	GD1	0.79371	3.73200	50	80	90	0.0360528	0.064317	0.087718	0.844907	0.034000
19	GD1	0.49785	4.00312	50	80	90	0.0339161	0.057826	0.078206	0.860526	0.028900
20	GD1	0.18050	4.29394	50	80	90	0.0319583	0.052215	0.069992	0.878896	0.024850
21	GD1	0.33928	4.77025	50	80	90	0.0283193	0.045202	0.059743	0.912840	0.014450
22	GD1	1.72839	2.91972	50	80	90	0.0448234	0.092803	0.130540	0.806459	0.017000
23	GD1	1.37596	3.24360	50	80	90	0.0407232	0.077820	0.108519	0.819617	0.029000
24	GD1	1.11882	3.47924	50	80	90	0.0382803	0.069596	0.096270	0.831080	0.034000
25	GD1	0.84300	3.73200	50	80	90	0.0353880	0.052476	0.085872	0.844453	0.040000

26	GD1	0.54714	4.00312	50	80	90	0.0338664	0.058314	0.078511	0.860165	0.034000
27	GD1	0.22979	4.29394	50	80	90	0.0319306	0.060925	0.068598	0.878644	0.029000
28	GD1	0.28998	4.77025	50	80	90	0.0293160	0.044315	0.058722	0.912783	0.017000
29	GD1	1.77968	2.91972	50	80	90	0.0449620	0.069234	0.126913	0.805636	0.014450
30	GD1	1.42525	3.24360	50	80	90	0.0407890	0.075249	0.105714	0.819812	0.024850
31	GD1	1.16811	3.47924	50	80	90	0.0363237	0.067481	0.083922	0.831347	0.028900
32	GD1	0.89229	3.73200	50	80	90	0.0380447	0.080716	0.083718	0.844844	0.034000
33	GD1	0.59543	4.00312	50	80	90	0.0339404	0.054874	0.074895	0.860673	0.028900
34	GD1	0.27808	4.28394	50	80	90	0.0320002	0.049816	0.087274	0.879282	0.024850
35	GD1	0.24069	4.77025	50	80	90	0.0293762	0.043476	0.057758	0.913648	0.014450
36	GD1	1.82797	2.91972	50	80	90	0.0452714	0.085996	0.123417	0.806392	0.012325
37	GD1	1.47455	3.24380	50	80	90	0.0411137	0.072776	0.103019	0.820413	0.021025
38	GD1	1.21741	3.47924	50	80	90	0.0386006	0.065416	0.091670	0.832460	0.024650
39	GD1	0.94158	3.73200	50	80	90	0.0362793	0.059034	0.081849	0.848082	0.029000
40	GD1	0.64573	4.00312	50	80	90	0.0341379	0.53502	0.073358	0.862050	0.024850
41	GD1	0.32838	4.29394	50	80	90	0.0321653	0.048707	0.086017	0.880814	0.021025
42	GD1	0.19140	4.77025	50	80	90	0.0295001	0.042884	0.058850	0.915442	0.012325
43	GD1	1.90191	2.91972	50	80	90	0.0465627	0.081330	0.118398	0.809145	0.007225
44	GD1	1.54848	3.24360	50	80	90	0.0420800	0.069250	0.099164	0.823834	0.012325
45	GD1	1.29134	3.47924	50	80	90	0.0393930	0.162508	0.088461	0.835884	0.014450
46	GD1	1.01552	3.73200	50	80	90	0.0369281	0.058852	0.079195	0.849534	0.017000
47	GD1	0.71967	4.00312	50	80	90	0.0346660	0.051588	0.071179	0.865758	0.014450
48	GD1	0.40231	4.29344	50	80	90	0.0325926	0.047147	0.064248	0.884800	0.012325
49	GD1	0.11746	4.77025	50	80	90	0.0298071	0.041578	0.055582	0.919895	0.007225

[a] The underlined distribution is the central distribution.

Table 5 Weighted Averages of the Standard Errors of the Logarithmic 50th, 80th, and 90th Percentiles and the Slope over All the Distributions in the Sensitivity Analysis

	Design=GD1				Design=GD5		
Percent	IDPCT	NPCT	Sortsum	Percent	IDPCT	NPCT	Sortsum
50	SEFVX50	49	0.036863	50	SEFVX50	49	0.037063
80	SEFVX80	49	0.065796	80	SEFVX80	49	0.064222
90	SEFVX90	49	0.090660	90	SEFVX90	49	0.087923
B1	SEFVX81	49	0.850717	B1	SEFVX81	49	0.820809
	Design=GD10				Design=GD6		
50	SEFVX50	49	0.038451	50	SEFVX50	49	0.03609
80	SEFVX80	49	0.058843	80	SEFVX80	49	0.08256
90	SEFVX90	49	0.077879	90	SEFVX90	49	0.11852
B1	SEFVX81	49	0.704621	B1	SEFVX81	49	1.14917
	Design=GD2				Design=GD7		
50	SEFVX50	49	0.037861	50	SEFVX50	49	0.039233
80	SEFVX80	49	0.061135	80	SEFVX80	49	0.058390
90	SEFVX90	49	0.082221	90	SEFVX90	49	0.076571
B1	SEFVX81	49	0.759807	B1	SEFVX81	49	0.693325
	Design=GD3				Design=GD8		
50	SEFVX50	49	0.038780	50	SEFVX50	49	0.038148
80	SEFVX80	49	0.058818	80	SEFVX80	49	0.059842
90	SEFVX90	49	0.077645	90	SEFVX90	49	0.079798
B1	SEFVX81	49	0.705694	B1	SEFVX81	49	0.728632
	Design=GD4				Design=GD9		
50	SEFVX50	49	0.037343	50	SEFVX50	49	0.040943
80	SEFVX80	49	0.062219	80	SEFVX80	49	0.056355
90	SEFVX90	49	0.084367	90	SEFVX90	49	0.071733
B1	SEFVX81	49	0.778833	B1	SEFVX81	49	0.623474

Table 6 Minima and Maxima of the Standard Errors of the Logarithmic 50th, 80th, and 90th Percentiles and the Slope over All the Distributions in the Sensitivity Analysis

	Design=GD1				Design=GD5		
	N	Minimum	Maximum		*N*	Minimum	Maximum
SEFVX50	49	0.029316	0.047555	SEFVX50	49	0.029622	0.047440
SEFVX80	49	0.041578	0.105432	SEFVX80	49	0.041387	0.101758
SEFVX90	49	0.055582	0.144400	SEFVX90	49	0.054838	0.138902
SEFVX81	49	0.805459	0.919895	SEFVX81	49	0.772841	0.894420
	Design=GD10				Design=GD6		
SEFVX50	49	0.031554	0.047595	SEFVX50	49	0.02775	0.04980
SEFVX80	49	0.041651	0.087573	SEFVX80	49	0.04551	0.14178
SEFVX90	49	0.053014	0.117208	SEFVX90	49	0.08528	0.19805
SEFVX81	49	0.641773	0.799141	SEFVX81	49	1.12243	1.19243
	Design=GD2				Design=GD7		
SEFVX50	49	0.030646	0.047480	SEFVX50	49	0.032382	0.048034
SEFVX80	49	0.041790	0.092691	SEFVX80	49	0.042927	0.083840
SEFVX90	49	0.054465	0.125116	SEFVX90	49	0.054734	0.111264
SEFVX81	49	0.690568	0.861523	SEFVX81	49	0.805445	0.82605
	Design=GD3				Design=GD8		
SEFVX50	49	0.031852	0.047782	SEFVX50	49	0.031101	0.047525
SEFVX80	49	0.042300	0.086001	SEFVX80	49	0.041628	0.089953
SEFVX90	49	0.054073	0.114733	SEFVX90	49	0.053529	0.120888
SEFVX81	49	0.627240	0.822425	SEFVX81	49	0.664329	0.824324
	Design=GD4				Design=GD9		
SEFVX50	49	0.030076	0.047356	SEFVX50	49	0.034806	0.048910
SEFVX80	49	0.041038	0.097405	SEFVX80	49	0.044264	0.077431
SEFVX90	49	0.053542	0.132328	SEFVX90	49	0.054499	0.100846
SEFVX81	49	0.733219	0.849374	SEFVX81	49	0.539006	0.755271

over all the 49 distributions in the sensitivity analysis; the distributions closer to the central distribution receive the greater weight. Table 6 displays the minima and the maxima of these standard errors over these same distributions. The maxima can be regarded as worst cases over the range of distributions considered plausible based on the current information.

Table 5 shows that the weighted averages of the standard errors of the $\log_{10}$ (LD_{50}) are similar across all the target allocations considered. This is not surprising since they were all selected to be symmetric about the a priori 50 percentile. Design GD6 is the smallest and design GD9 is the largest. By contrast, the standard errors of the $\log_{10}$ (LD_{90}) and the slope vary to a greater extent across the target allocations considered. Design GD9 is the smallest, and design GD6 is the largest. Similar considerations hold for the maxima of the standard errors. Designs GD3 and GD10 are compromises between the two extremes.

To utilize this information for a stagewise dose allocation, the numbers of stages and the number of animals per stage would be decided upon and design GD3, for example, appropriately scaled down, would be run for the first stage. Following the first stage the dose-response distribution estimate would be updated and the sensitivity analysis would be carried out, as above, to determine which second-stage dose allocations best augment the first-stage doses, in light of what has been learned from the first stage about the dose-response distribution. This procedure would be iterated following each stage of experimentation.

G. SAS Computer Program to Carry Out the Stagewise, Adaptive Dose Allocation Procedures

The procedures that have been discussed in previous sections have been implemented in a SAS computer program. Tables 1 to 6 are based on outputs from this program. The program is based on the two-parameter probit model. This section summarizes the various inputs to, calculations by, and outputs from the program.

A. Inputs to program

1. Experimental results from previous stages (including or excluding historical results)
2. Alternative candidate designs for next stage $(m_1, d_1), \ldots, (m_H, d_H)$ (m_j animals to be tested at dose d_j, $j = 1, \ldots, H$)
3. Estimates $\hat{\beta}_0$ and $\hat{\beta}_1$ of slope and intercept of probit dose response distribution based on experimental results from previous stages (including or excluding historical results) and variances and covariance of these estimates.

B. Program calculations (for each candidate design)

1. Old (local) information matrix, I, based on previously obtained experimental results and on dose-response distribution parameter values
2. New (expected) information matrix, J, based on anticipated results from next stage
3. Total information matrix, $T = I + J$
4. Expected variance–covariance matrix of parameters following next stage, $V = (T)^{-1}$

C. Sensitivity analysis to compare the candidate designs

1. Sensitivity analysis results are expressed in terms of expected precision of estimation of percentiles of interest (e.g., p_1 = 50th and p_2 = 95th percentiles as well as expected precision of estimation of the slope).
2. Let B1 = $\ln(\hat{\beta}_1)$ and let Z = $\hat{\beta}_0 - 5 + \hat{\beta}_1 a$, where a is selected so that B1 and Z are (asymptotically) uncorrelated. Let σ_B and σ_Z denote the standard errors of these quantities.
3. Perturb B1 and Z to B1 $\pm 1.75\sigma_B$, B1 $\pm 1.0\sigma_B$, B1 $\pm 0.5\sigma_B$, B1; Z$\pm 1.75\sigma_Z$, Z$\pm 1.0\sigma_Z$, Z$\pm 0.5\sigma_Z$, Z.
4. Form 49 pairs of seven perturbed B1 values with sever perturbed Z values. Each pair of perturbed B1 and Z values determines a unique dose-response distribution.
5. Evaluate the anticipated standard errors of the percentile and slope estimates for each candidate design and perturbed dose-response distribution.
6. Calculate weighted averages of the standard errors, using weights determined from the discretized bivariate normal distribution.
7. Designs with the smallest average standard errors for each percentile are the most sensitive for all the percentiles of interest. Often no single design will be most sensitive for all the percentiles of interest. In that event a compromise design must be used, which is nearly as good as the most sensitive at each endpoint of interest.

III. CASE STUDY OF THE APPLICATION OF THE STAGEWISE, ADAPTIVE DOSE ALLOCATION STRATEGY

In this section we discuss in detail a case study of the effectiveness of the stagewise, adaptive dose allocation strategy in a particular application. The case study illustrates how the components of the process, which were discussed individually in Section II, interface with one another. In Section IV we describe briefly the application of the methodology to a number of other programs, with varying results.

A. Background

An animal study was undertaken to assess the effectiveness of the drug, atropine, in alleviating toxic effects associated with exposure to a particular toxicant. Earlier studies had suggested that this drug would be extremely effective when administered in sufficiently high doses. The primary objective of the current study was to determine the ED_{95}, the minimum atropine dose necessary to result in a positive response in 95% of the experimental animals when administered in conjunction with fixed dose levels and schedules of several other drugs. The challenge dose of toxicant also remained constant throughout the study. A secondary objective was to assess the global shape of the dose-response relation in terms of its slope and ED_{50}.

It was assumed that all animals would have toxic effects if given no atropine and that no animals would have toxic effects if given sufficiently high doses. That is, the assumed dose-response relation increases from 0% response at zero dose to 100% response as the dose increases without limit. It was also assumed that the dose-response relation could be described by a two-parameter model [i.e., equation (1)], at least out to the 95th percentile. The validity of the probit model assumption permits utilization of the information obtained from the central portion of the dose-response region to make inferences concerning the 95th percentile. Without such a modeling assumption there would be no possibility of estimating the ED_{95} with adequate precision, based on the responses from the limited number of animals that were available for this program.

B. Design Strategy Prior to the Experiment

Resource constraints dictated at a maximum of 50 animals would be available for the experimental program. The precision of estimation of the ED_{95} and of the general shape of the dose-response distribution depends solely and heavily on the animal dose allocations to the dose-response distribution percentiles. As discussed earlier in the chapter, this dependency of the design sensitivity on the percentile allocation can be studied prior to the experiment, without knowing the true underlying dose-response relation.

Computer simulations were carried out to estimate the precision of estimation of the ED_{95}, the ED_{50}, and the slope as a function of the percentile dose allocation. Multiple candidate designs were generated, involving equal as well as unequal allocations to doses. In selecting candidate designs, conflicting considerations needed to be accounted for. That is, observations taken at doses below the ED_{50} would be expected to provide relatively little information about the extreme upper percentiles, such as the ED_{95}. Observations taken at extreme upper percentiles of the dose-response distribution provide very little information per observation to determine the shape of the dose-response distribution or to distinguish among the 90th, 95th, 99th, and so on, percentiles. A study design to accommodate both the primary and secondary study objectives thus needs to be concentrated in the upper portion of the dose-response region, but spread out over a sufficiently wide range of percentiles that at least the upper half of the dose-response distribution might be determined relatively precisely. It was thus decided to consider a class of dose allocations that emphasize the upper half of the dose-response distributions, that includes percentiles between the 50th and the 95th, and that allocates larger numbers of animals to the higher design percentiles than to the lower. The alternative candidate target designs considered are summarized in Table 7.

Each of the 23 target designs shown in Table 7 corresponds to the division of 50 animals among $k = 3$, 4, or 5 dose levels. The response probabilities corresponding to these doses are indicated by Q. For example, target design 20 consists of $k = 5$ dose levels, selected as the 10th, 30th, 50th, 70th, and 90th percentiles of the underlying dose-response distribution. Since the distribution parameters β_0 and β_1 are not known, $\beta_0 - 5$ is arbitrarily set at 0 and β_1 is arbitrarily set at 1 for purposes of comparing the target designs. The variable L10DOSE corresponds to the common logarithm of the dose associated with the specified percentile for this standardized distribution. For each design two dose allocations are considered, an equal allocation and an unequal. The equal allocation places the same number of animals at each dose. The unequal allocation is specified by the variable N2. The rationale for the unequal allocation is that the expected number of nonresponders, $N2(1 - Q/100)$, be constant at each dose in the design. For example, for design 20, $N2(1 - Q/100) = 2.7975$ for all doses. This requires that larger numbers of animals be placed at the higher percentiles than at the lower and results in approximately equal coefficients of variation for estimation of each of the higher percentiles, no matter how far out in the upper tail they may be. Note that for planning purposes the sample sizes do not necessarily have to be integer valued; this is the case for the designs in Table 7.

Table 8 summarizes the expected sensitivities (based on the Fisher information) associated with each of the target designs shown in Table 7. The target designs with equal sample allocation are indicated by the suffix "eq," those with unequal allocation by the suffix "uneq." These will be referred to simply as "E" or "U" in subsequent discussion.

The results in Table 8 show that for each target design (1 to 23), the unequal sample allocation results in a lower standard error for estimating the ED_{95} than the equal allocation; the equal sample allocation results in a lower standard error for estimating the ED_{50} than the unequal allocation. Designs 18 and 20 (E or U) have the smallest standard errors for estimating the slope; they correspond to the largest spreads among distribution percentiles of all the designs considered.

Table 7 Alternative Candidate Target Design Dose Allocations

K	Q	L10DOSE	N2	NSURV2
		Index = 1		
3	75	0.675	8.5217	4.8913
3	85	1.037	10.8694	9.2390
3	95	1.645	32.6083	30.9779
		Index = 2		
3	55	0.126	4.2373	2.3305
3	75	0.675	7.6272	5.7204
3	95	1.645	38.1359	36.2291
		Index = 3		
3	70	0.524	9.0911	6.3638
3	80	0.842	13.6388	10.9093
3	90	1.282	27.2732	24.5459
		Index = 4		
3	50	0.000	6.5219	3.2609
3	70	0.524	10.8698	7.8089
3	90	1.282	32.6094	29.3485
		Index = 5		
3	60	0.263	11.5388	5.9233
3	70	0.524	15.3851	10.7696
3	80	0.842	23.0778	18.4621
		Index = 6		
3	40	−0.263	9.0906	3.6362
3	60	0.263	13.6359	8.1815
3	80	0.842	27.2717	21.8174
		Index = 7		
3	50	0.000	12.7665	6.3833
3	60	0.263	15.9581	9.5749
3	70	0.524	21.2775	14.8943

K	Q	L10DOSE	N2	NSURV2
		Index = 14		
4	50	0.000	7.7924	3.8962
4	60	0.263	9.7405	5.8443
4	70	0.524	12.9874	9.0911
4	80	0.842	19.4810	15.5848
		Index = 15		
4	20	−0.842	5.9998	1.2000
4	40	−0.263	7.9997	3.1999
4	60	0.263	11.9996	7.1998
4	80	0.842	23.9992	19.1994
		Index = 16		
4	40	−0.263	8.7719	3.5088
4	50	0.000	10.5263	5.2632
4	60	0.263	13.1579	7.8947
4	70	0.524	17.5439	12.2807
		Index = 17		
5	55	0.126	3.1084	1.7096
5	65	0.385	3.9965	2.5977
5	75	0.675	5.5950	4.1963
5	85	1.037	9.3251	7.9263
5	95	1.645	27.9752	26.5764
		Index = 18		
5	15	−1.037	2.0328	0.3049
5	35	−0.385	2.6583	0.9304
5	55	0.128	3.8398	2.1119
5	75	0.975	6.9119	5.1837
5	95	1.645	34.5578	32.8299

		Index = 8		
3	30	−0.524	10.5832	3.1690
3	50	0.000	14.7885	7.3943
3	70	0.524	24.6475	17.2533
		Index = 9		
3	40	−0.263	13.5128	5.4051
3	50	0.000	16.2153	8.1077
3	60	0.263	20.2692	12.1615
		Index = 10		
4	65	0.385	4.2613	2.7699
4	75	0.675	5.9659	4.4744
4	85	1.037	9.9431	8.4517
4	90	1.282	29.8294	26.8464
		Index = 11		
4	35	−0.385	2.7709	0.9698
4	55	0.128	4.0024	2.2013
4	75	0.875	7.2044	5.4033
4	95	1.645	36.0218	34.2207
		Index = 12		
4	80	0.263	6.0001	3.6001
4	70	0.524	8.0001	5.5001
4	80	0.842	12.0002	9.6002
4	90	1.282	24.0004	21.6003
		Index = 13		
4	30	−0.524	4.2613	1.2784
4	50	0.000	5.9659	2.9829
4	70	0.524	9.9431	6.9602
4	90	1.282	29.8294	26.8464
		Index = 19		
5	50	0.000	4.3795	2.1898
5	60	0.263	5.4745	3.2847
5	70	0.524	7.2984	5.1096
5	80	0.842	10.9491	8.7593
5	90	1.282	21.8981	19.7083
		Index = 20		
5	10	−1.282	3.1084	0.3108
5	30	−0.524	3.9965	1.1989
5	50	0.000	5.5950	2.7975
5	70	0.524	9.3251	6.5275
5	90	1.282	27.9752	25.1776
		Index = 21		
5	40	−0.263	5.7471	2.2989
5	50	0.000	6.8966	3.4483
5	60	0.263	8.6207	5.1724
5	70	0.524	11.4943	8.0460
5	80	0.842	17.2414	13.7931
		Index = 22		
5	10	−1.282	4.6142	0.4814
5	30	−0.524	5.9326	1.7798
5	50	0.000	8.3058	4.1528
5	80	0.263	10.3821	6.2292
5	80	0.842	20.7641	16.6113
		Index = 23		
5	30	−0.524	6.5357	1.9607
5	40	−0.263	7.6250	3.0500
5	50	0.000	9.1500	4.5750
5	60	0.283	11.4375	6.8625
5	70	0.524	15.2499	10.6750

Table 8 Predicted Standard Errors of Estimate of ED_{95}, ED_{50}, and Slope Based on the Alternative Candidate Target Design Dose Allocations in Table 7

Index	SEEC95	SEEC50	SESLP
1eq	0.47219	0.662873	0.631506
2eq	0.48617	0.308383	0.392556
3eq	0.61114	0.806465	0.696348
4eq	0.51119	0.274955	0.403856
5eq	0.92870	0.460760	0.808332
6eq	0.62328	0.211660	0.422847
7eq	1.19583	0.281425	0.849588
8eq	0.73973	0.183303	0.435860
9eq	1.38531	0.178606	0.835105
10eq	0.49468	0.459565	0.520096
11eq	0.47725	0.220454	0.319637
12eq	0.59078	0.412795	0.558211
13eq	0.49780	0.204695	0.318591
14eq	0.79146	0.294958	0.607207
15eq	0.55955	0.189737	0.320000
16eq	0.96291	0.195959	0.621450
17eq	0.50469	0.341321	0.447772
18eq	0.47040	0.203715	0.267021
19eq	0.57031	0.300666	0.465833
20eq	0.47770	0.200998	0.263439
21eq	0.70968	0.219089	0.488774
22eq	0.54948	0.194422	0.301330
23eq	0.83991	0.181659	0.498498
1uneq	0.35953	0.824257	0.631189
2uneq	0.33581	0.529717	0.414808
3uneq	0.52655	0.701855	0.897496
4uneq	0.40827	0.403113	0.418091
5uneq	0.87841	0.512840	0.810309
6uneq	0.56214	0.270000	0.437721
7uneq	1.16913	0.313528	0.857496
8uneq	0.69895	0.194422	0.449110
9uneq	1.36540	0.181108	0.840892
10uneq	0.36514	0.613514	0.506754
11uneq	0.33744	0.407922	0.335410
12uneq	0.48997	0.508724	0.550000
13uneq	0.38682	0.306105	0.330806
14uneq	0.73293	0.349857	0.809426
15uneq	0.49097	0.216584	0.335559
16uneq	0.92778	0.219773	0.828649
17uneq	0.36662	0.493964	0.432551
18uneq	0.33726	0.351283	0.291033
19uneq	0.46386	0.397995	0.458694
20uneq	0.37184	0.268514	0.283725
21uneq	0.64599	0.288328	0.492443
22uneq	0.49173	0.207605	0.322025
23uneq	0.79790	0.189737	0.505371

It can be concluded from Table 8 that designs 1U and 17U, which are concentrated in the upper portion of the dose-response distribution, are relatively precise for estimating the ED_{95} but are relatively imprecise for estimating the ED_{50}. By contrast, designs 7U and 9U, which are concentrated in the central portion of the dose-response distribution and which have relatively narrow spread among percentiles, are relatively precise for estimating the ED_{50} but are relatively imprecise for estimating the ED_{95} or the slope. Designs 18U, 20U and 22U are reasonable compromise designs; they are relatively precise for estimating each of the ED_{50}, the ED_{95}, and the slope. In summary, designs 11U, 13U, 18U, and 20U are reasonable compromise designs if estimation of the ED_{95} is the most important goal. Designs 15U and 22U sacrifice some precision for estimating the ED_{95} but provide enhanced precision for estimating the ED_{50}. It should be noted that the designs 2U, 11U, and 18U, which provide the relatively best sensitivities for estimating the ED_{95}, all suggest placing considerable numbers of animals in the region of the ED_{95}.

C. Development of the A Priori Distribution

An earlier study had been carried out using the same toxicant and the same combination drug therapy regimen. In the earlier study, however, unlike the current study, the atropine dose was held constant while the toxicant dose was varied. Portions of the earlier study were carried out at atropine doses of 0.00, 0.095, and 0.40 mg/kg.

Two-parameter probit dose-response relations in toxicant doses were fitted to the portions of the data in the earlier study at each of the atropine doses. The response probabilities at the toxicant dose corresponding to the current study were estimated from each portion of the data. These estimates and their associated standard errors are as follows:

Atropine dose (mg/kg)	*N*	Response probability	Standard error	NEQV	NRSPEQ
0.00	48	0.00	0.00		
0.095	12	0.088	0.218	1.684	0.148
0.400	36	0.955	0.050	17.34	16.56

The columns NEQV and NRSPEQ correspond to an *equivalent sample size* and an *equivalent number of responses* for each atropine dose. They are calculated by equating the estimated response probability, q, to NRSPEQ/NEQV and the standard error to $[q(1 - q)/\text{NEQV}]^{1/2}$

"Equivalent sample sizes" and "equivalent numbers of responses" were used as if they were real data for stage 0 of the current experiment, when planning subsequent stages. Note that a fundamental assumption is being made that the prior, stage 0 results are relevant to the results that are anticipated to be obtained from the current study. The appropriateness of the dose selection made in the early stages of the current study depends very heavily on this assumption.

A two-parameter probit model [equation (1)] was fitted to the stage 0 results at atropine doses of 0.095 and 0.400. The estimated intercept and slope were $\hat{\beta}_0 = 8.640$ and $\hat{\beta}_1 = 4.885$, respectively. Initial percentile estimates were determined from the a priori probit model. These were used to arrive at a design for stage 1 of the current study.

D. Choice of Doses for Stage 1

It was decided to divide the total experimental sample size of $N = 50$ into five stages with 10 animals tested per stage. This decision represented a compromise between design flexibility and logistical convenience. The goal of the first stage was to obtain an initial, overall estimate of the dose response relation. This suggested that a global, LD_{50} type of design with widely spaced doses be used. Design 20E is among the best of the designs considered for estimating the ED_{50} and slope (Table 8) and does not degrade precision for estimating the ED_{95} too severely. Since the principal interest lies in the upper half of the dose-response distribution, it was decided to delete the 10th percentile tests from design 20E and shift them to the 80th percentile. A suggested first-stage design was thus to test two animals at each of the estimated 30th, 50th, 70th, 80th and 90th percentiles, the percentiles being estimated based on the a priori distribution. The percentiles, estimated atropine doses, and sample sizes for the 10-animal first-stage design are shown below.

Percentile	Atropine dose (mg/kg)	Number tested
30	0.14	2
50	0.18	2
70	0.23	2
80	0.26	2
90	0.33	2

E. Intermediate Experimental Results: Choice of Doses for Stages 2 and 3

This section briefly summarizes the use of stage 1 and stage 2 experimental results, in conjunction with the stagewise, adaptive design approach to select doses for stages 2 and 3. Section III.F describes in somewhat greater detail the use of the sensitivity analysis procedures to arrive at a dose allocation for stage 4, based on the results observed up through stage 3.

The stage 1 results are shown in Table 9. They are compatible with the a priori predictions. There is a graded dose response, from no response at the relatively low doses to complete response at the higher doses. To update the a priori distribution, a two-parameter probit model was fitted to the combined "data" from stages 0 and 1 (Table 9). The model fitted the data. The estimated slope was 7.17 (2.19) and the estimated 10th, 30th, 50th, 70th, 90th, and 95th percentiles were 0.15, 0.19, 0.22, 0.26, 0.33, and 0.375 mg/kg, respectively. These estimated percentiles are in agreement with those based on stage 0.

Table 9 Experimental Results from Stages 1, 2, 3, and 4[a]

Group	Stage	Dose	*N*	NRESP
Atropine	0	0.095	1.684	0.148
Atropine	0	0.400	17.340	16.560
Atropine	1	0.140	2.000	0.000
Atropine	1	0.180	2.000	0.000
Atropine	1	0.230	2.000	1.000
Atropine	1	0.260	2.000	2.000
Atropine	1	0.330	2.000	2.000
Atropine	2	0.190	2.000	1.000
Atropine	2	0.220	2.000	1.000
Atropine	2	0.250	2.000	1.000
Atropine	2	0.290	2.000	1.000
Atropine	2	0.330	2.000	0.000
Atropine	3	0.310	2.000	0.000
Atropine	3	0.350	2.000	1.000
Atropine	3	0.390	3.000	2.000
Atropine	3	0.450	3.000	2.000
Atropine	4	0.770	3.000	2.000
Atropine	4	1.200	3.000	2.000

[a] Stage 0 corresponds to the a priori distribution, based on historical data.

To select doses for stage 2, the percentile estimates based on the probit fit to the combined stage 0,1 results were used to associate doses with the percentiles (Q) of the target designs in Table 7.

Eight of the best (of 46) previously considered target designs for estimation of the ED_{95}, the ED_{50}, and the slope were evaluated for their expected sensitivity to estimate the ED_{95} and the ED_{50}, based on the anticipated stage 2 results, over and above the attained stage 0 and stage 1 results (i.e., designs 11E, 13E, 18E, 20E, 15U, 18U, 20U, 22U). All eight target designs resulted in similar expected sensitivities for estimating the ED_{95} and similar sensitivities for the ED_{50}. Design 20U was chosen since it was felt that a global design was still called for.

At the conclusion of stage 2, a total of 20 animals would have been tested in the current program (stages 1 and 2) and the equivalent of 19 "animals" from the historical data. The dose allocation for target designs 20U was scaled down from $N = 50$ to $N = 39$ and the sample sizes were rounded to the nearest integer. Table 10 shows the resulting target allocation (NTARGET) for $N = 38$ animals (stages 0, 1, and 2). The current dose allocation (stages 0 and 1) is indicated by NCURR. Ten of the 29 tests correspond to stage 1; 19 are based on historical data. Comparisons of NCURR with NTARGET show that the current allocation falls increasingly short of the target allocations as the distribution percentiles increase.

The suggested stage 2 dose allocation thus places 8 of 10 animals at doses at or above the estimated 50th percentile. This is indicated as NNEW in Table 10. The 4 animals allocated to the 70th percentile dose are divided between the 65th and 80th percentiles to further increase the number of animals tested in the upper tail. The resulting dose allocation is similar to but slightly higher than that for stage 1. This reflects the agreement between the stage 1 results and the a priori assumptions.

The stage 2 results are shown in Table 9. They are less optimistic than what had been anticipated based on the a priori assumptions and the stage 1 results.

Table 10 Selection of Doses for Stage 2 Based on Target Design 20U

Percentile	Target allocation dose	NTARGET	NCURR	NNEW	
10th	0.15 (or less)	2	3.684		
30th	0.19	3	2	2	
50th	0.22	4	2	2	
70th	0.26	7	2	4	{ 65 0.25 2 80 0.29 2
90th	0.33 (or more)	22	19.34	2	
		38	29.0		

Dose 0.33 is the estimated 90th percentile, yet neither of the two animals tested there responded. Doses 0.25 and 0.29 are the estimated 65th and 80th percentiles, respectively, yet just two of the four animals tested there responded.

Probit models were fitted to the results from various subsets of stages 0, 1, and 2. The stage 0 results were statistically compatible with those of stages 1 and 2 combined. There was, however, statistical evidence ($\alpha = 0.03$) that the stage 2 results were not compatible with those of stages 0 and 1 combined.

Despite the statistically significant difference between stage 2 and the earlier stages it was decided to retain the stage 2 results in the dose-selection process for stage 3. This is because the stage 2 results were considered to be fully valid. Questions arose about the appropriateness of the a priori assumptions; however, it was decided to retain the stage 0 results in the dose selection process because they were compatible with the combined stage 1 and 2 results. Dose-response distribution percentiles for the dose allocation in stage 3 were estimated from a probit model fit to the data from stages 0, 1, and 2 combined. The model fitted the data. The estimated slope was 5.861 (1.732), which was flatter than that following stage 1. The estimated 10th, 30th, 50th, 70th, 90th and 95th percentiles were 0.14, 0.19, 0.24, 0.29, 0.39, and 0.45 mg/kg, respectively. The estimates of the upper percentiles, particularly the 90th and 95th were somewhat higher than those following stage 1. The uncertainties in these estimates, particularly the upper confidence bounds, were substantial.

To select doses for stage 3, the percentile estimates based on the probit fit to the combined stage 0, 1, 2 results were used to associate doses with the percentiles of the target designs in Table 7. Twelve of the target designs in Table 7 were compared based on the anticipated stage 3 results, over and above the attained stages 0, 1, and 2 results. All 12 target designs resulted in similar expected sensitivities for estimating the ED_{95} and the ED_{50}. For each of the designs the expected variabilities for the ED_{95} exceeded those that were calculated following stage 1. Designs 13U, 18U, and 20U appeared similar and best for estimating the ED_{95}; design 18U was chosen.

At the conclusion of stage 3, a total of 30 animals would have been tested in the current program (stages 1, 2, and 3) in addition to the 19 "animals" from the historical data. The dose allocation for target design 18U and $N = 50$ animals thus did not need to be scaled down. Table 11 shows this target allocation (NTARGET). The current dose allocation (stages 0, 1, and 2) is indicated by NCURR. Comparison of NCURR with NTARGET shows that the current allocation exceeds the target allocation at the estimated 55th percentile and below, is about in line with the target allocation of the estimated 75th percentile, and falls short of the target allocation at the 95th percentile.

The suggested stage 3 dose allocation thus places 8 of the 10 animals in the proximity of the estimated 90th percentile. This dose allocation is indicated as

Table 11 Selection of Doses for Stage 3 Based on Target Design 18U

Percentile	Target allocation dose	NTARGET	NCURR	NNEW	
15th	0.16 (or less)	2	3.684		
35th	0.20	3	6		
55th	0.25	4	6		
75th	0.31	7	6	2	
95th	0.45(or more)	34	17.34	8	{ 85 0.35 2 90 0.39 3 95 0.45 3
		50	39.0		

NNEW in Table 11. An a priori assumption was that the ED_{95} was bounded from above by 0.40 mg/kg. Although the stage 2 test results appeared to contradict this, it was felt (based on toxicological judgment) that there was still not enough evidence to totally disregard the assumption. The 8 animals allocated to dose 0.45 mg/kg were thus spread among three doses, 0.35, 0.39, and 0.45 mg/kg, in order to obtain further information about the dose-response relation in the neighborhood of 0.40 mg/kg. This illustrates how the dose allocations that are arrived at incorporate toxicological judgment to evaluate and possibly modify the results of the formal calculations.

The stage 3 results are shown in Table 9. The observed response rates are much more pessimistic than what had been anticipated based on the a priori and stage 1 results. Stages 2 and 3 suggest that the dose-response Table 11 distribution may be very flat at doses above 0.20 mg/kg. It may even have an upper asymptote substantially less than 1.0.

The stagewise, adaptive design approach has thus led, midway during the study, to fundamental questions being raised concerning the appropriateness of the a priori assumptions underlying the design of the study.

F. Sensitivity Analysis of Alternative Candidate Dose Allocations to Select Doses for Stage 4

The stage 2 and 3 results raised questions concerning the applicability of the historical data for dose selection. To determine which portions of the data should be used for selecting doses for stage 4, probit dose response models were fitted to the data from various subsets of stages 0, 1, 2, and 3. Likelihood ratio tests were carried out to compare the compatibility of fits from different combinations of stages. The results of these fits are summarized below.

Stages	Slope (std. err)	−2 log likelihood	ED_{95}
0, 1, 2, 3	4.58 (1.45)	51.861	0.58
1, 2, 3	2.72 (1.75)	38.986	1.20
0, 2, 3	4.04 (1.77)	43.082	0.66
2, 3	0.96 (2.44)	27.368	22.03
0, 1	7.17 (2.29)	14.306	0.38
0	4.88 (2.35)	7.365	0.39

To carry out the likelihood ratio tests, the difference of the −2 log likelihood values from the full model and the submodel (−2 log λ) are compared to a chi-square distribution with 2 d.f. The results of these tests are:

Stage 0 vs. stages 1, 2, and 3

$$-2 \log \lambda = 51.861 - (7.365 + 38.986) = 5.510, p = 0.064$$

Stage 0 vs. stages 2 and 3

$$-2 \log \lambda = 43.082 = (7.365 = 27.368) = 8.349, p = 0.015$$

Stages 0 and 1 vs. stages 2 and 3

$$-2 \log \lambda = 51.861 - (14.306 + 27.368) = 10.187\, p = 0.006$$

In addition stage 1 is marginally significantly different from stages 2 and 3 combined ($p = 0.04$).

It was concluded that the stage 0 results are incompatible with those of stages 2 and 3 and should be deleted from further consideration. The stage 4 dose allocations should be planned using either the results from stages 1, 2, and 3 combined or stages 2 and 3 combined. It was felt that the results from stages 2 and 3 were too imprecise to be used by themselves for further dose planning. The slope flattens out very considerably at the higher doses and is imprecisely determined. The stage 1 results represent valid data on toxicological groups, despite the marginal statistical indications of differences from stages 2 and 3. It was thus decided to use the combined stage 1, 2, and 3 results for planning the doses in stage 4.

Table 12 displays the results of a probit model fit to the combined results from stages 1, 2, and 3; Table 13 displays the percentile estimates based on this fit. The estimated ED_{90} is 0.88 mg/kg and the estimated ED_{95} is 1.20 mg/kg. These percentiles are two to three times the dose level, 0.40, that was thought a priori to be an upper bound on the ED_{95}. The shallow slope, in combination with a relatively large standard error 2.72 (1.75), preclude the determination of finite-length confidence intervals by Fieller's method.

Table 8 shows that design 18U is among the most sensitive of the designs considered for estimating the ED_{95}, while still providing reasonable estimation

Table 12 Probit Model Fit to Combined Results from Stages 1, 2, and 3

Nonlinear least squares summary statistics: Dependent variable NDEAD

Source	D.F.	Weighted SS	Weighted MS
Regression	2	30.025301598	15.012650799
Residual	12	10.856570401	0.904714200
Uncorrected total	14	40.881871999	
(Corrected total)	13	16.598191158	
Sum of loss		38.985747155	

		Asymptotic	Asymptotic 95% confidence interval	
Parameter	Estimate	Std. error[a]	Lower	Upper
B1	2.723913299	1.7518998319	−1.0931541534	6.5409807517
B01	6.429245440	0.9986883178	4.2532873150	8.6052035645

Asymptotic correlation matrix of the parameters

CORR	B1	B01
B1	1.0000	0.9719
B01	0.9719	1.000

[a] Standard errors computed using SIGSQ = 1.

of the ED_{50}. Design 18U was thus chosen as an initial target design for stage 4. Table 7 displays the percentiles and the relative allocation of animals to those percentiles for design 18U. Table 13 displays the doses corresponding to those percentiles.

The dose allocation corresponding to target design 18U, scaled down to $N = 40$ animals, is shown in the NTARGET column of Table 14. The current allocation, based on stages 1, 2, and 3, is shown in the NCURR column. Comparison of NCURR with NTARGET shows that the current allocation exceeds the target allocation at the lower distribution percentiles but falls short at the upper percentiles, particularly in the region of the estimated 95th percentile. The suggested stage 4 dose allocation thus needs to be concentrated in the upper percentiles. The formal allocation places 8 of the 10 animals at the estimated 95th percentile, 1.20 mg/kg. Based on toxicological judgment, however, the formal allocation was modified so that these 8 animals were allocated to multiple doses, geometrically spaced between the 75th and 95th percentiles. The modification was made because of the uncertainty in the percentile estimates. Even after the surprisingly pessimistic results in stages 2 and 3 it was

Table 13 Percentile Estimates Based on Probit Model Fit to Combined Results from Stages 1, 2, and 3

Probability	Log10 (dose)	Dose
0.01	−1.37873923	0.04180813
0.02	−1.27866411	0.05264243
0.03	−1.21516966	0.06092988
0.04	−1.16740526	0.06801344
0.05	−1.12855260	0.07437850
0.06	−1.09548288	0.08026332
0.07	−1.06648722	0.08580504
0.08	−1.04052505	0.09109089
0.09	−1.01591350	0.09618038
0.10	−0.99517903	0.10111625
0.15	−0.90519252	0.12439630
0.20	−0.83367409	0.14666480
0.25	−0.77231765	0.16892050
0.30	−0.71721787	0.19177073
0.35	−0.66615933	0.21569530
0.40	−0.81770995	0.24115154
0.45	−0.57083462	0.26863672
0.50	−0.52470248	0.29874285
0.55	−0.47857034	0.33222297
0.60	−0.43169501	0.37008799
0.65	−0.38324563	0.41376559
0.70	−0.33218729	0.46538535
0.75	−0.27708731	0.52833903
0.80	−0.21573086	0.80851198
0.85	−0.14421244	0.71744326
0.90	−0.05422593	0.88262063
0.91	−0.03249146	0.92791574
0.92	−0.00887991	0.97978087
0.93	0.01708226	1.04011715
0.94	0.04607792	1.11193122
0.96	0.11800030	1.31220079
0.97	0.16576470	1.46475402
0.98	0.22925915	1.69534914
0.99	0.32933427	2.13468730

felt that 1.20 mg/kg, being more than three times the a priori upper bound of 0.40, was perhaps well beyond the ED_{95}. If 8 of 8 animals survived at that dose, there would be little information about the region between 0.40 and

Table 14 Determination of Stage 4 Dose Allocation Based on Approximation to Target Design 18U

Percentile	Target allocation dose	NTARGET	NCURR	NNEW	
15th	0.12 (or less)	2	2		
35th	0.22	2	12		
55th	0.33	3	13		
75th	0.53	6	3	2	0.62 2 0.77 2
95th	1.20 (or more)	27		8	0.96 2 1.20 2
		40	30		

1.20. It was thus felt that a more conservative posture of exploring a range of doses beween 0.40 and 1.20 would better focus in on the ED_{95}. Even the modified dose allocation, however, represents a more aggressive increase in doses than those selected in previous stages.

At the end of stage 3 there were serious doubts about the validity of the a priori assumptions. The dose-response relation flattened out considerably at the higher doses relative to a priori expectations. The slope of the probit fit based on stages 1, 2, and 3 combined was 2.72 (1.75); that based on stages 2 and 3 combined was 0.96 (2.44). Questions arose as to whether an ED_{95} even existed. The response rate might never exceed 70%, for example, no matter how high the atropine dose was raised.

Because of these doubts about the validity of the a priori assumptions, the stage 4 sample size was reduced from 10 animals to 6. These animals would be tested at the highest atropine dose levels. Alternative target allocations of 6 animals to one, two, or three dose levels were evaluated by the sensitivity analysis program. The prior distribution for the sensitivity analysis is that shown in Table 12, based on a probit model fit to the combined results from stages 1, 2, and 3. The data from the previous stages that enter into the attained (local) information are those from stages 1, 2, and 3, displayed in Table 9.

Alternative target allocations of 6 animals to one, two, or three dose levels are shown in Table 15 and the summary results of the sensitivity evaluations are shown in Table 16. Examination of the detailed evaluations for each distribution in the sensitivity analysis shows that the expected sensitivity varies widely with the distributions in the sensitivity analysis. There is much uncertainty in the estimate of the dose-response distribution slope [$\hat{\beta}_1 = 2.72$, std err$(\hat{\beta}_1) = 1.75$]. The precision of the ED_{95} estimate is very sensitive to β_1 and varies over an order of magnitude as β_1 varies.

Table 15 Sensitivity Analysis of Candidate Designs for Stage 4: Proposed Doses and Numbers of Subjects

Design ID	Dose 1	Number of subjects per dose 1	Dose 2	Number of subjects per dose 2	Dose 3	Number of subjects per dose 3
ATR1	1.20	6				
ATR2	0.96	3	1.20	3		
ATR3	0.78	3	0.90	3		
ATR4	0.75	3	0.80	3		
ATR5	0.64	3	0.70	3		
ATR6	0.77	2	0.96	2	1.20	2
ATR7	0.67	2	0.78	2	0.90	2
ATR8	0.70	2	0.75	2	0.80	2
ATR9	0.59	2	0.64	2	0.70	2

Target designs ATR1, ATR2, and ATR6 have the lowest weighted averages of standard errors of estimating the ED_{95}. These are the only designs, of the nine considered, that allocate animals to doses 0.96 and 1.20. These designs also have the lowest maximum standard errors, over all the distributions in the sensitivity analysis. This suggests that the stage 4 test doses should be increased substantially relative to the previous stages.

Design ATR1 has the lowest average standard error, but was considered impractical since it is concentrated at a single dose, almost three times that of the previous high dose. The stage 4 allocation was chosen to be a compromise between design ATR1 and ATR6:

Percentile	Dose	N
87th	0.77	3
95th	1.20	3

Note that the stagewise design process has led to the use of doses twice to three times those originally anticipated prior to stage 1.

Table 9 shows that the stage 4 test results were no different than the stage 3 results, despite the use of atropine doses that were two to three times higher. The slope estimate decreased to 1.41 and the ED90 and ED_{95} estimates increased to 2.75 and 4.98, respectively. This is toxicologically quite unreasonable since an atropine dose of 0.40 was shown to be quite efficacious in previous studies.

Table 16 Sensitivity Analysis Evaluation of Candidate Designs for Stage 4: Weighted Averages of Standard Errors of the 50th, 80th, and 95th Percentiles and the Slope over the Designs in the Sensitivity Analysis

	Design = ATR1				Design = ATR4				Design = ATR7		
Percent	PCT	NPCT	Sortsum	Percent	PCT	NPCT	Sortsum	Percent	PCT	NPCT	Sortsum
50	50	49	0.13720	50	50	49	0.14859	50	50	49	0.14162
80	80	49	0.32772	80	80	49	0.41013	80	80	49	0.36227
95	95	49	0.60734	95	95	49	0.76057	95	95	49	0.67207
81	B1	49	1.39058	81	B1	49	1.38785	81	B1	49	1.37854
	Design = ATR2				Design = ATR5				Design = ATR8		
50	50	49	0.13924	50	50	49	0.15472	50	50	49	0.14985
80	80	49	0.34406	80	80	49	0.44916	80	80	49	0.41840
95	95	49	0.63810	95	95	49	0.83178	95	95	49	0.77572
81	B1	49	1.38158	81	B1	49	1.41429	81	B1	49	1.39259
	Design = ATR3				Design = ATR6				Design = ATR9		
50	50	49	0.14580	50	50	49	0.14162	50	50	49	0.15668
80	80	49	0.39143	80	80	49	0.36227	80	80	49	0.46118
95	95	49	0.72617	95	95	49	0.67207	95	95	49	0.85356
81	B1	49	1.38077	81	B1	49	1.37854	81	B1	49	1.42542

At this point it was felt that an ED_{95} dose level might never be attainable. Perhaps a limited threshold response rate exists well below 95 percent. The experiment was thus stopped after $N = 36$ animals and efforts were begun to identify the reason(s) for disagreement of the current results with the historical.

The stagewise, adaptive design approach permitted considerable flexibility to respond to unanticipated test results. The test doses were raised to substantially higher levels than what had been anticipated prior to the study. When even this did not bring about the anticipated level of response, the stagewise approach permitted early termination of the study, thereby conserving time and resources.

IV. ADDITIONAL EXAMPLES OF THE APPLICATION OF THE STAGEWISE, ADAPTIVE DOSE ALLOCATION STRATEGY

The stagewise, adaptive dose allocation strategy has been applied in the design stages of a number of test programs. In some programs the flexibility of the adaptive approach permitted midstudy modifications to be made, in response to early stage results that were quite different from what had been anticipated prior to the start of the experiment. In other programs, where the a priori assumptions were predictive of the experimental results, the stagewise dose allocation helped to assure that tests were carried out in the appropriate portions of the dose-response region, based on the study objectives. This resulted in more efficient use of the available experimental resources. Several of these programs are discussed briefly in this section.

A. Studies Where the A Priori Assumptions Were Contradicted

In the case study that was discussed in detail in Section III, the study results proved to be very different from and much more pessimistic than the a priori assumptions. On the basis of historical data there was strong confidence that an atropine dose of 0.40 mg/kg would be an upper bound on the ED_{95} value; the purpose of the study was to determine how far the dose could be reduced to attain the ED_{95}. Instead, the study demonstrated a 30 to 40% nonresponse rate at atropine doses two to three times higher than the a priori "upper bound." The stagewise, adaptive dose allocation procedure permitted test doses to be increased continually from stage to stage, in response to increasingly more pessimistic results. These pessimistic warnings appeared early in the study and persisted. It was finally decided that the ED_{95} may not even exist. The stagewise design thus permitted the study to be terminated early, with a consequent savings of experimental resources. Furthermore, the negative results led to a search for and eventual resolution of the reasons that the a priori assumptions were contradicted. This led to a discovery of important differences in the characteristics of experimental animals originating from different sources, which prior to the study had been thought to be equivalent.

The stagewise, adaptive dose allocation procedure was applied in another study in which atropine was administered as part of a combination drug regimen to alleviate the effects of a particular toxicant. Four groups were tested in parallel: one with no drug treatment, one with atropine and pralidoxime chloride administered after exposure to the toxicant, and two with (different doses of) pyridostigmine bromide administered before exposure followed by atropine and pralidoxime chloride after exposure to the toxicant. The original study protocol specified that the atropine dose be fixed at 0.095 mg/kg. It was anticipated that preexposure treatment with pyridostigmine bromide would result in moderate improvements in efficacy, as compared to postexposure treatment only.

The study was designed in a stagewise fashion with eight stages. Each stage consisted of multiple animals from each treatment group being tested in parallel. The toxicant test doses were selected in adaptive fashion across stages, separately for each treatment group. The study objective was to estimate and compare the ED_{50} and other distribution percentiles from each of the groups.

After two stages were completed, intermediate statistical analyses indicted that contrary to a priori expectations the regimens, including pyridostigmine bromide pretreatment, showed little or no difference in treatment efficacy relative to the regimen with postexposure treatment only. The flexibility of the stagewise approach permitted the study to be stopped temporarily, to consider possible explanations for the unanticipated results and appropriate courses of action. It was decided to quadruple the atropine dose, from 0.095 mg/kg to 0.40 mg/kg.

The study was resumed at the higher atropine dose. The efficacy of the pretreatment regimen went from essentially nil at the lower atropine dose to substantially greater than anticipated at the higher atropine dose. The a priori expectation for the ratio of the ED_{50} values with and without pretreatment was in the range of 8 to 10. At the lower atropine dose the observed ratio was less than 2. At the higher atropine dose the ratio exceeded 40. The adaptive dose allocation strategy permitted toxicant doses to be consistently increased from stage to stage as the intermediate results appeared increasingly favorable. By the end of the study, the toxicant doses were more than an order of magnitude higher than what had been anticipated a priori.

B. Studies Where the A Priori Assumptions Were Confirmed

The stagewise, adaptive dose allocation procedure was applied to a study in which a substantial number of treatment regimens were compared simultaneously, in terms of their efficacy to alleviate toxicant effects. The study objective was to compare the ED_{50} and the ED_{84} values among treatment regimens.

The early stages of the program consisted of pilot experiments with relatively small numbers of animals that received either no treatment or the standard treatment regimen. These animals were tested in the classical up–down fashion to gain initial information about the centers and slopes of the dose-response distributions. The flexibility of the stagewise approach permits such data to be considered as the first stage and to be utilized both to plan the dose selection in the later stages and as part of the combined results.

The stagewise design permitted early culling of treatment regimens for which strong statistical evidence of relative ineffectiveness existed midway during the study. It also permitted early stopping in the event that one or more of the treatment regimens was substantially more effective than the remainder. The stagewise conduct of the study permitted the final results to be anticipated after just half or fewer of the animals had been tested.

The stagewise, adaptive design procedure was applied in another study that was carried out in a species for which no prior data existed pertaining to the treatment regimen, the toxicant, or the route of administration to be used in the current study. The study objective was to compare the efficacies of two alternative drug delivery systems in terms of the ED_{50} values and slopes of their associated toxicant dose-response distributions.

The a priori dose-response distribution was necessarily based on previous studies that had been carried out in different species. A working assumption was made that the dose-response relations would be similar among species. It turned out after the fact that the dose-response slopes were in fact similar across species. The ED_{50} (on a body weight basis) for the current study would have been better approximated if the historical ED_{50} had been adjusted by a surface area correction. Namely, if species 2 is heavier than species 1, a working assumption might be that the ED_{50} for species 1 needs to be scaled down by a factor $(W_1/W_2)^{1/3}$ to predict that for species 2, where W_1 and W_2 are the average body weights for the two species.

As with the study previously discussed, the stagewise design permitted early stopping in the event that strong statistical evidence was present midway during the study that one delivery system was substantially more efficacious than the other.

In yet another application of the stagewise, adaptive design approach it was desired to estimate the LD_{50} and the slope for animals that were exposed to graded doses of a particular toxicant. The dose-response distribution was to be estimated based on a very small number of animals, so it was essential that the animals be tested at doses representing appropriate regions of the (unknown) dose-response relation. Previous studies had been carried out on the same species, but on animals from a different source, and there were indications of substantial differences in response between the different groups of animals.

The a priori dose-response distribution was based on the results of an initial up–down pilot experiment, carried out with one animal at a time. After several animals had been tested in this manner, the assumption was made of a common dose-response slope with the historical data but a very different LD_{50}. This common slopes assumption, although not verifiable early in the experiment, permitted an initial dose-response distribution for the current study to be fitted based on just a handful of animals. This distribution in turn served as a prior distribution for planning later stages of the current study and proved to be a good predictor of the final results. The stagewise adaptive dose allocation process permitted the final study results to be anticipated very early in the study. The LD_{50} estimated based on the results from just $N = 8$ animals differed from the final estimate by just 7.4%.

C. Application of the Sensitivity Analysis Procedure for Study Planning

An example is discussed in Section II that illustrates how the sensitivity analysis calculation may be used for planning purposes. A study is to be undertaken to determine the 48-hour lethality following exposure to a toxicant and treatment with a single, standard regimen. The primary objective is to estimate the 50th percentile of the underlying dose-response distribution; secondary objectives are to estimate the 90th percentile and the slope. This study is in support of the design of a standardized screening program in which candidate treatment regimens will be challenged with the above LD_{50} dose of toxicant and compared with the standard treatment regimen for efficacy.

To make efficient use of the available experimental resources it is necessary that the animals be tested at appropriate regions of the dose-response distribution. Alternative target designs were considered, each design corresponding to the allocation of $N = 100$ animals to doses that represent specified percentiles of the a priori dose-response distribution. It was demonstrated that with appropriate allocation of doses the LD_{50} could be determined with acceptable precision based on just one-half to one-third the number of animals required for a classical single-stage, fixed-dose design.

The stagewise, adaptive dose allocation process was applied to the design of another study in which flexibility in the selection of doses was very important. Two different endpoints, lethality and immobilization, were of equal interest. It was not known how similar or how disparate the dose-response relations for these two endpoints would be. In the former case a single set of doses might suffice for both endpoints; in the latter case the experimental resources would need to be divided to carry out essentially two separate experiments. A compromise between these two extremes is the most likely situation. The dose allocation therefore needs to be carried out in a stagewise fashion, as information about the similarity of these two dose-response relations is accumulated.

V. DISCUSSION AND AREAS FOR FURTHER EXTENSION

In this chapter we have considered the needs for and the theory and methodology underlying a stagewise, adaptive approach to dose allocation in dose-response studies with quantal responses. The design methodology has been implemented in a special-purpose computer program that runs on the SAS statistical computing system.

The methods are flexible. They adapt to changes in the current estimates of the underlying dose-response relations as new experimental results are obtained. They permit the use of information external to the study and appropriate structure internal to the study to estimate and to update the a priori dose-response distribution that is the basis for dose selection in subsequent stages and for sensitivity evaluation of the alternative candidate designs. The methods allow for successive modifications in test dose levels, well above or beyond a priori expectations. They also allow for early termination of the entire study or of particular treatment regimens within the study if the observed results are substantially better or worse than what had been anticipated prior to the study. They can be adapted to meet many different design objectives.

The design approach incorporates toxicological judgment into all decisions concerning dose selection. The models and the sensitivity analysis calculations are regarded as vehicles for systematizing the statistical and toxicological interpretation of the intermediate study results and their implications about future results; they are not used as a substitute for scientific judgment.

The stagewise, adaptive design approach has been applied in a number of programs, either completed or in the planning stages. In some programs the experimental outcomes agreed with a priori expectations. In other programs the experimental outcomes turned out to be somewhat different than what had been anticipated prior to the study, either somewhat better or somewhat worse.

In either event the stagewise, adaptive approach led to the selection of test doses in subsequent stages that moved rapidly toward the appropriate regions of the dose-responses. This flexibility has provided the ability to make a priori unanticipated adjustments to experimental procedures or to the entire experiment, where needed.

A detailed, example case study was presented of the application of the methods in a study in which the a priori assumptions turned out to be incorrect. The stagewise, adaptive approach led to the early termination of the study. It also led to further investigations concerning the reasons for the unexpected results, which in turn led to discoveries of various characteristics of the animal model that were unanticipated prior to the experiment. Other applications of the methods were more briefly summarized.

The methodology discussed in this chapter is based on various assumptions. A number of these assumptions, consequences of using the methods, and various areas for extension, are discussed below.

1. The specific design procedures discussed in this paper are appropriate for quantal responses and for dose-response relations that can be described by simple, two-parameter probit models. The basic ideas, however, are much more generally applicable. The probit model can be generalized to have a nonzero background level and an asymptote less than 1. For example, the four-parameter model

$$P(d) = a + (b - a)\Phi(\beta_0 - 5 + \beta_1 x)$$

ranges between a and b. Setting $a = 0$, $b = 1$ reduces to equation (1). Such a model would be appropriate when longer-term responses are utilized, so that background response is of concern. If a morbidity response such as absence of convulsions after administration of dose d of a drug were of interest, the above-extended model might be appropriate. Some animals might not convulse, even with the absence of drug; other animals might convulse, even with the highest doses of drug deliverable. Other extensions of model (1) could be the incorporation of nonlinear dose effects in the probit scale, possibly even nonmonotonic effects, or the incorporation of stage effects or covariates. The quantal response could be extended to a categorical response with more than two categories, to a count response, or to a continuous response.

2. One advantage of the stagewise design approach is the opportunity for early termination of (portions of) the study if the results are substantially better or substantially worse than what had been anticipated prior to the study. Such a decision is based on a multiplicity of statistical inferences across groups and across stages. The error probabilities associated with the various early termination decision need to be divided among these decision points. A substantial

literature on simultaneous inference methods (Miller, 1966) and subset selection methods (Gibbons et al., 1977) is available. A substantial literature is also available on stopping rules for group sequential clinical trials (Geller and Pocock, 1987). Consideration needs to be given as to how best to apply such methods to the stagewise dose-response experimental design problem.

3. The design procedures discussed in this chapter lead to very different dose allocations than classical single-stage "LD_{50} study" designs. Classical designs utilize relatively small numbers of discrete doses with relatively large numbers of animals per dose. By contrast, the current design procedures lead to designs that utilize relatively large numbers of doses with relatively small numbers of animals per dose. It is possible that each animal in the study might be tested at a different dose. Standard probit analysis computer programs cannot be used to fit probit models to these dose-response data due to the nonstandard dose allocations and due to a number of other nonstandard aspects of the model specifications. Specialized procedures, based on nonlinear regression analyses, have been developed to fit dose-response models to these data. These procedures have been implemented in a series of computer programs based on the general-purpose nonlinear regression procedure in the SAS statistical computing system (SAS Institute, 1985).

4. Although the experimental design is carried out in stages, the basic probit model in equation (1) does not incorporate stage-to-stage variation (i.e., stage "effects"). Possible causes of such stage effects might be systematic drift in experimental conditions, isolated outlying responses, or random variation. The presence and nature of possible stage-to-stage variation needs to be determined and adjusted for when updating the prior distribution to be used for planning the subsequent experimental stages. The specialized model-fitting procedures that are mentioned in paragraph 3 include a test for stage-to-stage variation based on the studentized residuals from the fitted probit model (1). The statistical sensitivity of this test for stage effects needs to be studied. Rough calculations were carried out to gain some intuition about the performance of the test and are briefly discussed below. They should by no means be regarded as an in-depth examination of its properties. Model (1) can be rewritten as

$$E(y_{ij}) = \alpha_0 + \beta_1(x_{ij} - \bar{x}) \qquad i = 1, \ldots, I; \qquad j = 1, \ldots, n_i \tag{15}$$

where $E(y) = \Phi^{-1}(P(d))$, $x = \log_{10}(d)$, $k = \Sigma_i n_i$, $\bar{x} = (\Sigma_{ij} x_{ij})/k$, and $\alpha_0 = \beta_0 - 5 + \beta_1\bar{x}$. The index ij corresponds to the jth observation in the ith stage.

Two types of stage effects are considered, a systematic linear drift across stages, γi, and a random stage effect, γT_i. The random stage effects T_i are assumed to be independent and identically distributed with mean μ and variance σ_T^2. The models incorporating systematic linear drift and random stage effects can be written as

$$y_{ij} = \alpha_0 + \beta_1(x_{ij} - \bar{x}) + \gamma i + \epsilon_{ij} \tag{16}$$

and

$$y_{ij} = \alpha_0 + \beta_1(x_{ij} - \bar{x}) + \gamma T_i + \epsilon_{ij} \tag{17}$$

respectively. The random error ϵ_{ij} has an asymptotic variance, based on binomial distribution theory and propagation of errors, that is a function of the mean. The probit models are thus fitted to the data by an iteratively reweighted least squares procedure. For purposes of the rough calculations, however, merely to gain intuition about the characteristics of the tests on residuals, it was assumed that the ϵ_{ij}'s have constant variance σ_ϵ^2 that is known. The characteristics of ordinary (i.e., unweighted) least-squares estimates in models (16) and (17) were studied.

First consider model (16). Assume that the logarithmic doses, x_{ij}, have correlation ρ with the stage number. The correlation ρ would tend to be close to ± 1 in those cases when the doses increased monotonically or decreased monotonically with stage. Let $\hat{\beta}_1$ denote the least squares estimate of β_1. It can be shown that

$$E(\hat{\beta}_1) = \beta_1 + \gamma\rho \left[\frac{\Sigma_i n_i (i - \bar{i})^2}{\Sigma_{ij}(x_{ij} - \bar{x})^2} \right]^{1/2} \tag{18}$$

Equation (18) shows that if the doses are uncorrelated with the stage, the slope estimate is unbiased by systematic linear drift. Otherwise, the bias is proportional to the extent of the drift, γ, and the extent of the correlation, ρ. Let r_{ij} denote the residual from the fit to model (15), assuming that (16) is true. To detect a linear drift across stages, based on the residuals, the model

$$r_{ij} = \theta(i - \bar{i}) + \delta \tag{19}$$

can be fitted. Let $\hat{\theta}$ denote the least squares estimate of θ. It can be shown that

$$E(\hat{\theta}) = \gamma(1 - \rho^2) \tag{20}$$

Thus when ρ is close to 0, the linear drift across stages can be detected from the residuals. However, as ρ approaches ± 1, the residuals will reflect less and less of the drift. The calculations above imply that when linear drift across stages is present and when the doses are highly correlated with stage, the probit model slope estimate is biased by the drift and the stage effect cannot be detected by examination of the residuals. When the doses are uncorrelated with stage, this is not the case.

Next consider model (17), with random stage effects, T_i, that are assumed to be uncorrelated with dose. It can be shown that

$$\hat{\beta}_0 = \beta_0 + \gamma\bar{T} + \bar{\epsilon} \tag{21}$$

$$E(\hat{\beta}_1) = \beta_1 \tag{22}$$

and

$$r_{ij} = \gamma(T_i - \bar{T}) + \epsilon^* \tag{23}$$

Equations (21) to (23) show that the overall level of the estimated dose response is biased by the average of the stage effects, the slope estimate is not biased, and the stage effects can be detected from the residuals.

In summary, it is desirable to have as little stage-to-stage variation in experimental conditions as possible when using the stagewise, adaptive dose allocation procedure. Most applications of the stagewise design procedure would be expected to occur within a single study, carried out by a single investigator, in a single laboratory, over a contiguous and relatively short period of time. These represent the best of circumstances for maintaining constant experimental conditions across stages. If a study is expected to run over several seasons and the animal response is known to have a seasonal component, the seasonal component of response needs to be included in the models as a covariate, and adjusted for.

If stage effects cannot be totally, or at least nearly, eliminated by controlling the sources of experimental variation across stages, one or more positive control dose conditions might be included in the design to at least provide estimates of the stage effects in order to adjust for them. These doses would be repeated across stages and would provide direct comparisons across stages—therefore direct estimates of stage effects. This, however, is an alternative design objective from that discussed in Section II. The portion of the experimental resources allocated to detecting stage-to-stage variation detracts from the resources available for meeting the principal design objectives: estimating the specified percentiles of the dose-response distributions and comparing these across distributions. This, in turn, degrades the sensitivity of such inferences.

The adaptive aspects of the dose allocation procedures do in fact sometimes lead to high correlations between the dose allocation and stage. This occurs most frequently in studies where the a priori assumptions are contradicted by the study results. The studies discussed in Sections III and IV.A provide examples of this occurrence. In the first study the atropine dose was increased substantially from stage to stage, particularly in the later stages. In the second study the toxicant dose was increased substantially from stage to stage in both treatment groups that included pretreatment with pyridostigmine bromide. In both cases, therefore, the validity of the inferences concerning the nonefficacy or efficacy, respectively, of the drug regimens could be influenced by the constancy of experimental conditions across stages.

5. The data analysis procedures do not explicitly account for the stagewise, sequential manner in which the doses were selected. Mehta et al. (1988) demonstrate in the context of treatment allocation in the much simpler two-sample problems that accounting for the specific treatment allocation rule in the comparison of the treatments is not important if the study population is homogeneous across time (i.e., no stage effects) but becomes more and more important as the extent of time drifts in the population increases. Jennison and Turnbull (1983), Tsiatis et al. (1984), and Mehta et al. (1988) discuss hypothesis-testing and confidence-interval procedures for one- and two-sample problems that explicitly account for the sequential treatment allocation and sequential stopping rules.

The problem is substantially more difficult in the dose-response estimation case. It is conjectured, on the basis of Mehta et al.'s results, that utilizing the standard likelihood methods of analysis is appropriate either in the absence of stage effects or if stage effects are appropriately included in and adjusted for in the dose-response models. This problem, however, has not been studied and needs to be considered in detail.

ACKNOWLEDGMENT

This work was supported by the U.S. Army Medical Research and Development Command under Contract DAMD17-83-C-3129.

APPENDIX: DETERMINATION OF THE DISTRIBUTIONS THAT ENTER INTO THE SENSITIVITY ANALYSIS

The distributions in the sensitivity analysis are selected based on the parameters β_0 and β_1 of the prior distribution and the variance–covariance matrix of this distribution, as specified in equation (10). These five parameters are used to form a relatively crude prior distribution on the underlying dose-response distribution, which is a discretized form of a biavariate normal distribution. The procedure for constructing the prior distribution is discussed below.

Assume that the variance–covariance matrix specified in equation (10) is the actual, known variance–covariance and assume that $\hat{\beta}_0$ and $\hat{\beta}_1$ have a joint, bivariate normal distribution with this variance–covariance. Let

$$a = \frac{-c_{01}}{v_1} \tag{A.1}$$

$$Z = \hat{\beta}_0 - 5 + \hat{\beta}_1 a \tag{A.2}$$

$$\mathrm{B1} = \ln(\hat{\beta}_1) \tag{A.3}$$

The value of a has been chosen so that $\mathrm{cov}(Z,\hat{\beta}_1) = 0$. It can be shown by a simple propagation of errors argument that cov(Z,B1) is approximately 0. Therefore, Z and B1 have an approximate bivariate normal distribution with correlation 0 and are therefore approximately independent. The standard errors of Z and B1 are approximately

$$\sigma_Z \equiv \text{std err}(Z) \doteq (v_0 + 2ac_{01} + a^2 v_1)^{1/2} \tag{A.4}$$

$$\sigma_B \equiv \text{std err}(\mathrm{B1}) \doteq \frac{v_1^{1/2}}{\beta_1} \tag{A.5}$$

Perturb Z to Z $\pm 0.5\,\sigma_z$, $Z \pm 1.0\sigma_z$, $Z \pm 1.75\sigma_z$. Similarly, perturb B1 to B1 $\pm 0.5\sigma_B$, $\mathrm{B1} \pm 1.0\sigma_B$, $\mathrm{B1} \pm 1.75\sigma_B$. The seven values, Z and its six perturbations, are treated as a discretized normal distribution with seven levels; similarly for B1 and its six perturbations. The probabilities associated with each of these seven values are approximations to the areas under a standard normal distribution between boundaries that are midway between the seven values: $(-\infty,-1.375)$, $(-1.375,-0.75)$, $(-0.75,-0.25)$, $(-0.25,0.25)$, $(0.25,0.75)$, $(0.75,1.375)$, and $(1.375,\infty)$. The probabilities associated with these intervals are 0.085, 0.145, 0.17, 0.20, 0.17, 0.145, and 0.085, respectively. Since Z and B1 are approximately independent and normally distributed, the probabilities associated with pairs of perturbed Z and B1 values are simply the products of the probabilities associated with each value individually. This generates a 49-point bivariate distribution, each point of which represents a possible underlying dose-response distribution. The probabilities associated with the distributions are largest for the more central distributions and smallest for the more extreme distributions. For example, a probability of 0.040 is associated with the pair of central values Z, B1, while a probability of 0.0072 is associated with the pair of extreme values $Z + 1.75\sigma_z$, $\mathrm{B1} + 1.75\sigma_B$.

REFERENCES

Abdelbasit, K. M., and Plackett, R. L. (1983). Experimental design for binary data. *J. Am. Stat. Assoc. 78*: 90–98.

Dixon, W. J. (1965). The up-and-down method for small samples. *J. Am. Stat. Assoc. 60*: 967–978.

Geller, N. L., and Pocock, S. J. (1987). Interim analyses in randomized clinical trials: ramifications and guidelines for practitioners. *Biometrics 43*: 213–223.

Gibbons, J. D., Olkin, I., and Sobel, M. (1977). *Selecting and Ordering Populations: A New Statistical Methodology*, Wiley, New York.

Hsi, B. P. (1969). The multiple sample up-and-down method in bioassay. *J. Am. Stat. Assoc. 64*: 147–162.

Jennison, C., and Turnbull, B. W. (1983). Confidence intervals for a binomial parameter following a multistage test with application to Mil-Std 105D and medical trials. *Technometrics 25*: 49–58.

Lai, T. L., and Robbins, H. (1978). Adaptive design in regression and control. *Proc. Natl. Acad. Sci. USA 75*: 1068–1070.

Lai, T. L., and Robbins, H. (1979). Adaptive design and stochastic approximation. *Ann. Stat. 7*: 1196–1221.

McLeish, D., and Tosh, D. (1983). The estimation of extreme quantiles in logit bioassay. *Biometrika 70*: 625–632.

Mehta, C. R., Patel, W. R., and Wei, L. J. (1988). Constructing exact significance tests with restricted randomization rules. *Biometrika 75*: 295–302.

Miller, R. G., Jr. (1966). *Simultaneous Statistical Inference*, McGraw-Hill, New York.

SAS (1985). *SAS User's Guide: Statistics,* Version 5 ed., SAS Institute, Cary, N.C.

Tsiatis, A. A., Rosner, G. L., and Mehta, C. R. (1984). Exact confidence intervals following a group sequential test. *Biometrics 40*: 797–803.

Tsutakawa, R. K. (1980). Selection of dose levels for estimating a percentage point of a logistic quantal response curve. *Appl. Stat. 29*: 25–33.

Wetherill, G. B., Chen, H., and Vasudeva, R. B. (1966). Sequential estimation of quantal response curves: a new method of estimation. *Biometrika 53*: 439–454.

5

Stagewise, Group Sequential Experimental Designs for Comparisons of Quantal Response Levels Obtained with Candidate Treatment Regimens Versus Those with a Concurrent Control or a Specified Standard

Paul I. Feder, Carl T. Olson, David W. Hobson, M. Claire Matthews, and R. L. Joiner*

Battelle, Columbus, Ohio

I. INTRODUCTION

Battelle's Medical Research and Evaluation Facility designs and conducts experiments to assess the efficacy of candidate decontaminants, barriers, and drug therapies in mitigating the effects of exposure to various classes of toxic chemical substances. A number of these evaluation programs involve the application of standardized screening protocols that are run repeatedly to compare the efficacy of newly developed candidate treatments with the current standard treatment. Responses measured in these standardized screens may be continuous, such as red blood cell acetylcholinesterase inhibition level, may be ordered categorically, such as severity of signs (absent, mild, moderate, severe), or may be dichotomous, such as presence or absence of mortality or morbidity.

The statistical methods discussed in this chapter pertain to the dichotomous response situation. Each animal's response is scored as 0 or 1 (survival or death, absence or presence of a specified sign, etc.). Let p_1 denote the proportion of animals in the entire population whose response would be category 1

*Current affiliation: TSI Redfield Laboratories, Redfield, Arkansas

(e.g., death) when treated with the standard therapy. This is the *population response rate* (e.g., population lethality rate) associated with the standard treatment. Let p_2 denote the population response rate associated with the candidate treatment. The efficacy of the candidate treatment relative to the standard treatment is evaluated by comparing p_2 with p_1. In the situation of an adverse response such as lethality, the candidate treatment is as good as or better than the standard if $p_2 \leqslant p_1$; it is inferior to the standard if $p_2 > p_1$.

The screening studies are designed to identify those candidate treatments that are statistically significantly inferior to the standard. These candidate treatments are eliminated from consideration; all others are evaluated further in higher tiers of testing.

The evaluation of the efficacy of the candidate treatments relative to the standard is formulated statistically in a hypothesis-testing framework. The hypotheses $H_1: p_2 \leqslant p_1$ versus $H_2: p_2 > p_1$ are tested. The type 1 error (i.e., accepting H_2 when H_1 is correct) is set at level α. If H_1 is rejected in favor of H_2, the candidate treatment is not considered further. A principal statistical design objective is to have at least a specified level of power, $1 - \beta$, to reject H_1 when p_2 is at least a specified amount, δ, greater than p_1. Sufficient numbers of experimental subjects must be tested to attain the desired levels of type 1 error and power. As an example of this formulation, assume the lethality rate p_1 associated with the standard treatment regimen is approximately 0.50. If $p_2 \leqslant p_1 = 0.50$, it may be desirable to have probability no greater than $\alpha = 0.05$ of rejecting H_1. However, if $p_2 \geqslant 0.70$, it would be desirable to have power least $1 - \beta = 0.80$ for rejecting H_1.

Two distinct situations fall under this framework, the one-sample case and the two-sample case. In the one-sample case, p_1 is a known value. This situation arises if p_1 is an externally imposed standard. For example, it may be specified that animals exposed to a particular dose of a toxicant and given an acceptable candidate treatment regimen may have a lethality rate of no more than $p_1 = 0.15$. If p_2 is 0.15 or less, H_1 should be rejected with a probability of no more than $\alpha = 0.05$. If p_2 is 0.30 or greater, H_1 should be rejected with power at least $1 - \beta = 0.80$, and the treatment thus declared unacceptable. The one-sample case can also arise if there is a considerable amount of past experience with the screen, and thereby much historical data on the standard treatment. If experimental conditions and responses are stable over time, the historical data on the standard treatment can be pooled over very large numbers of animals, thereby resulting in an estimate of p_1 that is virtually error free. This situation occurs in phase II cancer clinical trials on human patients, in which a limited number of patients are treated with an experimental therapy, and their responses are compared with historical data from the many patients treated with the current standard therapy. It also occurs in a number of screening programs that are repeated frequently over time.

The two-sample case arises when the response rate attained from the candidate treatment is compared only with that attained from the concurrent control group. Schultz and Elfring (1986) suggest that the two-sample comparison be used when the screen is conducted only intermittently, when few historical data are available, or when testing conditions may not be stable over time. This situation occurs in phase III cancer clinical trials, where a more substantial number of patients are treated with an experimental therapy under very strict protocol and their responses are compared with those from a concurrent group treated with a standard therapy.

In screening programs with animals, it is important to use the smallest sample size possible to attain necessary levels of statistical sensitivity. Clinical experimentation with human subjects, such as clinical trials of cancer chemotherapeutic agents, involves the additional ethical concern to cease experimentation with a drug or treatment regimen as soon as there is evidence of a superior drug or treatment regimen.

Fixed-sample-size designs, fully sequential designs, and stagewise, group sequential designs are used for testing H_1 versus H_2. Fixed-sample-size designs are the simplest, both conceptually and logistically. They are, however, relatively inefficient; they require the largest sample sizes to attain specified levels of power. Fully sequential designs, in which decisions to stop or continue sampling are made after each observation, are the most efficient in terms of expected sample size, but temporally undesirable and logistically complicated. Wald and Wolfowitz (1948) proved that for all tests of H_1 versus H_2 with specified type I error, α, and power, $1 - \beta$, the Wald sequential probability ratio test (SPRT) has the smallest possible expected sample sizes under *both* H_1 and H_2 conditions. However, the SPRT procedure is operationally impractical because separate decisions must be made after each individual observation. Its boundary, being open, can sometimes require larger sample sizes than comparable fixed-sample-size procedures. The Wald SPRT is thus not recommended nor widely used for either drug screening or for clinical trials applications. Armitage (1975) discusses fully sequential designs with closed boundaries. These designs have upper bounds on the maximum possible sample sizes; however, they still require decisions after each observation, so are generally logistically impractical.

Stagewise, group sequential plans represent a compromise between fixed-sample-size plans and fully sequential plans. They involve placing specified numbers of animals on test at each stage, with a specified maximum number of stages. This a priori specified upper bound on the amount of experimentation required allows logistical considerations to be planned. Stagewise plans provide most of the sample size efficiency available with fully sequential plans, yet provide most of the simplicity of fixed-sample-size plans.

The gains in efficiency introduced by adding stages to the design are greatest for small numbers of stages. Even two-stage plans result in substantial decreases in the expected sample size necessary to accept or reject a hypothesis relative to fixed-sample-size plans. A two-stage plan may require the same number of animals as a fixed-sample-size plan for an individual screen since termination after the first stage is not always possible, but the savings in animals over a number of such screens may be substantial. Schultz et al. (1973) reported that a three-stage group sequential screening design required use of 16,240 mice to classify the effectiveness of 1548 compounds. A fixed-sample-size plan with very similar operating characteristics would have required 40,248 animals to accomplish the same task.

The stagewise designs illustrated in this chapter were not selected for optimal sample size reduction but for simplicity of interpretation. They are based on a stopping criterion proposed by Fleming (1982), under which if testing continues to the final stage, it arrives at the same decision that would have been obtained with a standard, single-stage procedure and the same sample size. This avoids the apparent ambiguity that sometimes arises when the stagewise procedure continues to the last stage and fails to reject the null hypothesis, yet if the stagewise nature of the design were ignored, the same test results would reject H_1 using a fixed-sample-size test. Investigators often have difficulty interpreting such results. The correspondence between the decision rules of the fixed-sample-size design and the last stage of the stagewise design is attained by having relatively conservative criteria for stopping the test in earlier stages. Alternative stagewise designs are available, such as those proposed by Pocock (1982) and co-workers, that reduce the average sample sizes even further than the designs illustrated in this paper. These alternative procedures, however, do not use the standard, single-stage decision rule after the last stage. Geller and Pocock (1987, 1988) and Chang et al. (1987) discuss a number of alternative testing criteria and associated stagewise testing strategies.

The considerations above imply that the specific designs discussed in this chapter should be regarded as representative of a class. They are not suggested for universal use, to the exclusion of other designs in the class. Rather, they demonstrate that even relatively simple, relatively easy to interpret, and relatively conservative plans result in substantial sample size reduction when compared with a standard, fixed-sample-size plan.

The specific experimental plan to be used for a particular study should depend on the design criteria for the individual test. Trade-offs are necessary among expected sample size, simplicity of interpretation after the last stage, anticipated estimation precision after the test has stopped, and ability to stratify test results on other secondary variables, as well as many other design considerations.

The results described in this chapter strongly suggest the utility of the routine use of stagewise, group sequential designs in standardized screening protocols. They do not, however, distinguish among the many design alternatives and resulting test plans available.

II. COMPARISON OF A CANDIDATE THERAPY RESPONSE RATE WITH A SPECIFIED STANDARD RATE (ONE-SAMPLE CASE)

Fixed-sample-size, sequential, and stagewise, group sequential plans are presented. The one-sample case arises in two contexts. The first context is when the standard rate is externally imposed. For example, one requirement for efficacy of a candidate therapy regimen may be that test animals exposed to a toxicant dose level of $2 \times LD_{50}$ for unprotected animals and subsequently treated with the test regimen experience at most a 15 percent lethality rate. The second context is when a candidate therapy regimen is to be compared with a standard therapy regimen for which considerable experience has been accumulated. For example, a second requirement for efficacy of a candidate therapy regimen may be that test animals exposed to a toxicant dose level of LD_{50} for animals treated with the standard regimen and subsequently treated with the candidate regimen test program experience a lethality rate no greater than that for animals given the standard regimen. If considerable past experience with the screen is available and if experimental conditions are stable over time, the lethality results for a given toxicant and standard treatment regimen can be pooled over time; the estimated lethality rate based on pooled results will be close to 50% and will have a very small standard error. The lethality rate observed in animals treated with the candidate therapy regimen will thus be compared with this 50% lethality yardstick.

A. Fixed-Sample-Size Plans

Sample sizes required to attain the desired type I error level α and power $1-\beta$ at alternatives p_1 or p_2 were calculated for the simplest type of design, a fixed-sample-size plan. These are shown in Table 1 for alternatives $p_1 = 0.15$ and $p_2 = 0.30$ and perturbations about these values. Type I error levels of $\alpha = 0.05$ and 0.10 and power levels of $1-\beta = 0.95$, 0.90, and 0.80 are shown. Values for alternatives (p_1, p_2) were chosen as (0.15, 0.30), (0.10, 0.30), (0.20, 0.30), (0.15, 0.35), and (0.15, 0.25). Required sample sizes and rejection criteria are shown for each combination. These sample sizes and critical values were obtained using a specialized computer program, ACCEPT (SUNY, 1984), that evaluates the properties of acceptance sampling plans for lot percent defective, based on quantal response data. This problem is directly analogous to the one-sample drug screening problem with dichotomous response. The calculations are either exact, based on the hypergeometric distribution (with "lot size" specified large enough to be essentially the binomial distribution), or are asymptotic, based on the large-sample normal distribution approximation to the hypergeometric distribution.

Table 1 shows that with N equal to approximately 40 animals, it is possible to attain, at best, approximately 80% power for testing $p_1 = 0.15$ versus

Table 1 Operating Characteristics of Fixed-Sample-Size Plans to Test $H_1: p \leqslant p_1$, Versus $H_2: p \geqslant p_2$ with Type I Error α and Power $1-\beta$ Based on Quantal Response Data

p_1	p_2	α (Approx)	$1-\beta$ (Approx)	N	S to Reject H_1
0.15	0.30	0.05	0.95	80	18
			0.90	62	15
			0.80	43	11
		0.10	0.95	66	15
			0.90	49	12
			0.80	37	9
0.10	0.30	0.05	0.95	41	8
			0.90	33	7
			0.80	27	4
		0.10	0.95	37	7
			0.90	25	5
			0.80	18	4
0.20	0.30	0.05	0.95	200	50
			0.90	156	40
			0.80	109	30
		0.10	0.95	161	40
			0.90	122	31
			0.80	81	22
0.15	0.35	0.05	0.95	48	12
			0.90	36	10
			0.80	28	8
		0.10	0.95	39	10
			0.90	32	8
			0.80	22	6
0.15	0.25	0.05	0.95	170	34
			0.90	131	27
			0.80	91	20
		0.10	0.95	137	27
			0.90	103	21
			0.80	68	15

Note:
S = Number of responses observed in *N* animals.

$p_2 = 0.30$. With N equal to approximately 25 animals, it is possible to attain approximately 80% power only if the alternative lethality level, p_2, is raised to 0.35 or if p_1 is lowered to 0.10.

B. Fully Sequential Plans

Fixed-sample-size procedures, although simplest logistically, are relatively inefficient in the number of animals needed. Greater sensitivity using fewer animals can be attained by using sequential plans for distinguishing between $p_1 = 0.15$ and $p_2 = 0.30$. A fully sequential plan, based on the Wald sequential probability ratio test (SPRT) (Wetherill, 1966, Chaps. 2–4), requires data analysis after each test to decide whether to continue. In addition, the boundary is "open," which means that some realizations of the test procedure might require extremely large sample sizes, perhaps somewhat larger than that of the fixed-sample-size procedure. For these reasons, a full SPRT testing procedure is *not* considered practical for most drug screening programs. The SPRT procedure, however, minimizes the average sample sizes needed to attain the specified type I error α and power $1 - \beta$ *simultaneously* when $p = p_1$ and when $p = p_2$. Thus if most of the candidate treatment regimens will either be very effective ($p < p_1$) or very ineffective ($p > p_2$), the SPRT would result in the most effective use of animals, on average. However, if many p values will lie midway between p_1 and p_2, the average sample size for the SPRT would be closer to that of the fixed-sample-size procedure.

Average sample sizes required to attain the desired type I error α and power $1 - \beta$ with the SPRT are shown in Table 2 for alternatives $p_1 = 0.15$ and $p_2 = 0.30$ and perturbations about these values. Average sample sizes associated with type I error levels $\alpha = 0.05$ and 0.10 and power levels $1 - \beta = 0.95$, 0.90, and 0.80 are shown. These values were calculated based on theoretical results in Wetherill (1966).

Comparison of Tables 1 and 2 shows that the average sample sizes at p_1 and p_2 with the sequential procedure are approximately half the corresponding fixed sample sizes. Even the worst-case maximum average sample sizes attained at p-values midway between p_1 and p_2 are no more than 80% of the required fixed sample sizes and sometimes substantially less. This demonstrates that the use of sequential procedures can reduce animal use over the course of a screening program by as much as one-half of the fixed-sample-size requirements.

The results in Table 2 should be regarded as indications of the potential maximal gains in efficiency that can be obtained from using sequential or stagewise test plans relative to fixed-sample-size procedures. The stagewise plans advocated herein have efficiencies in between those of the fixed-sample-size and fully sequential procedures.

C. Stagewise Plans

Stagewise plans have been developed as compromises between the efficiency of fully sequential plans and the logistical practicality of fixed-sample-size

Table 2 Operating Characteristics of Wald Sequential Probability Ratio Plans to Test $H_1: p \leqslant p_1$ Versus $H_2: p \geqslant p_2$ with Type I Error α and Power $1-\beta$ Based on Quantal Response Data

p_1	p_2	α	$1-\beta$	$E(N\|p_1)$	$E(N\|p_2)$	$\max_p E(N\|p)$	p_{max}
0.15	0.30	0.05	0.95	43.4	36.8	64.4	0.22
			0.90	32.7	33.0	48.4	0.22
			0.80	22.0	26.5	32.4	0.23
		0.10	0.95	38.9	27.7	49.2	0.20
			0.90	28.8	24.4	35.9	0.20
			0.80	18.8	18.9	23.2	0.22
0.10	0.30	0.05	0.95	22.8	17.2	31.4	0.17
			0.90	17.1	15.5	23.6	0.19
			0.80	11.5	12.4	15.6	0.19
		0.10	0.95	20.4	13.0	24.3	0.17
			0.90	15.1	11.4	17.7	0.17
			0.80	9.8	8.9	11.3	0.19
0.20	0.30	0.05	0.95	103.0	94.1	160.1	0.25
			0.90	77.5	84.4	120.2	0.25
			0.80	52.1	67.7	81.1	0.26
		0.10	0.95	92.3	70.8	121.2	0.24
			0.90	68.3	62.4	89.2	0.25
			0.80	44.5	48.4	57.8	0.25
0.15	0.35	0.05	0.95	26.3	21.7	38.1	0.24
			0.90	19.8	19.4	28.6	0.24
			0.80	13.3	15.6	19.1	0.26
		0.10	0.95	23.5	16.3	29.2	0.22
			0.90	17.4	14.4	21.3	0.22
			0.80	11.4	11.1	13.8	0.24
0.15	0.25	0.05	0.95	89.0	78.3	135.6	0.20
			0.90	67.0	70.2	101.8	0.20
			0.80	45.1	56.3	68.4	0.21
		0.10	0.95	79.8	58.9	103.1	0.19
			0.90	59.1	52.0	75.5	0.20
			0.80	38.5	40.3	48.9	0.20

Notes:

$E(N|p_1)$ = expected sample size required when $p = p_1$.

$E(N|p_2)$ = expected sample size required when $p = p_2$.

$\max_p E(N|p)$ = largest expected sample size required for p-value.

p_{max} = p-value that corresponds to largest expected number of animals required to differentiate H_1 from H_2.

plans. The test schedule is divided into a number of stages, specified prior to the outset of the program. At each stage a specified number of animals are placed on test. At the conclusion of each stage, the cumulative number of responses is updated and compared with prespecified acceptance and rejection points. If the observed number of responses is less than or equal to the acceptance level for that stage, $H_1: p > p_1$ is accepted. If the observed number of responses is greater than or equal to the rejection level for that stage, $H_2: p \geqslant p_2$ is accepted. If the observed number of responses lies between the acceptance and rejection levels, the test continues to the next stage.

Some pharmaceutical screening programs report that the overwhelming majority of tests ended after the first stage; indeed, this is the point of largest single increases in efficiency relative to fixed-sample-size procedures. Pocock (1982) demonstrates that average sample size decreases very little with plans having more than four or five stages.

At the same time, the stagewise plans provide much of the logistical practicality of the fixed-sample-size plans. The maximum number of stages, k, and the number of animals in the ith stage, n_i, are fixed. The n_i values can be equalized for logistical convenience without sacrificing much efficiency. Sometimes the sample size at the first stage is chosen to be larger than at the other stages to provide greater ability to estimate the response rate if the test stops early. A maximum number of animals to test is preestablished, which is usually no greater than that for the fixed-sample-size test.

Much has been published on the design and analysis of multiple-stage testing programs. J. R. Schultz and co-workers at The Upjohn Company have published a series of papers (Elfring and Schultz, 1973a; Schultz et al., 1973; Hearron et al., 1984; Schultz and Elfring, 1986) that present a unified approach for specifying and evaluating a class of group sequential designs. They discuss test procedures for comparing (1) the mean of a single binomial distribution against a specified level, (2) the means of two binomial distributions, and (3) the means of two continuous distributions.

A multistage plan for comparing the mean of a binomial distribution against a specified level is defined by specifying four parameters:

k	The maximum number of stages
$(n_1, n_2, \ldots, n_k)$	The numbers of animals tested at each stage
$(a_1, a_2, \ldots, a_k)$	The set of acceptance points
$(r_1, r_2, \ldots, r_k)$	The set of rejection points (with $r_k = a_k + 1$, so that the test must stop at stage k)

Let S_i denote the number of deaths observed in the ith stage and $\Sigma_{i=1}^{g} S_i$ the cumulative number of deaths observed up to and including the gth stage. At the gth stage,

$$\text{If } \sum_{i=1}^{g} S_i \leqslant a_g, \qquad \text{stop sampling and accept } H_1 : p \leqslant p_1.$$

$$\text{If } \sum_{i=1}^{g} S_i \geqslant r_g, \qquad \text{stop sampling and accept } H_2 : p \geqslant p_2.$$

$$\text{If } a_g < \sum_{i=1}^{g} S_i < r_g, \quad \text{continue to stage } g + 1.$$

The test parameters are chosen to approximately attain specified type I error level α when $p = p_1$ and specified power $1 - \beta$ when $p = p_2 > p_1$. Schultz et al. (1973) and Elfring and Schultz (1973a) explain the theory underlying these designs in greater detail.

Schultz et al. (1973) have written a series of interactive FORTRAN IV computer programs that evaluate the operating characteristics and average sample sizes of any specified stagewise design of this form, including problems 1 to 3 mentioned above. For problems 1 and 2 all calculations of size, power, and average sample size are based on exact binomial probabilities, using the direct method of sequential analysis described by Aroian (1968). These programs greatly facilitate the examination of alternative stagewise plans to find designs having the desired size and power characteristics.

Chang et al. (1987) have developed an algorithm to select an optimal stagewise design that requires the minimum average sample size for specified type I error, power, maximum sample size, and number of stages. Therneau et al. (1987a) have developed a series of interactive FORTRAN programs that evaluate, among other things, the operating characteristics and average sample sizes of any specified design. Their programs, like the programs of Schultz et al., are based on exact binomial calculations. The Schultz et al. programs evaluate the operating characteristics and average sample sizes for designs specified by the user. The programs of Therneau et al. will also do this, as well as obtain optimal designs (in terms of minimum average sample size) and provide exact confidence intervals of lethality rates that account for the fact that the random stopping time provides information about the lethality rate (Jennison and Turnbull, 1983). However, the Therneau et al. programs restrict attention to the one-sample problem, whereas the Schultz et al. programs also treat the two-sample problem.

Various researchers have suggested alternative strategies for selecting particular stagewise stopping criteria. Schultz et al. (1973) suggest starting with a fully sequential SPRT and modifying it to a multistage test of k stages. The properties of the modified plans are evaluated by the Schultz et al. or Therneau et al. computer programs and the design is further modified to the desired size and power characteristics.

Fleming (1982) suggests a stagewise test that employs the standard, fixed-sample-size test procedure at the last stage. This scheme allows for early stopping, yet provides exactly the same inferences as those of the fixed sample size test, on a sample-by-sample basis, if it proceeds to the last stage. As discussed in Section I, the Fleming designs' use of the standard single-stage test at the last stage simplifies the interpretation of results by preventing contradiction between the conclusions of a fixed-sample-size design and a stagewise design that extends to the last stage. The Fleming designs, however, require more substantial statistical evidence than other proposed stagewise designs for stopping at the early stages. The optimal designs proposed by Chang et al. (1987) or the designs proposed by Pocock (1982) or by Geller and Pocock (1988) might reduce the average sample size even more than the Fleming designs. These designs, however, do not use the single-stage test for data analysis after the last stage.

Table 3 displays the type I errors, powers, and average sample sizes of various one-, two-, and five-stage designs based on the stopping boundaries recommended by Fleming (1982; see Section 3 for details concerning his recommended acceptance and rejection points). In each case the null hypothesis is $H_1 : p_1 \leqslant p_2 \equiv 0.15$. Designs are chosen to have maximum sample sizes of 24, 25, or 40 animals, equally divided among one, two, and five stages. The nominal type I error is selected to be approximately 0.05 or 0.10; power and average sample size are shown for alternatives $p_2 = 0.30$, 0.35, or 0.40.

The actual significance levels of the designs in Table 3 differ from their nominal values of 0.05 or 0.10 because of the discreteness of the problem. The saving in average sample size, relative to a fixed-sample-size procedure, is substantial and increases as the true response rate becomes more extreme. The worst-case p with respect to average sample size and the corresponding worst-case average sample size are shown in the right-hand columns of the table.

Table 3 demonstrates that for $p_2 = 0.30$, a five-stage design with 8 animals per stage results in a 30 to 40% saving in average sample size relative to a fixed-sample-size procedure, without any sacrifice in power. This saving is even greater for larger values of p_2. A two-stage design results in about half or more of the sample size reduction of a five-stage design. Pocock (1982) finds little gain in efficiency beyond the fifth stage.

An indication of the relative gains in average sample size efficiency attained by adopting sequential or group sequential designs can be seen from the case $p_1 = 0.15$, $p_2 = 0.30$, $\alpha = 0.10$, $1 - \beta = 0.80$. The designs in Table 3 are seen to attain a power of approximately 0.80 for detecting $p_2 = 0.30$. A fully

Table 3 Operating Characteristics of Fleming Stagewise Group Sequential Plans to Test $H_1: p \leqslant p_1 \equiv 0.15$ Versus $H_2: p \geqslant p_2$ Based on Quantal Response Data

p_1	p_2	Number of stages	Number per stage	α	$1-\beta$	$E(N\|p_1)$	$E(N\|p_2)$	$\max_p E(N\|p)$	p_{max}
0.15	0.30	1	24	0.057	0.611	24	24	24	
		2	12	0.056	0.604	18.6	21.6	21.6	0.30
		5	5	0.037	0.500	16.0	17.7	18.0	0.25
		1	40	0.030	0.691	40	40	40	
		2	20	0.032	0.692	31.8	34.7	36.1	0.25
		5	8	0.038	0.683	24.3	27.6	28.8	0.25
		1	24	0.057	0.611	24	24	24	
		2	12	0.065	0.617	18.4	19.7	20.2	0.25
		5	5	0.079	0.634	14.2	16.6	16.7	0.25
		1	40	0.067	0.804	40	40	40	
		2	20	0.068	0.776	26.6	30.0	31.2	0.25
		5	8	0.091	0.793	24.0	23.8	26.2	0.20
0.15	0.35	1	24	0.057	0.789	24	24	Same plans as above	
		2	12	0.056	0.782	18.6	20.9		
		5	5	0.037	0.693	16.0	16.8		
		1	40	0.030	0.879	40	40		
		2	20	0.032	0.878	31.8	31.8		
		5	8	0.038	0.867	24.3	24.8		
		1	24	0.057	0.789	24	24		
		2	12	0.065	0.791	18.4	18.5		
		5	5	0.079	0.795	14.2	15.7		
		1	40	0.067	0.936	40	40		
		2	20	0.068	0.915	26.6	27.4		
		5	8	0.091	0.922	24.0	20.8		
0.15	0.40	1	24	0.057	0.904	24	24	Same plans as above	
		2	12	0.056	0.898	18.6	19.7		
		5	5	0.037	0.839	16.0	15.4		
		1	40	0.030	0.965	40	40		
		2	20	0.032	0.964	31.8	28.2		
		5	8	0.038	0.956	24.3	21.7		
		1	24	0.057	0.904	24	24		
		2	12	0.065	0.903	18.4	17.0		
		5	5	0.079	0.899	14.2	14.4		
		1	40	0.067	0.984	40	40		
		2	20	0.068	0.974	26.6	24.7		
		5	8	0.091	0.977	24.0	18.0		

Notes:

$E(N|p_1)$ = expected sample size required when $p = p_1$.

$E(N|p_2)$ = expected sample size required when $p = p_2$.

$\max_p E(N|p)$ = largest expected sample size required for p-value.

p_{max} = p-value that corresponds to largest expected number of animals required to differentiate H_1 from H_2.

sequential SPRT procedure that has essentially the same type I error and power at $p_1 = 0.15$ and $p_2 = 0.30$ is shown in Table 2. The average sample sizes for these designs are shown in Tables 2 and 3 to be:

Number of stages	Average N
1	40
2	27–30
5	24
SPRT	19

Thus the two-stage design can be regarded as about halfway between the fixed sample design and the fully sequential design in average sample size reduction; the five-stage design is about halfway between the two-stage design and the fully sequential design.

Similar conclusions can be drawn from the case $p_1 = 0.15$, $p_2 = 0.35$, $\alpha = 0.05$, $1 - \beta = 0.90$. The designs in Table 3 attain power a bit less than 0.90 for detecting $p_2 = 0.35$. An SPRT is shown in Table 2 with $\alpha = 0.05$ and $1 - \beta = 0.90$ at $p_1 = 0.15$ and $p_2 = 0.35$. The average sample sizes for these designs are:

Number of stages	Average N
1	40
2	32
5	25
SPRT	20

The relative sample size reductions are similar to those discussed above.

For applications in which it may be assumed that the standard therapy response rate is compatible with an anticipated 50%, the candidate therapy response rate can be compared with the 50% yardstick. The operating characteristics of the comparison procedures can be evaluated using the Therneau et al. programs, in direct analogy with the previous evaluations of the comparisons with the 15% yardstick.

Table 4 displays the type I errors, powers, and average sample sizes of various one-, two-, and five-stage designs based on the Fleming boundaries.

Table 4 Operating Characteristics of Fleming Stagewise Group Sequential Plans to Test $H_1: p \leqslant p_1 \equiv 0.50$ Versus $H_2: p \geqslant p_2$ Based on Quantal Response Data

p_1	p_2	Number of stages	N per stage	α	$1-\beta$	$E(N\mid p_1)$	$E(N\mid p_2)$	$\max_p E(N\mid p)$	p_{max}
0.50	0.65	1	24	0.032	0.358	24	24	24	
		2	12	0.032	0.355	16.6	20.9	21.6	0.70
		5	5	0.052	0.346	11.3	14.9	15.5	0.70
		1	40	0.040	0.572	40	40	40	
		2	20	0.041	0.566	28.1	35.2	35.2	0.65
		5	8	0.048	0.565	23.0	29.3	29.3	0.65
		1	24	0.076	0.526	24	24	24	
		2	12	0.078	0.514	16.4	19.6	19.6	0.65
		5	5	0.089	0.490	11.9	14.9	14.9	0.65
		1	40	0.077	0.695	40	40	40	
		2	20	0.080	0.682	27.8	32.7	32.7	0.65
		5	8	0.087	0.673	22.0	27.0	27.0	0.65
0.50	0.70	1	24	0.032	0.565	24	24	Same plans as above	
		2	12	0.032	0.560	16.6	21.6		
		5	5	0.052	0.532	11.3	15.5		
		1	40	0.040	0.807	40	40		
		2	20	0.041	0.801	28.1	34.3		
		5	8	0.048	0.795	23.0	28.0		
		1	24	0.076	0.725	24	24		
		2	12	0.078	0.710	16.4	19.6		
		5	5	0.089	0.676	11.9	14.8		
		1	40	0.077	0.885	40	40		
		2	20	0.080	0.873	27.8	30.7		
		5	8	0.087	0.861	22.0	25.3		

0.50	0.75	1	24	0.032	0.766	24	24	Same plans as above
		2	12	0.032	0.761	16.6	21.4	
		5	5	0.052	0.725	11.3	15.2	
		1	40	0.040	0.946	40	40	
		2	20	0.041	0.941	28.1	31.4	
		5	8	0.048	0.936	23.0	25.0	
		1	24	0.076	0.879	24	24	
		2	12	0.078	0.865	16.4	18.7	
		5	5	0.089	0.834	11.9	13.9	
		1	40	0.077	0.974	40	40	
		2	20	0.080	0.967	27.8	27.4	
		5	8	0.087	0.960	22.0	22.6	
0.50	0.80	1	24	0.032	0.911	24	24	Same plans as above
		2	12	0.032	0.907	16.6	20.5	
		5	5	0.052	0.878	11.3	14.0	
		1	40	0.040	0.992	40	40	
		2	20	0.041	0.991	28.1	27.4	
		5	8	0.048	0.989	23.0	21.2	
		1	24	0.076	0.964	24	24	
		2	12	0.078	0.956	16.4	17.1	
		5	5	0.089	0.936	11.9	12.3	
		1	40	0.077	0.997	40	40	
		2	20	0.080	0.995	27.8	23.9	
		5	8	0.087	0.993	22.0	19.9	

Notes:

$E(N|p_1)$ = expected sample size required when $p = p_1$.

$E(N|p_2)$ = expected sample size required when $p = p_2$.

$\max_p E(N|p)$ = largest expected sample size required for p-value.

p_{max} = p-value that corresponds to largest expected number of animals required to differentiate H_1 from H_2.

The null hypothesis is $H_1 : p \leqslant p_1 \equiv 0.50$. Designs are like those shown in Table 3 with respect to numbers of stages and sample size per stage. Power and sample sizes are shown for alternatives $p_2 \equiv 0.65, 0.70, 0.75$, and 0.80.

With a maximum of 40 animals and a type I error of $\alpha = 0.05$, a lethality rate of $p_2 = 0.70$ can be detected with probability 0.80 and a lethality rate of $p_2 = 0.75$ can be detected with probability 0.94. At $p_2 = 0.70$ the average sample sizes for the one-, two-, and five-stage designs are

Number of stages	Average N
1	40
2	28–34
5	23–28

At the lower end of the range of expected sample sizes (corresponding to $p_1 = 0.50$), the two-stage design provides about 70% of the average sample size reduction of the five-stage design. At the upper end of the range of expected sample sizes (corresponding to $p_2 = 0.70$), the two-stage design provides about 50% of the average sample size reduction of the five-stage design. In either case, the benefit of using a stagewise design with even a modest number of stages is obvious.

If the design is run in five stages with 8 animals per stage, the expected sample size is between 23 and 28 animals. This represents a 30 to 40 percent reduction in the required average number of animals relative to the fixed-sample-size procedure. A single-stage design with comparable sample size can detect $p_2 = 0.75$ with probability 0.77 and $p_2 = 0.8$ with probability 0.91. This is clearly a reduction in sensitivity relative to the five-stage procedure.

III. COMPARISON OF A CANDIDATE THERAPY RESPONSE RATE WITH A CONCURRENT STANDARD RATE (TWO-SAMPLE CASE)

Standardized screens often incorporate concurrent control groups that are treated with the standard therapy regimen. Commonly, an ED_{50} (effective dose for a particular response in 50% of those exposed) for animals given a standard therapy is selected, so that a response of approximately 50% is expected among the controls. If the expected occurs, the response rates observed with candidate treatment regimens are compared with a fixed 50% yardstick. This practice agrees with that recommended by Schultz and Elfring (1986), who state that each run should include both positive and negative standard controls.

When t different therapies are tested in a run, they recommend also including $\sqrt{t}$ positive control groups (e.g., standard therapy regimen) and $\sqrt{t}$ negative control groups (e.g., untreated animals). If any of the positive control groups have a response rate significantly greater than 50%, according to the first-stage criterion, Schultz and Elfring suggest that the entire run be repeated.

Schultz and Elfring also recommend that control charts be set up to check the validity of individual runs and to evaluate the short- and long-term run-to-run stability of the system. One-sample comparisons against fixed yardsticks (e.g., 50% lethality) and associated one-sample designs may be used when the run-to-run results are stable and no long-term trends in control response rates are observed. Two-sample comparisons with concurrent controls must be used when the extent of run-to-run variability in control group response rates is large enough to be both statistically and medically significant, or when the testing procedure is not conducted on a routine basis.

Schultz et al. (1973) have developed computer programs to evaluate the statistical characteristics of two-sample stagewise designs to test the equality of response rates between a candidate therapy and a concurrent control therapy. Either one- or two-sided alternatives can be tested. The discussion below deals with the one-sided alternative.

The approach follows that in Elfring and Schultz (1973a, Sec. 2). The standard therapy and candidate therapy response rates are denoted as p_1 and p_2, respectively. The standard rate, p_1, is estimated based on the response observed in the concurrent control group. The designs below involve equal sample sizes for the standard therapy regimen and for each of the candidate therapy regimens. This is not a theoretically necessary experimental design condition, nor is it always even preferred; however, the two-sample design computer programs of Schultz et al. assume equal sample sizes. Thus equal sample size allocations to the standard and candidate therapy groups are assumed for illustrative purposes in the evaluations below.

The test procedure is similar to that for the one-sample stagewise plans described above. The test is divided into an a priori specified number of stages. At each stage, equal numbers of animals are placed on test in each group. The subjects in each group are randomly paired, and each pair of responses is scored as follows:

Standard therapy outcome	Candidate therapy outcome	Score (X)	Probability
No response	Response	1	$(1 - p_1)p_2$
Response	Response	0	$p_1 p_2$
No response	No response	0	$(1 - p_1)(1 - p_2)$
Response	No response	−1	$p_1(1 - p_2)$

Thus

$$P(X = 1) = (1 - p_1)p_2 \equiv q_1$$
$$P(X = 0) = p_1 p_2 + (1 - p_1)(1 - p_2) \equiv q_2$$
$$P(X = -1) = p_1(1 - p_2) \equiv q_3$$

The scores within each stage are summed. The decision whether to stop after a particular stage or to continue to the next stage is based on the cumulative sum of scores across all past and current stages. Because the sum of the scores within a stage is merely the difference between the number of responses observed with the candidate therapy and the number observed with the standard therapy, the sum is invariant to the particular pairing that was carried out.

The test of the hypothesis $H_1 : p_2 \leqslant p_1$ versus the one-sided alternative $H_2 : p_2 > p_1$ is based on the cumulative sum of scores. The k-stage design is characterized by prespecified acceptance and rejection points $(a_1, a_2, \ldots, a_k)$ and $(r_1, r_2, \ldots, r_k)$, respectively, with $a_k = r_k - 1$ so that sampling must stop after the kth stage. The test proceeds analogously to the one-sample test described. At the gth stage, if the cumulative sum of scores is

$\leqslant a_g$	Stop sampling and accept $H_1 : p_1 \leqslant p_2$.
$\geqslant r_g$	Stop sampling and accept $H_2 : p_1 > p_2$.
$> a_g$ and $< r_g$	Continue to stage $g + 1$

Considerations for choice of the test parameters are analogous to those for the one-sample case.

Various researchers have suggested alternative strategies for selecting stopping boundaries $(a_1, a_2, \ldots, a_k)$ and $(r_1, r_2, \ldots, r_k)$. O'Brien and Fleming (1979) and Fleming (1982) suggest an approach to choosing boundaries that employs the fixed-sample-size test procedure at the last stage. As in the one-sample case, the Fleming designs simplify interpretation of results, but are more conservative about stopping early than other proposed stagewise designs. Pocock (1977, 1982) and Geller and Pocock (1987) review alternative suggestions that have been made in the literature. Some of these result in greater average sample size reduction than the Fleming approach, but they do not use the fixed-sample-size test procedure at the last stage.

Tables 5 and 6 display the type I errors, powers, and average sample sizes of various one-, two-, and five-stage designs based on the stopping boundaries derived in analogy with the approach suggested by Fleming (1982). Formulas for the acceptance and rejection boundaries appear in the appendix to this chapter. Table 5 pertains to the case $p_1 = 0.15$ and Table 6 pertains to the case $p_1 = 0.50$. Note that because the sample sizes indicated in these tables represent samples sizes *per group* per stage, the savings in average sample size relative to fixed-sample-size designs are, in fact, twice that shown in the tables.

The designs shown in Tables 5 and 6 have maximum sample sizes of 24, 25, or 40 animals, equally divided among one, two, and five stages, respectively. The power and average sample sizes are shown for alternatives $p_2 = 0.35$, 0.40, 0.45, and 0.50 in Table 5 and for alternatives $p_2 = 0.75$, 0.80, 0.85, and 0.90 in Table 6. The actual significance levels of the designs differ from the nominal values of 0.05 or 0.10 because of the discreteness of the problem. The worst-case p with respect to average sample size and the corresponding worst-case average sample size are shown in the right-hand columns of the table.

Table 5 indicates that for $p_2 = 0.35$, a five-stage design with 8 animals per stage results in a 30 to 40% reduction in average sample size relative to a fixed-sample-size procedure, with little decrease in power. This reduction is even greater for larger values of p_2.

Table 6 indicates that with a maximum of 40 animals and a type I error of $\alpha = 0.05$, a response rate of $p_2 = 0.80$ can be detected with probability better than 0.80, and a response rate of $p_2 = 0.85$ can be detected with probability better than 0.90. At $p_2 = 0.80$ the average sample sizes for the one-, two-, and five-stage designs are:

Number of stages	Average N
1	40
2	29–33
5	22–27

The five-stage design provides a 32 to 44% reduction in average sample size relative to the fixed sample procedure, with just a slight decrease in power (from 0.87 to 0.83). The two-stage design provides between 50 and 60% of the average sample size reduction of the five-stage design. This demonstrates, in agreement with the one-sample case, the increase in animal use efficiency that can be attained with even a modest number of stages.

IV. EXAMPLE

The protocols for the Medical Research and Evaluation Facility's first-stage screens specify that each candidate treatment be evaluated based on a sample size of $N = 24$ animals. The nominal response rate for the standard treatment

Table 5 Operating Characteristics of Fleming Two-Sample Group Sequential Plans to Test $H_1 : p_1 \leqslant p_2 \equiv 0.15$ Versus $H_2 : p_1 > p_2$ Based on Quantal Response Data

p_1	p_2	Number of stages	N/Group/ stage	α	$1 - \beta$	$E(N \mid p_1)$	$E(N \mid p_2)$	$\max_p E(N \mid P)$	p_{max}
0.15	0.35	1	24	0.034	0.542	24.0	24.0	24.0	
		2	12	0.034	0.532	16.6	20.0	20.0	0.35
		5	5	0.042	0.571	15.4	18.2	18.3	0.30
		1	40	0.042	0.747	40.0	40.0	40.0	
		2	20	0.044	0.749	31.6	33.4	35.2	0.25
		5	8	0.046	0.727	24.7	27.3	28.5	0.30
		1	24	0.077	0.673	24.0	24.0	24.0	
		2	12	0.078	0.650	16.4	18.3	18.5	0.30
		5	5	0.089	0.662	14.6	15.6	16.1	0.25
		1	40	0.078	0.824	40.0	40.0	40.0	
		2	20	0.081	0.803	27.8	29.6	31.4	0.25
		5	8	0.088	0.789	22.9	23.9	25.9	0.25
0.15	0.40	1	24	0.034	0.695	24.0	24.0	Same plans as above	
		2	12	0.034	0.682	16.6	19.8		
		5	5	0.042	0.716	15.4	17.5		
		1	40	0.042	0.880	40.0	40.0		
		2	20	0.044	0.879	31.6	31.0		
		5	8	0.046	0.859	24.7	25.3		
		1	24	0.077	0.801	24.0	24.0		
		2	12	0.078	0.775	16.4	17.7		
		5	5	0.089	0.782	14.6	14.8		
		1	40	0.078	0.924	40.0	40.0		
		2	20	0.081	0.905	27.8	27.5		
		5	8	0.088	0.893	22.9	21.9		

0.15	0.45	1	24	0.034	0.817	24.0	24.0	Same plans as above
		2	12	0.034	0.803	16.6	19.1	
		5	5	0.042	0.829	15.4	16.6	
		1	40	0.042	0.952	40.0	40.0	
		2	20	0.044	0.951	31.6	28.3	
		5	8	0.046	0.937	24.7	23.0	
		1	24	0.077	0.891	24.0	24.0	
		2	12	0.078	0.866	16.4	16.8	
		5	5	0.089	0.870	14.6	13.9	
		1	40	0.078	0.973	40.0	40.0	
		2	20	0.081	0.960	27.8	25.3	
		5	8	0.088	0.951	22.9	19.8	
0.15	0.50	1	24	0.034	0.902	24.0	24.0	Same plans as above
		2	12	0.034	0.889	16.6	18.1	
		5	5	0.042	0.906	15.4	15.4	
		1	40	0.042	0.985	40.0	40.0	
		2	20	0.044	0.983	31.6	25.7	
		5	8	0.046	0.976	24.7	20.8	
		1	24	0.077	0.947	24.0	24.0	
		2	12	0.078	0.927	16.4	15.9	
		5	5	0.089	0.927	14.6	12.8	
		1	40	0.078	0.992	40.0	40.0	
		2	20	0.081	0.985	27.8	23.4	
		5	8	0.088	0.980	22.9	17.9	

Notes:

$E(N|p_1)$ = expected sample size required when $p = p_1$.

$E(N|p_2)$ = expected sample size required when $p = p_2$.

$\max_p E(N|p)$ = largest expected sample size required for p-value.

p_{max} = p-value that corresponds to largest expected number of animals required to differentiate H_1 from H_2.

Table 6 Operating Characteristics of Fleming Type Two-Sample Group Sequential Plans to Test $H_1: p_1 \leqslant p_2 \equiv 0.50$ Versus $H_2: p_1 > p_2$ Based on Quantal Response Data

p_1	p_2	Number of stages	N/Group/ stage	α	$1-\beta$	$E(N\|p_1)$	$E(N\|p_2)$	$\max_p E(N\|p)$	p_{max}
0.5	0.75	1	24	0.030	0.443	24.0	24.0	24.0	
		2	12	0.029	0.425	15.2	20.2	21.1	0.85
		5	5	0.033	0.441	12.8	17.7	18.2	0.85
		1	40	0.046	0.727	40.0	40.0	40.0	
		2	20	0.048	0.721	28.6	34.7	35.0	0.70
		5	8	0.048	0.684	22.3	28.4	28.5	0.70
		1	24	0.097	0.681	24.0	24.0	24.0	
		2	12	0.101	0.666	16.6	19.2	19.3	0.70
		5	5	0.066	0.576	13.6	17.8	17.8	0.75
		1	40	0.073	0.799	40.0	40.0	40.0	
		2	20	0.076	0.790	28.4	32.5	33.4	0.70
		5	8	0.080	0.769	22.3	26.8	27.5	0.70
0.5	0.80	1	24	0.030	0.593	24.0	24.0	Same plans as above	
		2	12	0.029	0.572	15.2	20.8		
		5	5	0.033	0.587	12.8	18.2		
		1	40	0.046	0.867	40.0	40.0		
		2	20	0.048	0.862	28.6	33.3		
		5	8	0.048	0.830	22.3	27.3		
		1	24	0.097	0.806	24.0	24.0		
		2	12	0.101	0.791	16.6	18.8		
		5	5	0.066	0.715	13.6	17.7		
		1	40	0.073	0.912	40.0	40.0		
		2	20	0.076	0.904	28.4	30.7		
		5	8	0.080	0.887	22.3	25.3		

0.5	0.85	1	24	0.030	0.739	24.0	24.0	Same plans as above
		2	12	0.029	0.719	15.2	21.1	
		5	5	0.033	0.730	12.8	18.2	
		1	40	0.046	0.951	40.0	40.0	
		2	20	0.048	0.949	28.6	31.1	
		5	8	0.048	0.929	22.3	25.6	
		1	24	0.097	0.902	24.0	24.0	
		2	12	0.101	0.889	16.6	18.1	
		5	5	0.066	0.835	13.6	17.2	
		1	40	0.073	0.972	40.0	40.0	
		2	20	0.076	0.968	28.4	28.2	
		5	8	0.080	0.958	22.3	23.3	
0.5	0.90	1	24	0.030	0.861	24.0	24.0	Same plans as above
		2	12	0.029	0.846	15.2	21.0	
		5	5	0.033	0.853	12.8	17.8	
		1	40	0.046	0.989	40.0	40.0	
		2	20	0.048	0.987	28.6	28.3	
		5	8	0.048	0.979	22.3	23.4	
		1	24	0.097	0.962	24.0	24.0	
		2	12	0.101	0.954	16.6	17.0	
		5	5	0.066	0.924	13.6	16.3	
		1	40	0.073	0.994	40.0	40.0	
		2	20	0.076	0.993	28.4	25.5	
		5	8	0.080	0.990	22.3	21.2	

Notes:

$E(N|p_1)$ = expected sample size required when $p = p_1$.

$E(N|p_2)$ = expected sample size required when $p = p_2$.

$\max_p E(N|p)$ = largest expected sample size required for p-value.

p_{max} = p-value that corresponds to largest expected number of animals required to differentiate H_1 from H_2.

is 50%. If the attained standard treatment response rate is statistically compatible with the nominal ($\alpha = 0.05$), the screening procedure eliminates a candidate treatment from further testing if its response rate is statistically significantly greater than 50% at the $\alpha = 0.05$ level of significance.

If the attained standard treatment response is compatible with 50%, the null hypothesis, $H_0 : p \leqslant 0.50$ is tested for each candidate treatment. Let X denote the number of responses observed among the $N = 24$ animals. A fixed-sample-size design rejects H_0 ($\alpha = 0.05$) if X is 17 or greater. The operating characteristics for this test are:

Type I error	$\alpha = 0.032$
Power, $p = 0.75$	$1 - \beta = 0.766$
Power, $p = 0.80$	$1 - \beta = 0.911$

For logistical reasons the screening test is divided into three portions, with $N = 8$ animals tested within each portion. It would thus be simple to modify the fixed-sample-size test procedure to a three-stage test, with $N = 8$ animals per stage. The conduct and properties of this three-stage design were studied. The acceptance and rejection boundaries and the operating characteristics are as follows:

	Stage (k)		
	1	2	3
N	8	8	8
a_k	3	10	16
r_k	9	13	17

The specification of $a_1 = 3$, $r_1 = 9$ implies that H_0 can be accepted following stage 1, but not rejected. The acceptance and rejection boundaries following stage 3 coincide with the fixed-sample-size procedure.

The operating characteristics for this test are:

Type I error	$\alpha = 0.030$
Power, $p = 0.75$	$1 - \beta = 0.725$
Power, $p = 0.80$	$1 - \beta = 0.881$

$E(N \mid p = 0.50) = 13.8$
$E(N \mid p = 0.75) = 19.0$
$E(N \mid p = 0.80) = 18.5$

	Probability of stopping after stage:		
	1	2	3
$p = 0.50$	0.36	0.54	0.09
$p = 0.75$	0.03	0.57	0.40
$p = 0.80$	0.01	0.67	0.32

Under both the null hypothesis and alternatives of $p = 0.75$ or greater, the test has high probability of stopping after one or two stages. The type I error and power of the three-stage test differ only marginally from those of the corresponding fixed-sample-size test. Yet the reduction in expected sample size is

$p = 0.50$	43%
$p = 0.75$	21%
$p = 0.80$	23%

For extremely efficacious treatments ($p < 0.50$) or for extremely non-efficacious treatments ($p > 0.80$) the reductions in expected sample size would be even greater.

The fixed-sample-size test was carried out for a number of candidate treatments. The responses for five candidate treatments were reanalyzed using the three-stage procedure. The following results were obtained:

Candidate treatment	Cumulative responses	Three-stage test results	Fixed-sample test results
DP 36–88	1 1 4	Accept H_0, $N = 8$	Accept H_0, $N = 24$
DP 37–88	1 1 2	Accept H_0, $N = 8$	Accept H_0, $N = 24$
DP 38–88	1 1 1	Accept H_0, $N = 8$	Accept H_0, $N = 24$
CB 29–87–0.29	0 3 7	Accept H_0, $N = 8$	Accept H_0, $N = 24$
CB 29–87–0.68	1 2 3	Accept H_0, $N = 8$	Accept H_0, $N = 24$

In all five cases the three-stage test arrived at the same conclusion as the fixed-sample-size test, but based on one-third the number of animals. This clearly illustrates the efficiencies that can be obtained with stagewise, group sequential designs.

The fixed-sample-size procedure was also compared with the three-stage procedure for a series of tests with standard treatments. Denote the toxicant by 1, 2, or 3 and the test series by A, B, ... Thus 2-E would represent test series E with toxicant 2. The following results were obtained:

Standard treatment series	Cumulative responses	Three-stage test results	Fixed-sample test results
1-A	7 11 13	Accept H_0, $N = 24$	Accept H_0, $N = 24$
1-B	7 13 20	Reject H_0, $N = 16$	Reject H_0, $N = 24$
1-C	5 11 16	Accept H_0, $N = 24$	Accept H_0, $N = 24$
2-A	1 5 8	Accept H_0, $N = 8$	Accept H_0, $N = 24$
2-B	5 9 13	Accept H_0, $N = 16$	Accept H_0, $N = 24$
2-C	3 6 8	Accept H_0, $N = 8$	Accept H_0, $N = 24$
2-D	1 4 11	Accept H_0, $N = 8$	Accept H_0, $N = 24$
2-E	4 7 12	Accept H_0, $N = 16$	Accept H_0, $N = 24$
2-F	3 7 10	Accept H_0, $N = 8$	Accept H_0, $N = 24$
2-G	2 6 8	Accept H_0, $N = 8$	Accept H_0, $N = 24$
2-H	1 6 10	Accept H_0, $N = 8$	Accept H_0, $N = 24$
3-A	3 4 8	Accept H_0, $N = 8$	Accept H_0, $N = 24$
3-B	5 9 12	Accept H_0, $N = 16$	Accept H_0, $N = 24$
3-C	4 7 12	Accept H_0, $N = 16$	Accept H_0, $N = 24$
3-D	7 12 17	Reject H_0, $N = 24$	Reject H_0, $N = 24$
3-E	5 11 16	Accept H_0, $N = 24$	Accept H_0, $N = 24$
3-F	2 7 13	Accept H_0, $N = 8$	Accept H_0, $N = 24$

The results of the three-stage test and the fixed-sample-size test agree in all 17 cases. The average sample sizes for the three-stage tests are:

Toxicant	Number of tests	Average N	Percent reduction
1	3	21.3	11.1
2	8	10	58.3
3	6	16	33.3
Pooled	17	14.1	41.2

The overall reduction in sample size is 41.2%, which closely agrees with the predicted 43% reduction when $p = 0.50$. This again illustrates the efficiencies that can be attained with stagewise, group sequential designs.

V. DISCUSSION

The use of stagewise designs for standardized screening programs to evaluate the efficacy of candidate drugs and medical devices to mitigate the effects of exposure to various toxic substances has been demonstrated. These designs retain the sensitivity of the fixed sample designs while allowing a substantial reduction in the number of animals required. The conservative five-stage designs resulted in 30 to 40% average sample size reduction, depending on the acceptable response rates. Designs have been proposed in the statistics literature that provide even greater sample size reduction.

The greatest percent reduction in sample size is realized when going from a fixed-size design to a two-stage design. A two-stage design can result in an average sample size reduction of 20% or more relative to a fixed-sample-size design. Investigators have suggested that little sample size efficiency is gained beyond five stages.

The foregoing implies that stagewise designs will be logistically feasible in many common testing situations. The number of stages, the number of animals per stage, and the elapsed time between stages can be anticipated and therefore accommodated. The principal requirement for the feasibility of a stagewise or sequential plan is that responses be available fairly soon after treatment, so that the decision whether to stop or to continue to the next stage can be made in a timely fashion.

Because the designs discussed above are conservative about early stopping, they require larger average sample sizes than other stagewise plans might. The choice of a stagewise test for a particular testing program depends on many design criteria. Simplicity of execution (e.g., equal-sized stages), simplicity of interpretation (e.g., applicability of a standard, fixed sample test after the last stage), and/or ability to estimate response rates precisely after terminating the test may compete with the desire to reduce the average sample size to the minimum possible. Some investigators have suggested that the test should include a larger first stage so that it will not terminate before sufficient data are obtained for precise estimates.

The previous discussion was concerned with the construction of testing rules to test a hypothesis in a stagewise fashion. After the testing has stopped and a decision has been reached, more information (e.g., an estimate of some function of the response rates) may be required from the test than a simple decision to accept or reject. Berry and Ho (1988) propose a compromise, a one-sided stopping boundary, in the one-sample case. When the interim test results demonstrate that the candidate treatment is inferior to the standard, testing should be stopped early. When the interim test results indicate that the candidate treatment is as good as or superior to the standard, the test will be continued to the final stage to obtain more precise estimates of its efficacy. Their design thus trades expected sample size for better estimates of the response rates of the favorable candidate treatments. Jennison and Turnbull (1983), Tsiatis et al. (1984), and Kim and DeMets (1987) propose procedures for constructing confidence intervals on response parameters following termination of a stagewise test. They present computational procedures and computer programs for constructing the intervals.

Jennison and Turnbull (1983) point out the one-to-one correspondence between the one-sample drug screening/medical trials testing problem and the acceptance sampling problem. This suggests that the acceptance sampling literature is an additional source of information concerning design options, analysis procedures, and available computer programs.

ACKNOWLEDGMENT

This work was supported by the U.S. Army Medical Research and Development Command under contract DAMD17–83–C–3129.

APPENDIX: ACCEPTANCE AND REJECTION BOUNDARIES FOR TWO-SAMPLE, ONE-SIDED *K*-STAGE GROUP SEQUENTIAL TESTING DESIGNS

The one-sided hypothesis to be tested is $H_1 : p_2 \leqslant p_1 \equiv p$ versus $H_2 : p_2 > p_1$. The type I error is specified as α (e.g., $\alpha = 0.05$) when $p_2 = p_1$, and the power is specified as $1 - \beta$ (e.g., $1 - \beta = 0.80$) when $p_2 = p_1 + \Delta$. The specification of p_1, α, and Δ imply a sample size N for a fixed-sample-size design having these characteristics. The sample sizes, N per group, in the evaluations in Section III are set at $N = 24$, 25, or 40, values that are practical for screening programs and that are used in the one-sample evaluations in Section II.

Under H_1, $p_2 = p_1 = p$ (specified). Let S_1 and S_2 denote the number of responses in N animals per group, for groups 1 and 2, respectively. Let $Z_{1-\alpha}$ denote the upper $(1 - \alpha)$th percentile of the standard normal distribution. The fixed-sample-size test with N animals per group rejects H_1 if

$$Y_N \equiv \frac{S_2 - S_1}{[2Np(1 - p)]^{1/2}} \geqslant Z_{1-\alpha} \tag{A1}$$

It can be shown that under the assumption that Y_N is approximately normally distributed, the test specified in equation (A1) has power $1 - \alpha$ when $p_2 = \tilde{p}_A \equiv p + \Delta_A$, where

$$\Delta_A = \frac{2Z_{1-\alpha}[2Np(1-p)]^{½} + Z_{1-\alpha}^2(1-2p)}{N + Z_{1-\alpha}^2} \tag{A2}$$

In analogy with Fleming (1982), consider a k-stage design with $n \equiv N/k$ subjects/group/stage. Let $S_{g,1}$ and $S_{g,2}$ denote the cumulative numbers of responses after g stages, in groups 1 and 2, respectively. Fleming's suggested procedure is:

Reject H_1 in favor of H_2 after stage g ($g = 1, 2, \ldots, k$) if

$$\left(\frac{gn}{N}\right)^{½} \frac{S_{g,2} - S_{g,1}}{[2gnp(1-p)]^{½}} \geqslant Z_{1-\alpha} \tag{A.3}$$

Reject H_2 in favor of H_1 after stage g ($g = 1, 2, \ldots, k - 1$) if

$$\left(\frac{gn}{N}\right)^{½} \frac{S_{g,2} - S_{g,1} - gn\Delta_A}{[gnp(1-p) + gn\tilde{p}_A(1-\tilde{p}_A)]^{½}} \leqslant -Z_{1-\alpha} \tag{A.4}$$

where Δ_A and $\tilde{p}_A$ are defined in equation (A2). Reject H_2 after stage k if equation (A3) is not satisfied. Following Fleming, equations (A3) and (A4) lead to the rejection and acceptance boundaries:

$$r_g = [Z_{1-\alpha}[2Np(1-p)]^{½}]^* + 1 \qquad g = 1, \ldots, k \tag{A5}$$

$$a_g = [gn\Delta_A - Z_{1-\alpha}[Np(1-p)] + N\tilde{p}_A(1-\tilde{p}_A)]^{½*} \qquad g = 1, \ldots, k-1 \tag{A6}$$

$$a_k = r_k - 1$$

where $[x]^*$ represents the nearest integer to x, and Δ_A and $\tilde{p}_A$ are defined in equation (A2)

As an example of these boundary calculations, consider the case $p = 0.15$, $N = 40$, $\alpha = 0.05$, and $k = 1$, 2, and 5.

$$\begin{aligned} k &= 1: \quad a_1 = 5 & r_1 &= 6 \\ k &= 2: \quad (a_1, a_2) = (-1, 5) & (r_1, r_2) &= (6, 6) \\ k &= 5: \quad (a_1, a_2, a_3, a_4, a_5) & &= (-4, -2, 1, 3, 5) \\ & \quad\;\; (r_1, r_2, r_3, r_4, r_5) & &= (6, 6, 6, 6, 6) \end{aligned}$$

These boundaries result in the operating characteristics shown in Table 5. Note that the *final* stage boundaries are the same as those for the fixed-sample-size boundaries, irrespective of the number of stages in the design.

REFERENCES

Armitage, P. (1975). *Sequential Medical Trials,* Wiley, New York.

Aroian, L. A. (1968). Sequential analysis, direct method. *Technometrics 10*: 125–132.

Berry, D. A., and Ho, C. H. (1988). One-sided sequential stopping boundaries for clinical trials: a decision-theoretic approach. *Biometrics 44*: 219–227.

Chang, M. N., Therneau, T. M., Wieand, H. S. and Cha, S. S. (1987). Designs for group sequential phase II clinical trials. *Biometrics 43*: 865–874.

Elfring, G. L., and Schultz, J. R. (1973a). Group sequential designs for clinical trials, *Biometrics 29*: 471–477.

Elfring, G. L., and Schultz, J. R. (1973b). *FORTRAN IV Time Sharing Computer Programs for the Evaluation of One-Sample and Two-Sample Group Sequential Designs.*

Fleming, T. R., (1982). One-sample multiple testing procedure for phase II clinical trials. *Biometrics 38*: 143–151.

Geller, N. L., and Pocock, S. J. (1987). Interim analysis in randomized clinical trials: ramifications and guidelines for practitioners. *Biometrics 43*: 213–223.

Geller, N. L., and Pocock, S. J. (1988). Design and analysis of clinical trials with group sequential stopping rules. Chapter 11 in *Biopharmaceutical Statistics for Drug Development* (Karl E. Peace, ed.), Marcel Dekker, New York.

Hearron, A. E., Elfring, G. L., and Schultz, J. R. (1984). Biopharmaceutical applications of group sequential designs. *Commun. Stat. Theory Methods 19*:2419–2450.

Jennison, C., and Turnbull, B. W. (1983). Confidence intervals for a binomial parameter following a multistage test with applications to MIL-STD 105D and medical trials. *Technometrics 25*: 49–58.

Kim, K., and DeMets, D. L. (1987). Confidence intervals following group sequential tests in clinical trials. *Biometrics 43*: 857–864.

O'Brien, P. C., and Fleming, T. R. (1979). A multiple testing procedure for clinical trials. *Biometrics 35*: 549–556.

Pocock, S. J. (1977). Group sequential methods in the design and analysis of clinical trials. *Biometrika 64*: 191–199.

Pocock, S. J. (1982). Interim analyses for randomized clinical trials: the group sequential approach. *Biometrics 38*: 153–162.

Schultz, J. R., and Elfring, G. L. (1986). Sequential procedures in practice: nonclinical applications. *Proceedings of the Biopharmaceutical Section, American Statistical Association.*

Schultz, J. R., Nichol, F. R., Elfring, G. L., and Weed, S. D. (1973). Multiple-stage procedures for drug screening. *Biometrics 29*: 293–300.

SUNY (1984). *ACCEPT, A Computer Program for the Design of Acceptance Sampling Plans,* Center for Statistics, Quality Control, and Design, State University of New York at Binghamton, Binghamton, N.Y.

Therneau, T. M., Wieand, H. S., and Cha, S. S. (1987a). *SUN Computer Program: Evaluate a Phase II Design for Various Values of P.* Mayo Clinic, Rochester, Minn.

Therneau, T. M., Wieand, H. S., and Chang, M. N. (1987b). *Time Sharing Computer Programs to Evaluate One-Sample Group Sequential Designs and to Enumerate Optimal Designs.*

Tsiatis, A. A., Rosner, G. T., and Mehta, C. R. (1984). Exact confidence intervals following a group sequential test. *Biometrics 40*: 797–803.

Wald, A., and Wolfowitz, J. (1948). Optimum character of the sequential probability ratio test. *Ann. Math. Stat. 19*: 326–339.

Wetherill, G. G. (1966). *Sequential Methods in Statistics,* Methuen, London.

III

APPLICATIONS IN ANTICANCER CLINICAL DRUG DEVELOPMENT

6

Application of a Sequential Screening/ Efficacy Design in an Advanced Colorectal Cancer Study

Samuel Wieand and Daniel J. Schaid

Mayo Clinic, Rochester, Minnesota

I. BACKGROUND

The sequential procedure discussed in this chapter was applied to a phase III trial for patients with advanced colorectal cancer. The trial was conducted by the North Central Cancer Treatment Group and the Mayo Clinic. To be eligible for the study, a patient had to have histological or cytological confirmation of unresectable or metastatic colorectal cancer. The study was initiated in 1983, at which time the standard regimen for these patients was 5FU alone, as various combination regimens had failed to result in an improvement in survival in earlier trials. The median survival for this group of patients was approximately 6 months with very few patients surviving beyond 2 years.

In the early 1980s, three other drugs, methotrexate, leucovorin, and cisplatinum, had shown promise when given with 5FU, in that they were associated with an increase in the proportion of tumors that shrunk or disappeared after therapy administration. From these drugs, five regimens were chosen, all of which had been promising in earlier trials, where tumor shrinkage was an endpoint. Details regarding the exact dosage and schedule for the regimens are discussed in detail in Poon et al. (1989). For simplicity, in this section the five combination regimens will be referred to as 5FU, cisplatin; 5FU, high-dose methotrexate; 5FU, low-dose methotrexate; 5FU, high-dose leucovorin; and 5FU, low-dose leucovorin. It is an important fact that the 5FU was given in higher doses with the low-dose methotrexate (low-dose leucovorin) than with the high-dose methotrexate (high-dose leucovorin) and that regimens were designed to be nearly equally toxic. Thus the 5FU/high-dose methotrexate regimen was not necessarily more dose intensive than the 5FU/low-dose methotrexate regimen, and there was no a priori belief regarding which of the two regimens would be better if they differed. The same statement applies to the two 5FU–leucovorin regimens.

II. PROTOCOL

The primary goal of the study was to be able to identify with near certainty any of the five combination chemotherapy regimens that offered a doubling in median survival when compared to 5FU alone in this group of advanced colorectal patients and to have a reasonably high probability of identifying a combination regimen that offered a 50% increase in median survival. A concurrent goal was to take advantage of the knowledge that had been gained midway through the trial so that we would discontinue accrual to less promising regimens.

The randomization schema we chose is shown in Figure 1. The endpoint used for the design was time to death. Sample size determination was based on the following goals.

1. To be able to identify any treatment that offered a 50% increase in median survival over 5FU alone with a probability of at least 0.75
2. To have no more than a 5% chance of claiming that at least one combined therapy regimen offered an improvement over 5FU alone if all six of the regimens were equivalent in effect

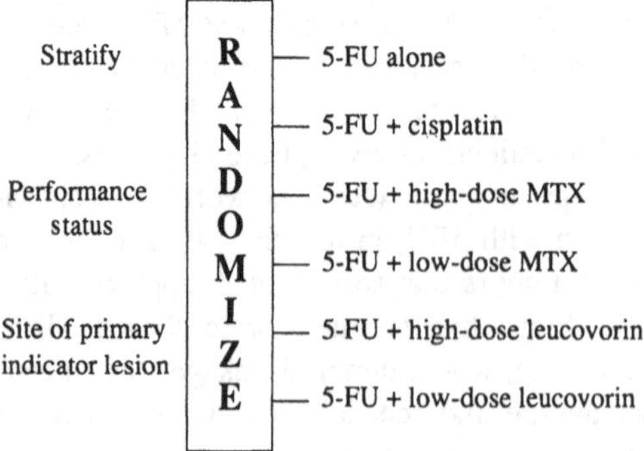

Figure 1 Treatment schema.

Another way of stating goals 1 and 2 is that we wanted the pairwise power for detecting a 50% improvement in median survival for an experimental regimen to be 0.75 and the global significance level for the trial to be 0.05. Thus the significance level was to be adjusted for multiple comparisons. We were aware of the possibility that some or all of the combination regimens might fail to offer an improvement over 5FU alone. This led us to consider a design that would allow us to do an analysis midway through a trial and, at that time, to stop accruing to the less effective combination chemotherapy regimens and to continue accruing only to promising regimens and to 5FU alone. If 5FU alone was clearly less efficacious than one of the experimental regimens, we wanted to have the possibility of stopping accrual to 5FU alone and discontinuing the trial.

We had just completed another trial that used 5FU and several combination regimens in a similar group of patients. Based on the results of that trial and the changes in the size of our cooperative group, we assumed that we would be able to accrue 140 patients per year and that the median survival for the 5FU alone arm would be about 6 months. For our power computations, we assumed that the patient survival would roughly follow an exponential distribution for both the control arm and the experimental regimens.

The decision rule that we implemented in order to carry out this trial was as follows:

1. Initially accrue 420 patients (70 per regimen).
2. At the time of the 420th entry, compute a logrank statistic for each combined therapy regimen versus the 5FU-alone regimen.
3. If a one-sided p-value > 0.15 for a comparison, discontinue accrual to the combined therapy regimen used in that comparison and conclude that the combined therapy regimen was not significantly better than 5FU alone.
4. If $p \leqslant 0.15$ for a comparison, accrue 70 more patients to the combined therapy regimen used in that comparison. If accrual is extended to any combined therapy regimen, accrue 70 more patients to the 5FU alone regimen.
5. If $p < 0.005$ in any comparison, consider discontinuing the trial and concluding that the combined therapy regimen used in that comparison offered an improvement in survival over 5FU alone.

If an experimental regimen went on to accrue 140 patients, the final analysis was to be performed approximately 1 year after the study closed. A regimen would be deemed effective if the normalized logrank statistic comparing the regimen to 5FU alone had a p-value < 0.01. Under the assumptions stated above, this decision rule would have a global significance level 0.06 and pairwise power 0.76 for detecting a 50% increase in median survival associated with a combined therapy regimen, and power of more than 0.99 for detecting a doubling in median survival associated with a combined therapy regimen.

One can give a more intuitive meaning to the decision rule. Rejecting the hypothesis using a test at p-value 0.01 is, under the assumption of proportional hazards, comparable to saying that at the end of the trial we would conclude that a combined therapy regimen offered an improvement over 5FU alone if the hazard associated with 5FU alone relative to that associated with the combined therapy regimen exceeded 1.34. Under the assumption of exponentiality this would be roughly equivalent to saying that the median survival observed for patients receiving the combined therapy regimen was at least one-third greater than the median survival observed for patients receiving 5FU alone. The interim analysis criteria would be equivalent to saying that we would stop accrual to a combined therapy regimen if at the first look the hazard associated with the 5FU only relative to that associated with the combined therapy regimen was less than 1.23. Stopping early and concluding that a combined therapy regimen was effective would take place if the hazard associated with 5FU alone relative to that associated with the combined therapy regimen exceeded 1.67.

This rule would greatly reduce the expected number of patients to be accrued if none of the combination therapy regimens offered an improvement over 5FU alone. As Figure 2 indicates, if none of the five combination therapy regimens offered an improvement, there would be more than a 60% chance that accrual would terminate at 420 patients, a more than 20% chance that exactly one combined therapy regimen would have a p-value < 0.15 and that the study would accrue 560 patients, and so on. A fixed-sample design with the same significance level and power would require the accrual of approximately 700 patients.

III. MONITORING AND DATA COLLECTION

The operations office and statistical center for the study were located at the Mayo Clinic. Patients were assigned treatment using an allocation method proposed by Pocock and Simon (1975). For the North Central Cancer Treatment Group (NCCTG) patients, data were submitted on forms designed at the operations office. During the period when patients were receiving therapy, forms were to be submitted for every treatment cycle, although the data manager could wait for two cycles to be completed before submitting data (the longest treatment cycle was 5 weeks). The forms required detail toxicity and outcome data. Once a patient experienced disease progression or was unable to comply with the protocol monitoring schedule, the NCCTG data managers were required to submit (to the operations office) an evaluation form every 3

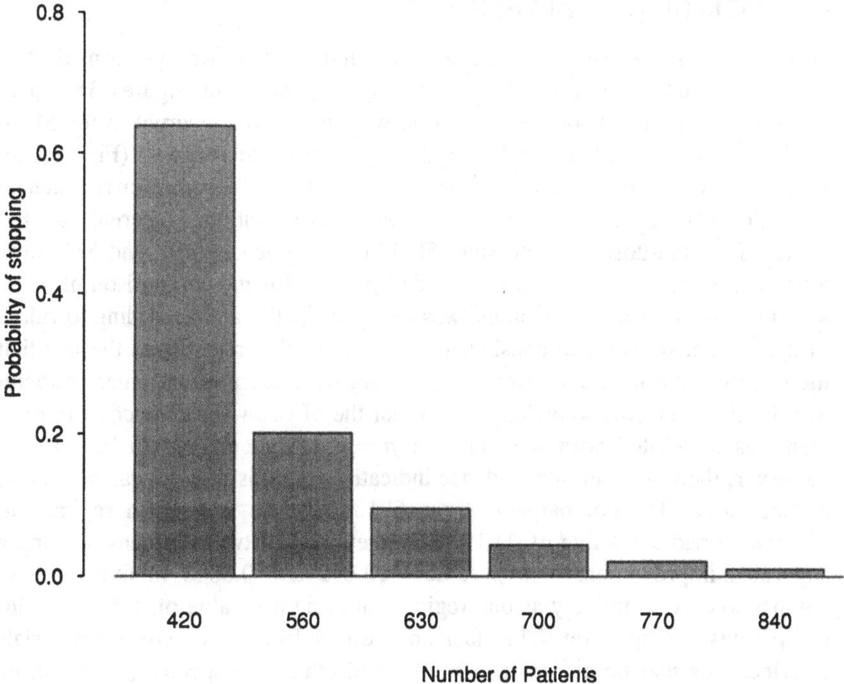

Figure 2 Probability of stopping for each possible sample size when the treatments are equivalent.

months which required a summary of the patient's disease and survival status. These forms were reviewed by a data monitor in the operations office and entered into a computer. Problem cases were reviewed by the Mayo study chairman (a physician) and the study statistician. For Mayo Clinic patients, data were entered into the computer directly from an oncology record that was part of the patient chart. Data entry was performed within 3 weeks of each patient evaluation. After a patient progressed or was unable to return for evaluations, survival information was obtained every 3 months from sources such as the local doctor or contact with the family.

In addition to routine quality edits, a summary of the data in the form of a statistical report was reviewed every 6 months by a monitoring committee consisting of the NCCTG study chairman, the Mayo Clinic study chairman, and the responsible statistician. The purpose of this review was to see if the protocol needed modification due to unsatisfactory toxicity patterns or accrual rates. The monitoring committee also performed the formal statistical evaluation according to the decision rule when 420 patients had been entered.

IV. STATISTICAL ANALYSES

When 420 patients had been accrued, the first analysis was performed. The survival curves and one-sided p-values were as shown in Figures 3a and b. According to part 3 of our decision rule we were to stop accrual to the 5FU–cisplatin regimen and the 5FU/low-dose methotrexate regimen (Figure 3b). Had the p-value for the comparison of 5FU/low-dose leucovorin regimen to 5FU alone been slightly larger, we would have continued accrual to 5FU alone, 5FU/high-dose methotrexate, 5FU/high-dose leucovorin, and 5FU/low-dose leucovorin. As it was, the one-sided p-value for the comparison of 5FU/low-dose leucovorin to 5FU alone was less than 0.005, and according to rule 5 of the design, we were to consider termination of the trial. Given the fact that there were multiple comparisons, this would have been an extremely difficult decision had our only knowledge been that the 5FU/low-dose leucovorin regimen was associated with a p-value of $p = 0.0048$ compared to 5FU alone. However, there was further evidence indicating that this finding was not due to chance alone. The comparison of the 5FU/high-dose leucovorin regimen to 5FU alone had a p-value of 0.012. The likelihood of two regimens offering a suggested improvement with p-values <0.012 and 0.0048 in five pairwise comparisons is as unlikely as one regimen offering a p-value of 0.005 in a single pairwise comparison. This fact and results from other concurrent trials convinced us that both from a scientific and ethical perspective, it would be inappropriate to continue accruing patients to 5FU alone, and the trial was terminated with the conclusion that 5FU was inferior to (at least) the 5FU/low-dose leucovorin regimen. A new design was proposed which permitted immediate continuation of accrual to the 5FU/high-dose methotrexate regimen and the two 5FU–leucovorin regimens as a second phase of the trial to be analyzed separately.

The results of the six-regimen trial were presented in Poon et al. (1989). At the time of the analyses presented in that manuscript, 88% of the patients had died. Follow-up for the patients who were still alive ranged from 14 to 41 months. The results of the survival comparisons were as shown in Figure 4. As can be seen, the apparent benefit associated with the combination regimens was less (statistically) significant than at the time of interim analysis. This is due primarily to the fact that virtually all the patients failed. The survival curves came back together, which is equivalent to saying that the assumption of proportional hazards, and in particular the assumption of exponentiality, did not hold. Nevertheless, the logrank statistics associated with both comparisons of a leucovorin regimen to 5FU alone remained significant at the 0.05 level and the conclusion in that manuscript was that 5FU–leucovorin in combination does offer an improvement in survival compared to 5FU alone. The most efficacious way of combining the drugs was still to be determined, as was the relationship of the 5FU–leucovorin regimens to the 5FU/high-dose methotrexate regimen.

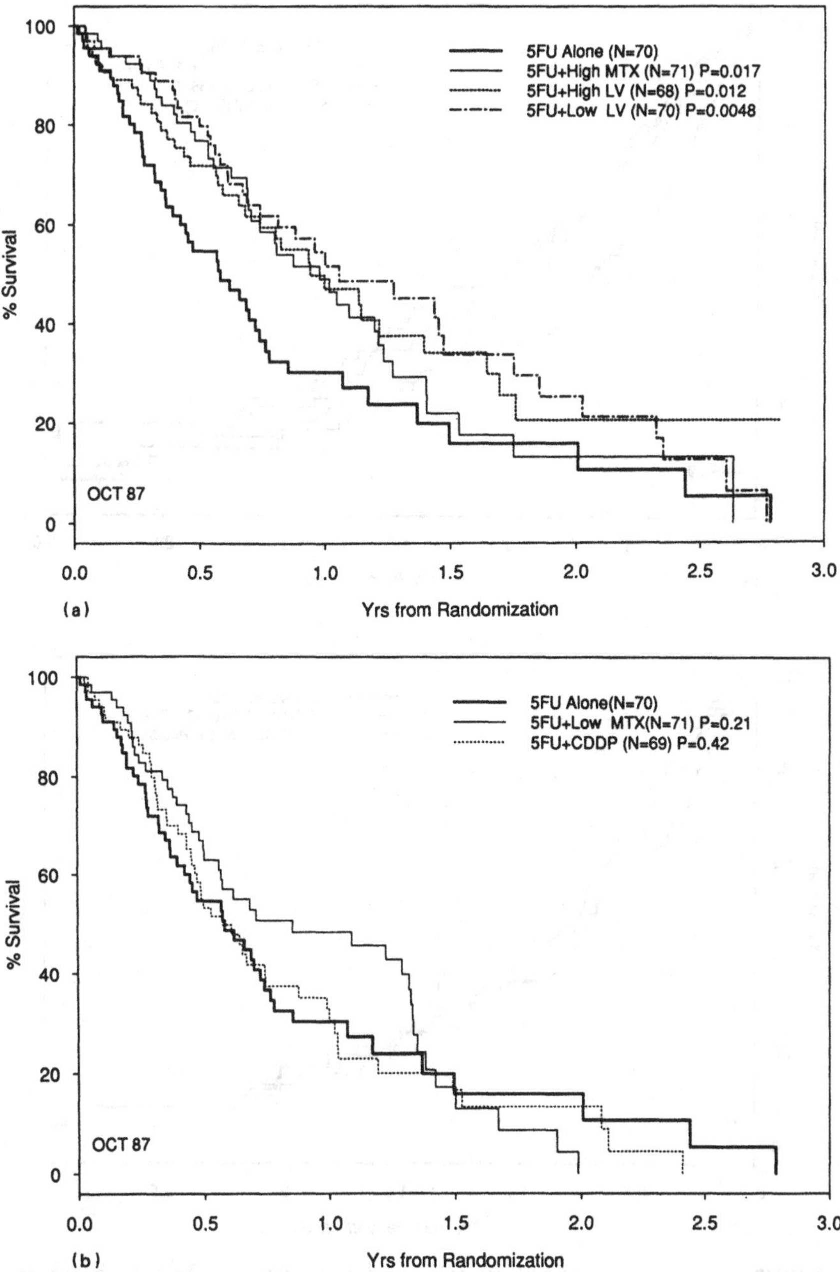

Figure 3 Survival curves and one-sided logrank p-values for the combination regimens versus 5FU alone at the time of the first analysis. Number of eligible patients are shown in parentheses.

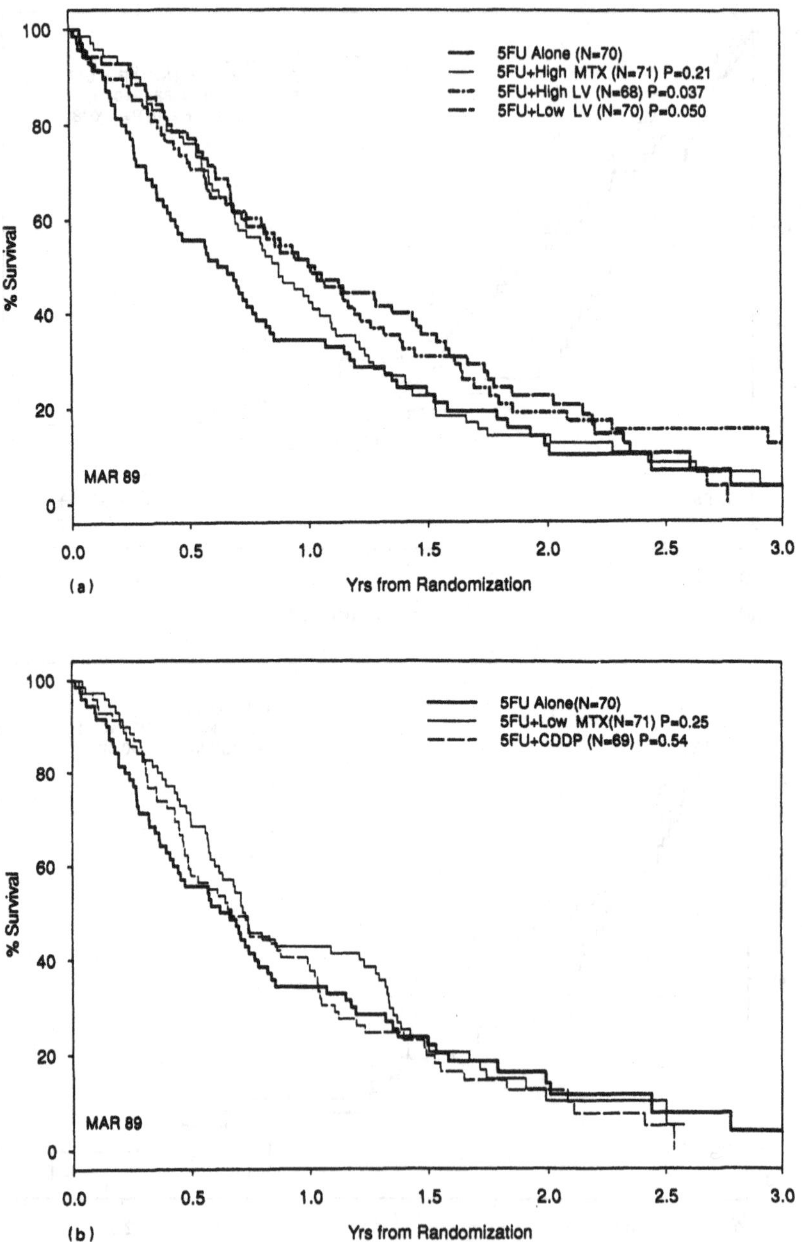

Figure 4 Survival curves and one-sided logrank p-values for the combination regimens versus 5FU alone at the time of final analysis. Number of eligible patients are shown in parentheses.

Secondary survival analyses were performed in accordance with the protocol design. These included multifactor analyses using the Cox proportional hazards model (Cox, 1972) and pairwise comparisons using the Gehan-Wilcoxon statistic (Gehan, 1965). Nontreatment covariates predictive of survival were performance score, tumor-related symptoms, and degree of tumor anaplasia. After adjustment for these three factors, the one-sided p-values associated with the 5FU/high-dose methotrexate, 5FU/high-dose leucovorin, and 5FU/low-dose leucovorin compared to 5FU alone were $p = 0.076$, $p = 0.051$, and $p = 0.051$, respectively. The p-values associated with the same comparisons using the Gehan-Wilcoxon statistics were $p = 0.032$, $p = 0.022$, and $p = 0.006$, respectively.

Analyses using endpoints such as progression-free survival, weight gain, improvement in performance score, and improvement in symptomatic status were also performed and, again, the 5FU/high-dose methotrexate regimen and the two 5FU–leucovorin regimens were associated with the most improvement compared to 5FU alone. Over 50% of the patients experienced some severe toxic reactions on each regimen, and none of the six regimens offered a significant reduction or increase in severe toxicities compared to 5FU alone.

V. CONCLUSION

The conclusion in the manuscript was that either 5FU–leucovorin regimen offered a therapeutic advance over 5FU alone, but that the most efficacious way of combining the two drugs was still to be determined, as was the relationship of the 5FU–leucovorin regimens to the 5FU/high-dose methotrexate regimen. The 5FU/low-dose methotrexate regimen and 5FU–cisplatin regimen were found not to offer a significant improvement in survival compared to 5FU alone, and use of the latter three regimens in this patient population appears to be unjustified.

VI. DISCUSSION

When we designed the trial, we did not expect any treatment to offer the advantage that 5FU/low-dose leucovorin did, and we thought the attractive feature of the design was that it would allow termination of less promising regimens (as 5FU–cisplatin and 5FU/low-dose methotrexate turned out to be) before going to the second stage. We have used the design in subsequent trials in advanced cancer and, in a current trial, we have dropped two experimental regimens and are in a second stage with only a standard regimen and one experimental regimen. There was no attempt at choosing a design that obtained the minimum expected sample size in this trial, but a method for doing this has since been developed and presented by Schaid et al. (1990).

The decision at the time the 420th patient entered was not based only on the design and was made with some reservations. There were several arguments against dropping the 5FU-only regimen. One was that when the decision rule was written, we expected to have 50 or more deaths on the 5FU-alone arm. In fact, there were only 46. With fewer deaths at the interim analysis than planned, the correlation between statistics computed at the interim and final analyses was smaller than accounted for, and hence may increase the α error. Another was that when other significant prognostic factors were included in the model, the one-sided p-value associated with 5FU/low-dose leucovorin (versus 5FU alone) was 0.01. Arguments in favor of discontinuing accrual to 5FU were compelling. Of course, one was that the p-value associated with the log-rank test was less than 0.005, so this design criterion was met. An equally compelling one was that both 5FU–leucovorin arms were showing a dramatic improvement over 5FU, and this was true when we looked at other endpoints to include progression-free interval, tumor shrinkage, improvement in symptoms, improvement in performance score, and weight gain. The decision to terminate accrual to 5FU alone was made when the three members of the monitoring committee and the NCCTG group chair gathered and reviewed the data. All of the points above were discussed.

Another issue we faced, which is always present when sequential decision rules are used in cancer trials, was how to present p-values. By the time the final draft of the manuscript was written, 18 months had elapsed and there had been considerably more deaths than at the time of interim analysis. We presented p-values based on the most current data. The issue of how to present point estimates, confidence intervals, and so on, following a sequential trial is discussed in a number of references, including Tsiatis et al. (1984), DeMets (1987), Kim and DeMets (1987), Kim (1989), and Jennison and Turnbull (1989). The issue is further complicated in cancer trials by the fact when a trial is terminated early, the data at the time the trial is analyzed for publication may be quite different than they were at the time the trial was terminated.

Another issue of some concern was that the decision rule was based on the assumption of proportional hazards, despite the possibility that nearly all of the patients would die before the final analysis would be performed. In this case, the curves were likely to come together (i.e., crossing hazards). Figure 5 illustrates the relative hazards, estimated by the Cox proportional hazards model (Cox, 1972), during 3-, 6-, and 12-month intervals for each of the five 5FU-combination regimens versus 5FU alone. These ratios are for the hazard rate of the 5FU alone divided by the hazard rate for combination regimens. Although the hazard ratios do not appear constant over the five time intervals, the standard errors are large and the estimated hazard ratios over the entire

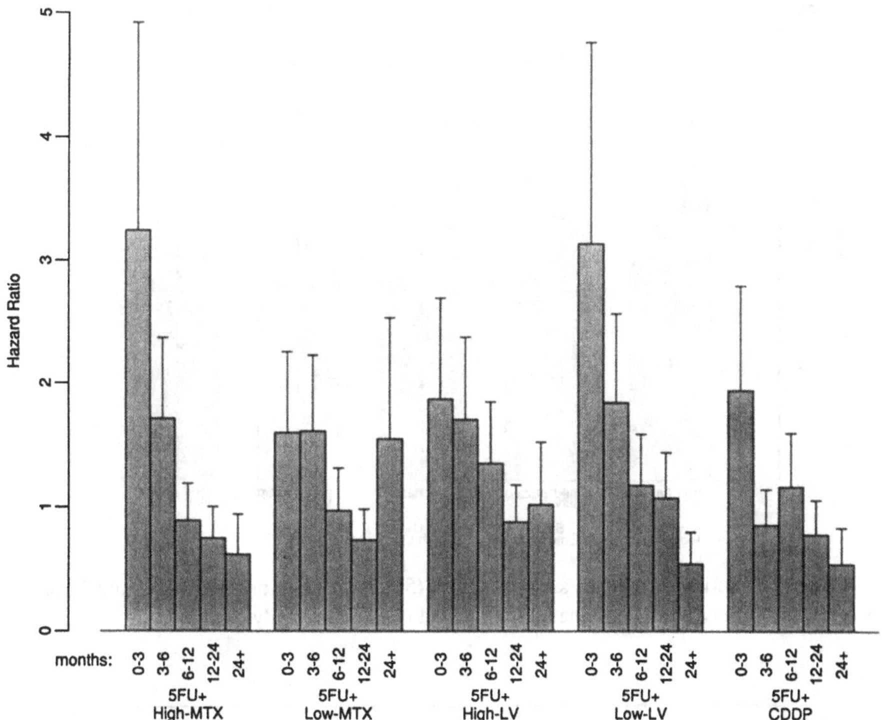

Figure 5 Estimated relative hazards (5FU only/5FU–combination) over five time intervals, with standard error bars.

duration of the study were considerably concordant with the ratios of the median survivals, as depicted in Figure 6. Hence the initial assumption that power computations based on hazard ratios is also applicable to ratios in median survivals seems to be a reasonable approximation.

We noted in Section IV that randomization was continued to the two 5FU–leucovorin regimens and to the 5FU/high-dose methotrexate regimen. Currently, 216 of 248 patients entered into this second phase of the trial have died and the current survival data are summarized in Figure 7. Given that the 5FU/high-dose methotrexate regimen was the third best arm on the first phase of the trial, these new results are highly supportive of the conclusion that 5FU–leucovorin combination therapy represents a true therapeutic advance in the treatment of advanced colorectal cancer.

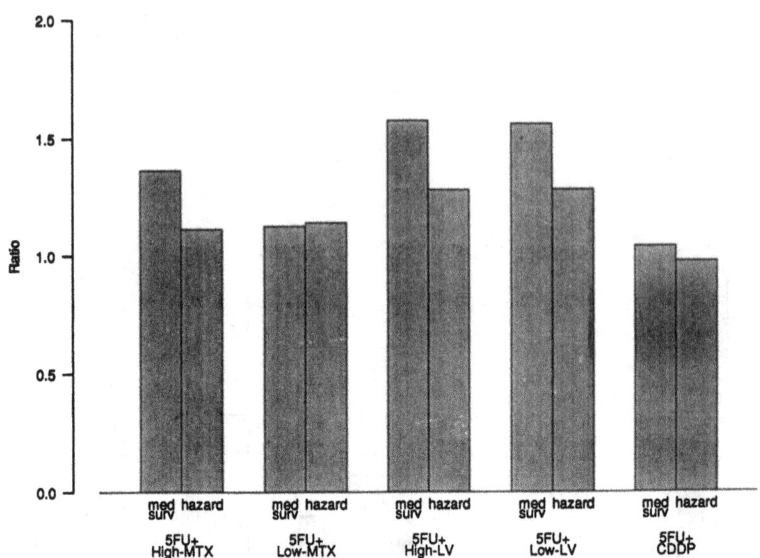

Figure 6 Ratios of median survival times (5FU–combination/5FU only) and hazard ratios (5FU only/5FU–combination) estimated over entire study duration.

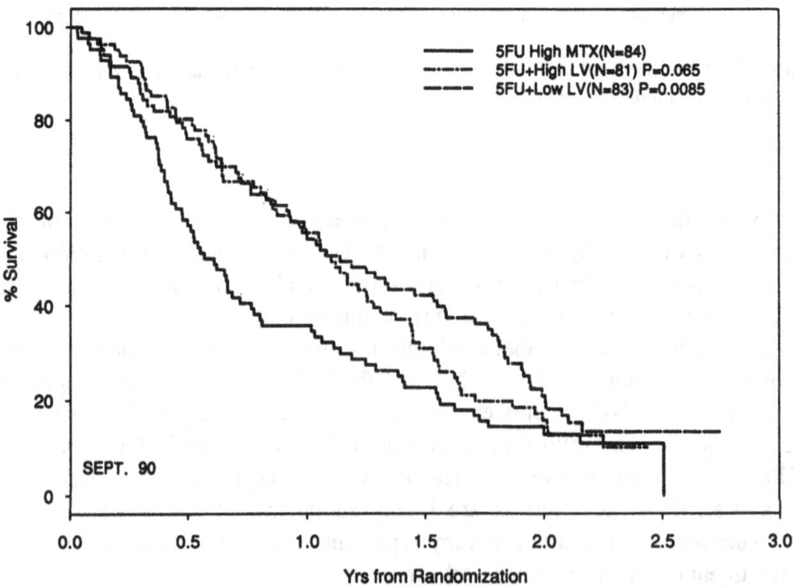

Figure 7 Survival curves and two-sided logrank *p*-values for the 5FU–leucovorin regimens versus 5FU/high-dose methotrexate in the second phase of the trial. Number of eligible patients are shown in parentheses.

REFERENCES

Cox, D. R. (1972). Regression models and life tables. *J. R. Stat. Soc. B 34:* 187–202.

DeMets, D. L. (1987). Practical aspects in data monitoring: a brief review. *Stat. Med. 6:* 753–760.

Gehan, E. A. (1965). A generalized Wilcoxon test for comparing arbitrarily singly-censored samples. *Biometrika 52:* 203–223.

Jennison, C., and Turnbull, B. W. (1989). Interim analyses: the repeated confidence interval approach. *J. R. Stat. Soc. B 51:* 305–361.

Kim, K. (1989). Point estimation following group sequential tests. *Biometrics 45:* 613–617.

Kim, K., and DeMets, D. L. (1987). Confidence intervals following group sequential tests in clinical trials. *Biometrics 43:* 857–864.

Pocock, S. J., and Simon, R. (1975). Sequential treatment assignment with balancing for prognostic factors in the controlled clinical trial. *Biometrics* 31: 103–115.

Poon, M. A., O'Connell, M. J., Moertel, C. G., Wieand, H. S., Cullinan, S. A., Everson, L. K., Krook, J. E., Mailliard, J. A., Laurie, J. A., Tschetter, L. K., and Wiesenfeld, M. (1989). Biochemical modulation of fluorouracil: evidence of significant improvement of survival and quality of life in patients with advanced colorectal carcinoma. *J. Clin. Oncol. 7:*(10): 1407–1418.

Schaid, D. J., Wieand, H. S., and Therneau, T. M. (1990). Optimal two-stage screening designs for survival comparisons. *Biometrika. 77*: 507–513.

Tsiatis, A. A., Rosner, G. L., and Mehta, C. R. (1984). Exact confidence intervals following a group sequential test. *Biometrics 40:* 797–803.

7

Group Sequential Methods in Multi-institutional Cancer Clinical Trials

A Case Study

Kathleen J. Propert

Harvard School of Public Health, Boston, Massachusetts

Kyungmann Kim

Harvard School of Public Health and Dana-Farber Cancer Institute, Boston, Massachusetts

I. BACKGROUND

We present a case study of a phase III clinical trial conducted by Cancer and Leukemia Group B (CALGB) to test two therapies for treatment of patients with a particular type of lung cancer. Details of the clinical aspects of this study are given elsewhere (Dillman et al., 1990). This study was terminated early before reaching accrual goals due to the appearance of treatment differences. Although this study did not originally have a group sequential design, group sequential methods were implemented after patient accrual began and used in the decision for early closure. We use this study to illustrate the use of such methods in assessing treatment differences over time and the role of a data monitoring committee (DMC) for such a trial in a multi-institutional cooperative group setting. We also review the development of sequential methods as applied to chronic disease clinical trials and discuss some of the methods of statistical inference that have been proposed in conjunction with these procedures.

CALGB is one of a number of multi-institutional cooperative groups that were formed in the 1950s to conduct large-scale cancer clinical trials. These cooperative groups allow many researchers and institutions to pool patients and resources. One advantage to this structure is that trials may be conducted in less time than would normally be required for a single institution, especially for rare forms of cancer. However, efficient coordination of data collection and analysis is crucial for such large groups to function effectively. For example, 22 main member institutions of CALGB and a number of affiliates participated in the phase III trial we report here. Protocol development, data management, and statistical support are centralized and there is a close working relationship among the study chairmen, statistician, and data managers on each study. This structure allows easy access to data and facilitates any decision-making process. Control over all aspects of study design, conduct, and analysis is particularly important in the case of a phase III trial in which ethical considerations lead to the need for careful monitoring.

Such phase III clinical trials compare the efficacy of two or more treatment programs in a sample of patients with a specific type and stage of cancer. In lung cancer, the primary endpoint of interest is usually survival, defined as the time from randomization to one of the treatment regimens to the time of death from any cause or to the last follow-up time. Patients who are known to be alive at the last follow-up are considered "censored." Until recently, these trials have generally had a fixed-sample design in which patients are simply accrued over time until some previously determined sample size is reached. For time-to-failure outcomes such as survival, this sample size is based on the number of failures, or deaths, required to ensure adequate power to detect a specified difference in the failure rates at a specified type I error level, α. The treatment difference of interest is usually defined as a difference in median survival or difference in survival at a particular time point, such as 3 years. Determination of the required sample size assumes that all patients are entered on the study and analysis occurs when a certain percentage of these patients have failed. Therefore, for a hypothesis test based on the fixed sample size to have the required power properties, patient accrual continues until the target sample size is reached and follow-up continues until the required number of failures has occurred. At this time the final analysis of the study is performed and the results are reported.

Even with such a fixed-sample design, most phase III cancer clinical trials are monitored during both the accrual and follow-up periods to evaluate study conduct and safety. Such monitoring is done through a series of interim analyses in which patient accrual, treatment-related toxicities, and efficacy are examined. In CALGB, these interim analyses are usually performed every 6 months to correspond to the CALGB semiannual meetings. As a result of these interim analyses, studies may be amended to remedy emerging problems, such as slow patient accrual or unexpected toxicities. Treatment comparisons with respect to efficacy outcomes such as survival are an integral part of this monitoring process. For example, if one treatment appears substantially better than another, early termination of patient accrual might be considered to avoid further treatment of patients with possibly inferior therapy. However, if a study is closed prematurely due to early differences that are later found to be attributable to usual statistical fluctuation, the power to detect real differences between treatments is reduced. The term *closure* refers either to closing a protocol to further patient accrual or, if the target sample size has been reached, to reporting results before the required number of failures has been observed. When the possibility of early closure based on hypothesis tests exists, statistical methods for fixed-sample designs no longer have the desired properties.

Group sequential methods provide a means of taking into account repeated looks at the data. This methodology leads to *stopping rules* or *boundaries* that define how large treatment differences must be at any particular interim analysis to indicate closure of the study. These stopping rules allow the overall type I error and power to be maintained, while allowing for early closure of the trial when large treatment differences are observed before the scheduled termination is reached. Use of these methods require an adjustment in the sample size (or amount of follow-up) required for the trial. Stopping rules have also been developed that allow early closure of a trial when there are no apparent treatment differences and thus negative studies may be detected earlier. The ethical issues involved in closing a trial for lack of treatment differences differ from those involved in early closure due to treatment differences. For example, if two therapies compared in a study prove to be equally efficacious and toxic, reasons for early closure may rest on issues such as cost considerations or the need to move on to study newer therapies, rather than on ethical considerations directly pertaining to patients on the study. To our knowledge, these "lower" boundaries are not yet widely used in cooperative group cancer research.

The use of group sequential methods to monitor phase III clinical trials has recently become standard in cancer cooperative groups. We now describe our experience of applying these methods in a CALGB phase III clinical trial. The design of this trial, conceived in 1983, did not originally incorporate group sequential methods. However, the emergence of apparent treatment differences coincided with the institution of new policy regarding monitoring and reporting of phase III trials, and therefore this trial was the first in CALGB to use these methods formally. Many of the decisions regarding the role of a data monitoring committee and the choice of sequential stopping rules on this trial were later adopted as standards for the conduct of phase III trials in CALGB.

II. STUDY DESIGN, OBJECTIVES, AND DATA COLLECTION PROCEDURES

The study we describe here was designed in 1983 to compare standard treatment with radiotherapy (RT) alone to an experimental treatment regimen of two courses of combination chemotherapy (CT) given prior to the standard radiotherapy as treatment for regional stage III non-small cell carcinoma of the lung. Carcinoma of the lung is the leading cause of cancer deaths in the United States. For treatment purposes, lung cancer is generally subdivided into two categories, based on the cell type presenting at diagnosis. The first type, small cell (or oat cell) anaplastic carcinoma, is strongly associated with smoking and accounts for roughly 30% of all lung cancers. Most other cell types are classified as non-small cell lung cancer (NSCLC), which includes adenocarcinoma, squamous cell carcinoma, and large cell anaplastic carcinoma. All cancers are usually classified further according to the extent or stage of disease so that therapies may be tailored to the particular disease stage. For example, lung cancer presenting as a small solitary pulmonary nodule may respond to treatment with surgery alone. However, patients with metastatic disease in which lymph nodes or other organs are involved usually require systemic therapy, which may include chemotherapeutic agents and/or radiation therapy.

Patients with NSCLC who have extensive disease in the chest but no demonstrable distant metastases are defined as having stage III NSCLC. Such patients are not generally considered curable by surgery alone. For many years, RT has been the treatment of choice for these patients, leading to a median survival of 9 to 11 months and a 3-year survival rate of less than 10%. In attempts to improve survival in these patients, clinical researchers in the early 1980s considered the possibility that RT alone might not be sufficient to eradicate micrometastatic disease. At that time there was also some evidence that platinum-based CT was beneficial in terms of survival in more advanced disease patients. Therefore, various systemic approaches to treatment of stage III patients, which included CT in conjunction with standard RT, were proposed. The current study was designed to compare the standard treatment (RT only), consisting of RT delivered over 6 weeks to the original tumor volume and involved regional lymph nodes, to an experimental treatment (CT + RT), which employed 5 weeks of cisplatin plus vinblastine prior to the RT. The RT on the experimental arm was identical in dose, schedule, and volume to that for the standard treatment. The rationale for the experimental therapy was that up-front systemic CT might lead to initial tumor shrinkage, which would then improve the local control provided by RT and also eliminate micrometastatic disease.

The patient population for this study was limited to patients with documented regional stage III (T_3) NSCLC. Patient eligibility criteria included no prior CT, RT, or total resection, performance status of 0 or 1, and weight loss of less than 5% in the 3-month interval prior to study entry. Standard CALGB eligibility criteria regarding laboratory values, other diseases, and so on, were also used. All eligible patients who began treatment and had follow-up data were included in the analyses. Eight percent of the patients on this study did not meet this criteria and were excluded from the analysis.

The primary objective of this study was to compare survival on the experimental treatment (CT + RT) to that on the standard treatment (RT only). Under the proportional hazards assumption, we can write a model for these data as

$$\lambda(t|z) = \lambda_0(t)\ \exp(\theta z)$$

where $\lambda_0(t)$ represents the baseline hazard at time t, z is a treatment indicator, and θ is the log hazard ratio. The null hypothesis of no treatment difference is H_0: $\theta = 0$; the alternative hypothesis that the two treatments differ with respect to survival (two-sided) is $H_1: \theta \neq 0$. If we let Δ be the hazard ratio [i.e., $\Delta = \exp(\theta)$], we can write $H_0: \Delta = 1$ and $H_1: \Delta \neq 1$.

The original fixed sample size for this trial was 240 patients (120 patients per treatment arm). This sample size was calculated to provide 80% power to detect a hazard ratio of 1.5:1 ($\Delta = 1.5$) assuming that the logrank test would be used at a two-sided significance level of $\alpha = 0.05$. This hazard ratio represents a 50% difference in median survival between the two groups. For example, if median survival for one therapy were 9 months, this sample size would give 80% power to detect a median survival of 13.5 months in the other arm, assuming an exponential distribution. Equivalently, we could detect a difference in the 1-year survival rate between 40 and 55%. By the formula (Schoenfeld, 1981)

$$\frac{[2(z_{\alpha/2} + z_{1-\beta})]^2}{(\log \Delta)^2}$$

where z_γ is the upper γ quantile of the standard normal distribution, a total of 190 failures on the two arms was required. The fixed sample size was calculated by assuming that the final analysis of the study would be performed after 80% of the patients had died, such that 190/0.8 or approximately 240 patients were required. Based on previous experience with the treatment of these patients in CALGB, the entire process from the entry of the first patient to the final analysis was expected to take 4½ years. Again note that when this study was designed in 1983, only this fixed sample size was used. Thus, although semiannual interim analyses were planned, the sample size was not adjusted to account for the possibility of early closure of the trial due to observed treatment differences.

Once the studies opened to patient accrual, after required laboratory and staging work had been done, each patient was randomly assigned to one of the two treatments and registered on study. At this time, the contributing institution was required to send in an "on-study" form which contained all relevant demographic, clinical, and prognostic information on the patient. Following each phase or cycle of treatment, a flow sheet describing the patient's course and an associated "follow-up" form were sent. Follow-up information was also required at disease progression or death, or if the patient terminated treatment for any reason such as excessive toxicity. At the completion of RT, a radiation therapy form was sent to the Quality Assurance Review Committee (QARC) in Providence, Rhode Island, which reviews the adequacy of RT on all CALGB protocols. All forms were initially reviewed by the study data manager at the CALGB Data Management Center, who coded the information into the clinical database. A query letter was sent to any institutions that had delinquent records. After review of patient data by the study data manager, case evaluation forms were generated and sent to the study chair for review. Evaluation of internal consistencies and validity of the clinical data were also checked by the study data manager, statistician, and study chairman through the mechanism of the semiannual interim reports. In addition to these internal quality control measures, all CALGB institutions are audited via a site visit at least once every three years. These audits are used to verify compliance with federal regulations and protocol requirements and entail detailed review of records for a random selection of patients. A total of 38 (21%) patients in this study, involving all participating institutions, had such review. Radiation therapy was monitored by QARC and also by an ad hoc committee of CALGB radiotherapists.

III. GROUP SEQUENTIAL METHODS AND STUDY MONITORING

The CALGB policies for interim monitoring and reporting of randomized trials were amended in 1986, coinciding with the emergence of treatment differences on the current study. Prior to that time, all CALGB members received summary reports of ongoing and recently closed trials twice a year. These reports contained comparisons of efficacy on phase III trials, including p-values; however, the treatments appeared in coded form as A, B, and so on. Such coding was designed to reduce the possibility that early differences might be interpreted in a way that would adversely affect patient accrual.

Under the new policies, based on those proposed by O'Fallon (1985) and later by Green et al. (1987), CALGB as a whole is provided only with summary efficacy results that combine all treatments on a study. It should be noted that unlike clinical trials in many other disease areas, physicians treating cancer patients on clinical trials are generally not blinded to the treatment a patient receives. This is because of the severe toxicity associated with cancer therapies. Part of the management of such treatment-related toxicities requires knowledge of the type of toxicities that might be expected, and therefore treatment-specific toxicities still appear separately for each treatment in interim reports.

A DMC is formed for each phase III study at the time of the first interim analysis. This committee receives the full interim analysis, including treatment comparisons when applicable. The treatments are presented in coded form. Under the original guidelines, each DMC met twice a year to discuss the interim results and determine if any action was required. More recently, the CALGB policy has been revised such that interim analyses are performed after approximately every 20% of the projected failures. This change was made to reduce the number of interim looks for slowly accruing studies or studies in diseases for which the failure rate is low. Eight persons served on the DMC for the current study: the two study chairmen representing medical oncology and radiotherapy, the Respiratory Disease Committee chairman and vice-chairman, the study statistician, the central data manager for the study, and two members of CALGB not directly involved in the study who would not have any direct personal interest in the research. This committee met five times between mid-1985 and the decision to close the study in the spring of 1987.

We briefly review here the group sequential methods that were considered for use in the current trial. A review of the development of these methods is given in Section V. The primary problem with multiple "looks" at a study when these looks may lead to early closure is that if the trial is simply terminated the first time the observed p-value exceeds the desired significance level α, the overall significance level of the study will exceed α. Group sequential methods specify the p-value that should be considered statistically significant at any one interim analysis in order to maintain the overall significance level at α. We shall refer to these values as *boundary significance levels.* Sequential stopping rules were originally designed for trials in which the outcome is observed instantaneously so that the result for each patient is known before the next patient is tested. When survival (or any time-to-failure outcome) is used to monitor a clinical trial, there is a delay in observing the event of interest, and the number of patients and the length of follow-up available for those patients changes over time. Also, practical considerations require that data be analyzed after groups of patients have been treated. Use of sequential methodology in this situation is thus more complicated.

Many stopping boundaries have been developed for chronic disease clinical trials. We briefly describe two commonly used boundaries, the Pocock (1977) and the O'Brien–Fleming (1979), which were considered for the evaluation of the current study. These methods were developed for studies with standard group sequential designs in which the number of interim analyses or looks at the data is specified in advance. At each interim analysis, the observed p-value is compared to the boundary significance level rather than to the overall significance level α. It is assumed that the interim analyses occur after equal numbers of failures. For example, for 190 failures and five planned interim looks, data analysis would occur after every 38 failures are observed.

Group sequential methods correct for the inflation in the type I error that occurs with multiple looks by apportioning the overall significance level over the interim analyses. Consider survival data, which are usually compared between two treatments using the logrank test written as $T = (O - E)/\sqrt{\text{var}[O]}$. Here O is the observed number of failures from one of the two treatment groups and E is the expected number of failures under the null hypothesis. With the Pocock boundary the study stops the first time that the standardized test statistic T above exceeds some constant value; a plot of the boundary values for the test statistic versus looks is flat. With the O'Brien–Fleming boundary, the study stops the first time the unstandardized test statistic $(O - E)$ exceeds some constant value; a plot of this boundary over the looks is decreasing. The constant value is chosen to ensure the desired overall significance level. To maintain the power of the test, the required number of patients must be increased over the fixed sample size. The Pocock boundary typically requires 15 to 25% increase in the sample size, whereas the O'Brien–Fleming boundary requires only a 3 to 5% increase.

In deciding on the appropriate boundary to use, whether the O'Brien–Fleming, Pocock, or some other boundary, a number of factors must be considered. First is the increase in sample size, which may represent a substantial number of patients in a large trial using boundaries such as the Pocock. Second, some boundaries have a level at the final analysis which is substantially different from α. Although such a level is statistically correct, it may be difficult to explain to nonstatisticians involved in the study. For example, for five looks with a two-sided $\alpha = 0.05$, the observed p-value at the final analysis must be less than 0.016 in order to reject the null hypothesis at the $\alpha = 0.05$ level using the Pocock boundary. A third consideration is that boundaries that are extremely conservative early in the monitoring process (i.e., require very small observed p-values in order to reject the null hypothesis) have the potential disadvantage of not allowing closure of the trial even when very large treatment differences are observed. For example, with five looks, the standard O'Brien–Fleming boundary requires an observed $p \leqslant 0.0006$ at the second look, after 40% of the failures have been observed. Many investigators would find it unethical to continue a trial with, say, $p = 0.001$, even though the O'Brien–Fleming boundary was not crossed. An alternative is to truncate the O'Brien–Fleming boundary at 3.0 standard deviations ($p < 0.0013$) and terminate the trial whenever the p-value is less than either the boundary significance level or 0.0013, whichever is larger. Such truncation does not appreciably affect the properties of the O'Brien–Fleming boundary (Lan and DeMets, 1983).

Both of the boundaries described above require that the number of looks be specified in advance and that the number of additional failures observed between interim analyses be constant. This is generally not feasible in cooperative group clinical trials with censored survival data in which the rate of patient accrual fluctuates, there is a waiting period to observe the event, and there may be a lag time in the submission of follow-up data. Lan and DeMets (1983) have suggested a procedure in which a *use function* is chosen that determines how the type I error is used up over time. For example, one such use function is

$$\alpha_3^*(t) = \alpha t$$

in which α is spent as a linear function of time, t. Here time is represented by the proportion of total failures that have occurred $(0 < t < 1)$. For instance, with observation of 38/190 failures, $t = 0.2$. The quantity t is sometimes called the *percent of information* or *information time* as it represents the amount of variance that is proportional to the number of failures for the logrank test under a proportional hazards alternative. Such functions allow more flexibility in the timing and frequency of interim analyses but in practice have the potential disadvantage of requiring software that can calculate the boundary significance levels after any arbitrary number of failures.

Lan and DeMets (1983) derived a use function that provides a continuous analog to the O'Brien–Fleming boundary,

$$\alpha_1^*(t) = 2 - 2\Phi\left(\frac{z_{\alpha/2}}{\sqrt{t}}\right)$$

and another which is a close approximation to the Pocock boundary,

$$\alpha_2^*(t) = \alpha \log[1 + (e - 1)t]$$

Alternative use functions such as

$$\alpha_4^*(t) = \alpha t^{1.5}$$

have also been proposed (Kim and DeMets, 1987a). The three boundaries above were considered for use in the current trial. In the next section we report the results of interim analyses of the current study, which led to the decision for early closure. As per CALGB policy at the time, the interim analyses were scheduled to correspond to the semiannual CALGB meetings rather than being based on the number of failures, and therefore the Lan–DeMets methodology was used (DeMets and Gail, 1985; Lan and DeMets, 1989a).

IV. RESULTS AND STATISTICAL ANALYSES

We now turn to the application of this methodology to the current study. We restrict discussion to the survival endpoint; details of the results for other outcome measures are reported elsewhere (Dillman et al., 1990). Patient accrual to this study began in May 1984. Initial accrual was slow and the first interim analysis was not performed until the fall of 1985. The sample size at this time (10 deaths in 50 eligible patients) was too small to allow any meaningful comparisons of survival by treatment. At the next regularly scheduled interim analysis in the spring of 1986, the logrank test of survival between the two treatments gave an observed $p = 0.021$. The Kaplan–Meier (1958) curves are shown in Figure 1; the median length of follow-up was 6 months. At this time, summary measures were presented to the CALGB as a whole and the treatment results were only provided to the study team (who later comprised part of the DMC). Although formal sequential procedures were not yet in place, the team decided at this time that these data did not represent compelling evidence of a true treatment difference because of the limited number of patients (16 deaths observed) and short follow-up. The DMC was formed at this time and it was decided that group sequential methods would be implemented beginning with the next scheduled analysis in August 1986.

Since this was the first study in CALGB to implement group sequential methods formally, at the time of the August 1986 analysis, the DMC had to decide how such procedures would be applied to this trial. Four boundaries were considered: the Pocock, the standard and truncated O'Brien–Fleming boundaries, and the boundaries generated by α_4^*. Table 1 summarizes the p-

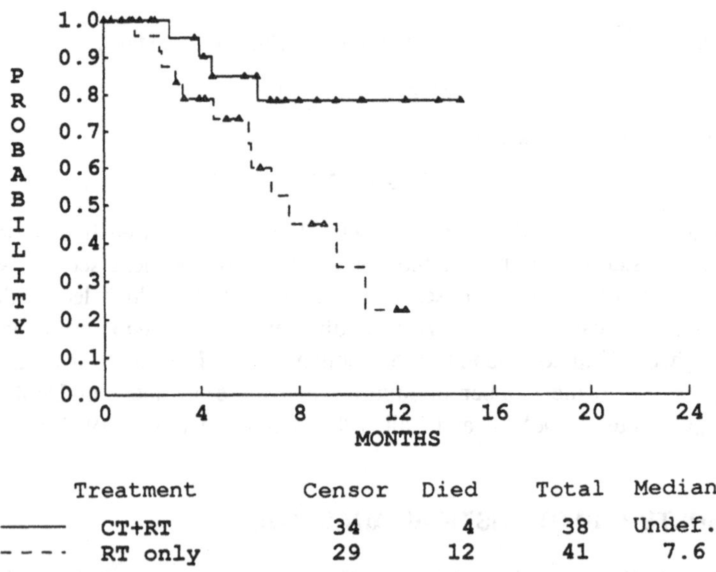

Figure 1 Survival comparison by treatment as of March 1986 ($p = 0.021$).

Table 1 Summary of Observed p-Values and Boundary Significance Levels Used in the Monitoring Process

Analysis date	Percent of information	Logrank p-value	Boundary significance levels: Truncated O'Brien–Fleming[a]	Pocock	$\alpha_4^*(t)$	Decision
Sept. 1985	5	—	0.0013	0.0041	0.0006	Keep open
Mar. 1986	8	0.021	0.0013	0.0034	0.0007	Keep open
Aug. 1986	18	0.0071	0.0013	0.0078	0.0027	Keep open
Oct. 1986	22	0.0015	0.0013	0.0061	0.0026	Keep open
Mar. 1987	29	0.0015[b]	0.0013	0.0081	0.0042	Close

[a] The standard O'Brien–Fleming boundary would give a boundary significance level of $p \leqslant 0.0001$ at each interim analysis shown.

[b] The p-value from the Cox model ($p = 0.0008$) was used in the decision for early termination of the study.

values observed at each interim analysis, the boundary significance levels calculated based on the percent of information available (number of failures observed/190 total failures planned), and the decisions of the DMC. As can be seen in the table, the standard O'Brien–Fleming boundary is very conservative early in the monitoring period, requiring p-values less than 0.0001 at all of these analyses as evidence of a true treatment different. The O'Brien–Fleming boundary truncated at 3.0 standard deviations allows closure if the observed p-value is less than 0.0013 at any interim look. The Pocock boundary would have allowed closure of the study much earlier. The α_4^* boundary is also conservative compared to the Pocock boundary but is more sensitive to early differences than is the O'Brien–Fleming boundary. All of these boundaries maintain an overall significance level of $\alpha = 0.05$.

Recall that use of the Pocock boundary requires 15 to 25% increase in the projected sample size in order to maintain the power at 80%, whereas the O'Brien–Fleming boundary only requires 3 to 5% increase. Since the study was not designed using group sequential methods, it was decided that the conservative O'Brien–Fleming approach which would minimize the additional patients required would be most appropriate. However, there was concern that the O'Brien–Fleming boundary was too conservative early in the monitoring period. The DMC members were uncomfortable with the possibility of continuing to accrue patients to a trial in which the treatment difference was associated with an observed significance of, say, $p = 0.0005$. Therefore, following the suggestion of Lan and DeMets (1983), the O'Brien–Fleming boundary truncated at 3.0 standard deviations (boundary significance level of 0.0013) was selected as the boundary to be used for all monitoring of the study. We have included the boundary values for the Pocock and α_4^* boundaries to illustrate how the decision process would have differed if these boundaries were used.

Figure 2 shows survival by treatment as it was presented to the DMC committee in August 1986. With 18% of the information and an observed $p = 0.0071$, the truncated O'Brien–Fleming boundary of 0.0013 was not crossed and the study remained open to patient accrual. Up to this point, the treatments were coded in the reports to the DMC, and officially, only the study statistician knew which was the apparently better therapy. It was decided, however, that these data should be unblinded to the committee members at this time, for two reasons. First, the combined therapy (CT/RT) was known to be more toxic than RT alone. There was concern that the observed treatment difference was due to mortality on the CT/RT arm associated with the CT-related toxicities, which would suggest a revision of the combined therapy. Second, survival on the inferior arm appeared to be worse than that generally reported for patients treated with standard RT. In fact, the RT alone arm had the inferior survival and it was decided that an evaluation of the adequacy of RT on the study should be instituted. Although such unblinding could potentially have introduced bias, it should be noted that many DMC members had daily contact with the data and were aware of the direction of observed trends.

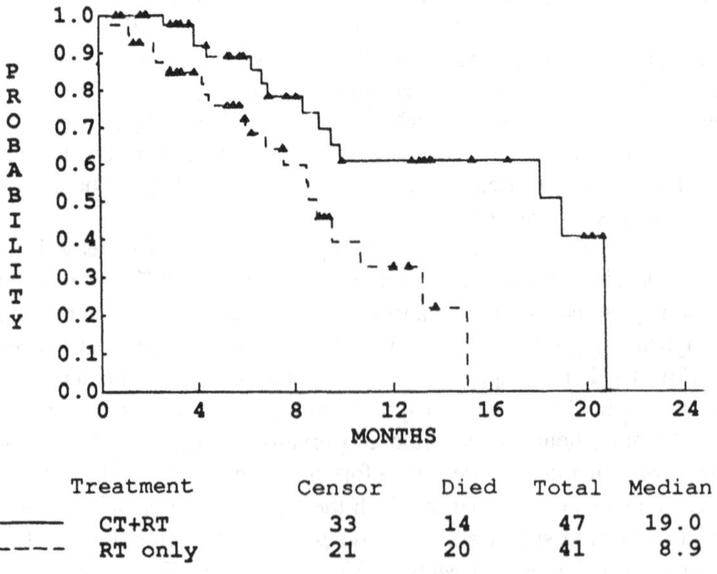

Figure 2 Survival comparison by treatment as of August 1986 ($p = 0.0071$).

We do not feel that this unblinding in any way compromised the ability of the DMC to make appropriate decisions regarding closure of the study. However, it remains the CALGB policy to present treatments in coded form to each DMC unless otherwise indicated.

As a result of the interim analysis as of August 1986, an additional interim analysis was scheduled 2 months later, for which a strong effort was made to collect the most up-to-date follow-up information available for patients on the study. Such data-driven looks have been shown not to change the properties of group sequential tests appreciably (Lan and DeMets, 1989b; Pampallona and Tsiatis, 1990a). By the October 1986 analysis, an additional eight failures had been observed, increasing the amount of information from 18% to 22%. With 4% more information, the observed significance for the comparison of survival by treatment had decreased to $p = 0.0015$, which almost touched the truncated O'Brien–Fleming boundary significance level of 0.0013. Despite the close proximity to the boundary, the DMC again decided that there was insufficient evidence to recommend closure of the study and that the next analysis would be performed as scheduled in March 1987.

The March 1987 interim analysis led to the decision to close the trial to further accrual. At this time, 163 out of the projected 240 patients had been accrued and follow-up data were available for 105 patients. The median length of follow-up was 8 months. Survival by treatment is shown in Figure 3. The

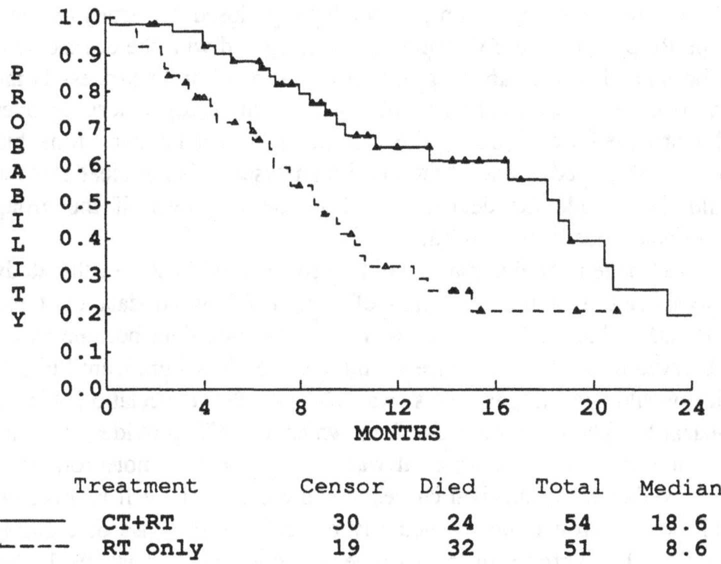

Figure 3 Survival comparison by treatment as of March 1987 ($p = 0.0015$).

observed p-value for this comparison was 0.0015 with a total of 56 failures representing 29% of the information. In response to concerns of the DMC that the observed treatment differences might be attributable to differences in the two treatment groups with respect to other prognostic factors, such as age or substage of disease, a comprehensive analysis including use of the Cox (1972) proportional hazards model was undertaken. The prognostic factors examined were comparable in the two treatment arms. The results of the Cox analysis, which controlled for various prognostic factors known for survival in NSCLC, gave $p = 0.0008$ for the treatment comparison. This analysis reaffirmed that the observed difference represented a real treatment effect. This adjusted p-value had crossed the truncated O'Brien–Fleming boundary and the DMC unanimously voted to close the study.

These data were presented to the Respiratory Core Committee, comprised of approximately 20 CALGB members who are primarily responsible for all decisions regarding CALGB lung cancer research. It is interesting to note that this group was initially reluctant to accept the recommendation of the DMC for early closure. The results were presented as we have presented them here, beginning with the analysis in the fall of 1985 and continuing up to March 1987. Although the DMC was unanimous in its recommendation and cited the compelling evidence of a real treatment effect, the Respiratory Core Committee members expressed their concern that the results were preliminary and that closure of the trial before reaching accrual goals would seriously affect the integrity of the study. This reaction was somewhat surprising to the DMC, which had expected some criticism for not having closed the study earlier. However, the Respiratory Core Committee finally agreed with the decision for closure. It became clear that an integral part of the monitoring process is the opportunity to observe the treatment difference in this study emerging over time. If the observed treatment differences had not evolved over time but instead suddenly appeared at one of the interim analyses, it is not clear that the DMC would have made the decision to close the trial even if the group sequential boundary had been crossed.

The observed benefit of this particular CT given prior to RT in the study remained significant with the collection of further follow-up data on these patients. The DMC had predicted that as more follow-up data became available, the observed treatment difference would become "less significant" in that the p-value would get larger. This was due to the expectation that a "crossing-hazards" phenomenon existed in which the CT provided only an initial early improvement in survival. It was expected that as more follow-up data became available, the survival curves would meet. As is well known, the fixed sample logrank test is not particularly powerful in the case of crossing hazards. In fact, this increase in the p-value was observed at analysis 1 year after the study closed. However, with even more follow-up, it was seen that

23% of the patients who received CT prior to RT were surviving at 3 years as compared to 11% of the patients who received RT alone, suggesting potential long-term benefit of the CT (Cox model $p = 0.0075$). A good discussion of the issues in using group sequential methods with nonproportional hazards is given in Fleming et al. (1984). As a result of the study reported here, the CALGB has recommended that protoadjuvant CT with cisplatin plus vinblastine prior to high-dose RT be used as treatment for good performance-status patients with stage III non-small cell lung cancer. Whether these results will hold in a less restricted population of patients remains to be seen. CALGB is currently studying other combined modality approaches to treatment of these patients.

V. DISCUSSION

We close by discussing some of the major issues in study design, analysis, and statistical inference arising from the use of group sequential methods in cancer clinical trials. First, we review some of the statistical literature that addresses the use of various two-sample linear rank test statistics in the context of sequential monitoring with censored survival data and discuss the rationale for the use function approach. Second, we focus on some of the less understood inferential issues that arise as a consequence of repeated applications of significance tests, such as what to report as the observed significance of the trial, how to report point and confidence interval estimates for the treatment difference following rejection of the null hypothesis, and how to adequately perform supplementary analysis of secondary outcomes following group sequential tests based on the primary outcome variable. Finally, we briefly review the implications for study design of group sequential tests.

Theory and methods for sequential analysis have been in the statistical literature since the late 1940s, beginning with the seminal work by Wald (1947). Most of these methods were targeted for industrial experiments such as quality control or acceptance sampling. Applications of sequential methods to clinical trials began to appear in the literature in the early 1950s. Armitage (1975) gives an excellent account of these applications. Unfortunately, methods developed by the early 1970s could not be applied to typical clinical trials in chronic diseases in which time to failure was the primary endpoint. These early methods were set up for continual monitoring of the data and applied to experiments in which responses were observed almost immediately. The administrative complexity of most clinical trials these days precludes continual monitoring. Instead, the accumulating data are analyzed in "groups" through a series of interim reports. Moreover, the primary endpoint of these studies is often some sort of time-to-event outcome, a response that is not instantaneously observed but rather prolonged over time.

Since the early 1970s major methodological advances have appeared in the literature that have made it feasible to design and analyze such clinical trials using sequential stopping rules. These methods are largely concerned with protecting the type I error probability from the effect of repeatedly applying significance tests. Pocock (1977) modified earlier work of Armitage et al. (1969) and McPherson and Armitage (1971) to the case of clinical trials in which patient response to treatment is available soon after entry and data are available on groups of patients at each analysis. These group sequential methods originally proposed by Pocock (1977) and O'Brien and Fleming (1979) require that the sequence of the test statistics computed over time (1) be multivariate normal, (2) have independent increments, and (3) have equal increments in variance.

Although these methods are very useful, their implementation in chronic disease clinical trials may be difficult. One constraint is that the number of repeated significance tests has to be specified in advance. Another constraint is the difficulty of ensuring that the amount of statistical information accumulated between each repeated analysis, expressed in terms of the variance of the test statistic, has to be constant. As mentioned previously, in cooperative group cancer clinical trials, it is almost impossible to select the times of interim monitoring to achieve this. However, the use function approach of Lan and DeMets (1983) removes these requirements by choosing a use function that essentially characterizes the rate at which the overall type I error probability is allocated over the repeated significance tests. Equivalently, the use function specifies how much of the overall significance level can be used as a function of the accumulating variance of the test statistic.

The effect of treatment on time-to-failure outcomes in clinical trials is generally analyzed using nonparametric linear rank tests such as the logrank test (Mantel, 1966; Peto, 1972), the modified Wilcoxon test (Gehan, 1965), or the generalized Wilcoxon test (Peto and Peto, 1972; Prentice, 1978). The advantage of these linear rank tests is that they are nonparametric, that is, the distribution of these test statistics under the null hypothesis does not depend on the actual shape of the survival distribution. This class of linear rank tests satisfies many of the foregoing requirements for group sequential methods. For these linear rank tests to be used in conjunction with group sequential methods, it is necessary that the joint distribution of these tests computed sequentially over time be determined. A number of authors have studied the properties of these tests. Tsiatis (1981) was among the first to investigate the joint distribution of the efficient scores test statistics for the proportional hazards model. Gail et al. (1981) investigated the asymptotic distribution of the sequentially computed logrank statistics via simulation. Later Tsiatis (1982) rigorously proved the asymptotic normality and the independence of the increments for the sequentially computed logrank test, the generalized Wilcoxon test (Peto and Peto,

1972), and G^ρ statistics suggested by Harrington and Fleming (1982). Slud and Wei (1982), on the other hand, showed that the asymptotic joint distributions for the modified Wilcoxon test do not have independent increments. Sellke and Siegmund (1983) showed the asymptotic distribution of the efficient scores test for the proportional hazard model using the counting process argument (Allen, 1975; Gill, 1980). Slud (1984) showed the same for a general linear rank statistics.

We now turn to issues of statistical inference, following group sequential tests, which are not well understood and often controversial. For fixed-sample-size studies, one usually reports the observed p-value as an indication of the degree of departure from the null hypothesis. The p-value is a probability of observing values of the test statistic as extreme as the observed one when the null hypothesis is true. In the fixed-sample design, it is clear how to define values of the test statistic that are more extreme. However, with repeated significance tests, it is not so clear how to order the sample space to provide an equivalent notion to the p-value. Several suggestions have been made. Fairbanks and Madsen (1982) proposed an ordering in the sample space under sequential sampling by defining early stopping to be more extreme than later stopping and larger absolute values of the test statistic at any one time to be more extreme than smaller values. Given these criteria (or a similarly defined ordering), the p-value may be determined by calculating the probability of seeing a value more extreme than the one observed. A second approach to reporting the statistical significance of a study is to report the value of the significance level that would have resulted in the group sequential boundary being crossed exactly at the observed value of the test statistic. Both of the methods above implicitly assume an underlying ordering of the sample space, and there seems to be no consensus among statisticians. Another simple solution when a boundary is crossed is to report only the overall significance level α with which the study was designed. However, this method may be less acceptable to nonstatisticians involved in the study.

In practice, we have generally taken a middle position and reported both the observed p-value at the time the boundary was crossed and the overall significance level α. However, even this becomes problematic in the case where time elapses between the time at which the boundary is crossed and the time of final reporting of results such as might occur if the final analysis is delayed until additional follow-up becomes available. In the current trial, the truncated O'Brien–Fleming boundary significance level of 0.0013 was met with an observed adjusted p-value of 0.0008 and 29% of the information, and the study was closed to further patient accrual. However, the final analysis of these data was delayed in order to retrieve as much information as possible on patients already treated. At the final analysis, the observed adjusted p-value was 0.0075. Although these two values are fairly close in this study, in other studies the observed logrank p-value may fluctuate quite a bit, especially in the presence of nonproportional hazards. There is again no consensus on what results to report when such additional follow-up is available. This problem is not unique to clinical trials employing sequential stopping rules but may occur in any trial where the amount of follow-up increases over time. It should be noted that in the current study, the failure rate was rapid compared to the accrual rate, such that closure of the study occurred before the target sample size was reached. More often, a boundary crossing occurs after patient accrual had been completed and indicates the time at which follow-up should be terminated and the results reported.

Although tests of hypotheses using group sequential methods are valuable tools for monitoring a clinical trial for early termination, it is often desirable also to report point and confidence interval estimates of the parameter(s) under consideration. Traditional methods for obtaining point estimates and confidence intervals, which ignore the possibility of early stopping, are known to be inappropriate when group sequential methods are used and result in biased estimates and incorrect coverage probabilities. Some authors have explored methods for estimation in this context. For example, Tsiatis et al. (1984) developed a procedure for constructing confidence intervals with exact coverage probabilities for a normal mean. Kim and DeMets (1987b) modified this exact procedure to be applicable to the use function approach. In addition, Kim (1989) proposed adjusted point estimators of a normal mean which were shown to be less biased than the naive point estimator. All of these methods are based on a seemingly natural ordering of the sample space as described above (Fairbanks and Madsen, 1982). Procedures with different ordering of the sample space were also proposed independently by Rosner and Tsiatis (1988) and Chang (1989).

Another problem is the analysis of secondary outcomes at the conclusion of a clinical trial. Although valid methods exist to deal with the endpoints actually used in the sequential design and analysis, very little has been written about analysis of secondary endpoints. For example, suppose that a clinical trial has been designed and carried out using group sequential methods with survival as the primary endpoint. However, in reporting the trial, supplementary endpoints such as tumor response rates or disease-free survival are of interest. Any analysis that ignores the sequential design of the study is potentially biased, and this holds for analyses of endpoints not used directly to determine whether the study should be terminated early. In most clinical trials, these endpoints are correlated with the primary response used in the sequential monitoring. Whitehead (1986) suggested two approaches to the analysis of secondary outcomes following termination of a study. The first approach is a conditional analysis based on the fact that the conditional distribution of the secondary endpoint, given that a study has been terminated when the test statistic for the primary outcome variable crosses a group sequential boundary, is independent of the sequential stopping rule. The second approach is an unconditional analysis in which the joint distribution of the primary outcome variable and the secondary response variable is used. The difficulty with both of these methods is the lack of knowledge of the joint distribution of the primary and secondary outcome variables. For example, in a typical phase III clinical trial for lung cancer, the primary outcome is survival and one important secondary outcome is the objective tumor response, which is an ordered categorical variable. There is no clear understanding of the joint distribution between the survival time and the objective response. Further research is needed on the effect that group sequential tests based on a single endpoint have on the fixed sample inference of secondary endpoints.

In this report, we have only considered group sequential methods for stopping early for treatment difference, mainly for ethical reasons. However, as mentioned earlier, there are occasions when one has to consider terminating the study earlier than scheduled for seeming lack of treatment difference. A number of recent articles have addressed the calculation of such "lower" boundaries. DeMets and Ware (1980, 1982) argued that the rationale for early stopping is not "symmetric" between treatment difference and the lack of it and proposed several asymmetric group sequential boundaries for one-sided tests of hypotheses. Emerson and Fleming (1989) proposed group sequential boundaries that are symmetric in their considerations of type I and II error probabilities, and Pampallona and Tsiatis (1990b) included asymmetric boundaries. Pampallona et al. (1990) considered the use function approach for stopping early for both treatment difference and for lack of such difference.

Whenever group sequential stopping rules are to be implemented in the conduct of a clinical trial, these rules should be taken into account from the very beginning during the design process to ensure that the required statistical properties are maintained. For designing fixed-sample-size or fixed-duration clinical trials with censored survival data, any of the procedures proposed by Bernstein and Lagakos (1978), Rubinstein et al. (1981), Schoenfeld (1981), or Schoenfeld and Richter (1982) can be used to calculate the fixed sample size. When group sequential methods are used, either a larger sample size or longer study duration (more follow-up) is required to maintain the desired power of the test. The necessary increase in the sample size may sometimes be determined using published tables. However, these tables are of limited usefulness for censored survival data since they do not generally take into account the patient accrual rates and the duration of additional patient follow-up and do not allow arbitrary scheduling of analysis times. Kim and Tsiatis (1990) developed a procedure for designing group sequential clinical trials with censored survival data. Under common assumptions that the patient survival distribution is exponential and the treatment comparison will be made by the logrank test, this procedure allows the power to be calculated based on the accrual and follow-up durations specified, or vice versa, using the use function approach. Kim (1990) extended this design procedure so that stratification, random censoring, and unequal patient allocation to the treatments are allowed.

Finally, turning to the current study, the impact of instituting group sequential methods in a study with a fixed sample design is not clear. In a study such as the one described here, it would be unethical not to allow the possibility of early closure. We feel that the choice of a conservative boundary such as O'Brien–Fleming or truncated O'Brien–Fleming is less problematic when these methods are implemented after the trial has begun. At the time of the closure of this study, all ongoing phase III trials in CALGB were redesigned to allow the prospective use of group sequential methods and all new studies now incorporate a group sequential design. The truncated O'Brien–Fleming boundary is used and formal interim analyses on phase III trials are now scheduled to correspond to approximately every 20% of the failures for a total of five looks.

ACKNOWLEDGMENTS

This work was supported in part by Grants CA-11789, CA-23318, CA-33601, and CA-52733, awarded by the National Cancer Institute, DHHS. The authors would like to thank the Cancer and Leukemia Group B, especially Robert Dillman, M.D., and Mark Green, M.D., for the use of their data.

REFERENCES

Allen, O. O. (1975). Statistical inference for a family of counting processes, Ph.D. thesis, University of California, Berkeley.

Armitage, P. (1975). *Sequential Medical Trials,* 2nd ed. Blackwell, Oxford.

Armitage, P., McPherson, C. K., and Rowe, B. C. (1969). *J. R. Stat. Soc. A 132:* 235.

Bernstein, D., and Lagakos, S. W. (1978). *J. Stat. Comput. Simulation 8:* 65.

Chang, M. N. (1969). *Biometrics 45:* 247.

Cox, D. R. (1972). *J. R. Stat. Soc. B 34:* 187.

DeMets, D. L., and Gail, M. H. (1985). *Biometrics 41*: 1039.

DeMets, D. L., and Ware, J. H. (1980). *Biometrika 67*: 651.

DeMets, D. L., and Ware, J. H. (1982). *Biometrika 69*: 661.

Dillman, R. O., Seagren, S. L., Propert, K. J., Guerra, J., Eaton, W. L., Perry, M. C., Carey, R. W., Frei, E. F., and Green, M. R. (1990). *N. Engl. J. Med. 323*: 940.

Emerson, S. S., and Fleming, T. R. (1989). *Biometrics 45*: 905.

Fairbanks, K., and Madsen, R. (1982). *Biometrika 69*: 69.

Fleming, T. R., Green, S. J., and Harrington, D. P. (1984). *Controlled Clin. Trials 5*: 55.

Gail, M. H., DeMets, D. L., and Slud, E. V. (1981). Simulation studies on increments of the two-sample logrank score test for survival time data, with application to group sequential boundaries. In *Survival Analysis,* IMS Lecture Notes, Monograph Series 2 (R. A. Johnson and J. Crowley, eds.). Institute of Mathematical Statistics, Hayward, Calif., pp. 287–301.

Gehan, E. A. (1965). *Biometrika 53*: 203.

Gill, R. D. (1980). *Censoring and Stochastic Integrals,* Mathematical Centre Tracts 124, Mathematisch Centrum, Amsterdam.

Green, S. J., Fleming, T. R., and O'Fallon, J. R. (1987). *J. Clin. Oncol. 5*: 1477.

Harrington, D. P., and Fleming, T. R. (1982). *Biometrika 69*: 133.

Kaplan, E. L., and Meier, P. (1958). *J. Am. Stat. Assoc. 53*: 457.

Kim, K. (1989). *Biometrics 45*: 613.

Kim, K. (1990). Design consideration for group sequential clinical trials with censored survival data adjusting for stratification (unpublished manuscript).

Kim, K., and DeMets, D. L. (1987a). *Biometrika 74*: 149.

Kim, K., and DeMets, D. L. (1987b). *Biometrics 43*: 857.

Kim, K., and Tsiatis, A. A. (1990). *Biometrics 46*: 81.

Lan, K. K. G., and DeMets, D. L. (1983). *Biometrika 70*: 659.

Lan, K. K. G., and DeMets, D. L. (1989a). *Stat. Med. 8*: 1191.

Lan, K. K. G., and DeMets, D. L. (1989b). *Biometrics 45*: 1017.

Mantel, N. (1966). *Cancer Chemother. Rep. 50*: 163.

McPherson, C. K., and Armitage, P. (1971). *J. R. Stat. Soc. A 134*: 15.

O'Brien, P. C., and Fleming, T. R. (1979). *Biometrics 35*: 549.

O'Fallon, J. R. (1985). *Cancer Treatment Rep. 69*: 1101.

Pampallona, S., and Tsiatis, A. A. (1990a). Group sequential trials with data-dependent interim analyses (unpublished manuscript).

Pampallona, S., and Tsiatis, A. A. (1990b). Group sequential designs for one-sided and two-sided hypothesis testing with provision for early stopping in favor of the null hypothesis (unpublished manuscript).

Pampallona, S., Tsiatis, A. A., and Kim, K. (1990). Type I and type II error probability spending functions for group sequential trials that allow for early stopping in favor of the null hypothesis (unpublished manuscript).

Peto, R. (1972). *Biometrika 59*: 472.

Peto, R., and Peto, J. (1972). *J. R. Stat. Soc. A 135*: 185.

Pocock, S. J. (1977). *Biometrika 64*: 191.

Prentice, R. L. (1978). *Biometrika 65*: 167.

Rosner, G. L., and Tsiatis, A. A. (1988). *Biometrika 75*: 723.

Rubinstein, L. V., Gail, M. H., and Santner, T. J. (1981). *J. Chronic Dis. 34*: 469.

Schoenfeld, D. A. (1981). *Biometrika 68*: 316.

Schoenfeld, D. A., and Richter, J. R. (1982) *Biometrics 38*: 163.

Sellke, T., and Siegmund, D. (1983). *Biometrika 70*: 315.

Slud, E. V. (1984). *Ann. Stat. 12*: 551.

Slud, E. V., and Wei, L. J. (1982). *J. Am. Stat. Assoc. 77*: 862.

Tsiatis, A. A. (1981). *Biometrika 68*: 311.

Tsiatis, A. A. (1982). *J. Am. Stat. Assoc. 77*: 885.

Tsiatis, A. A., Rosner, G. L., and Mehta, C. R. (1984). *Biometrics 40*: 797.

Wald, A. (1947). *Sequential Analysis.* Wiley, New York.

Whitehead, J. (1986). *Biometrics 42*: 461.

8

Group Sequential Trial of Two Combination Chemotherapy Regimens in Good-Risk Patients with Advanced Germ Cell Tumors

Nancy L. Geller

National Heart, Lung, and Blood Institute, National Institutes of Health, Bethesda, Maryland

George J. Bosl

Memorial Sloan-Kettering Cancer Center, New York, New York

I. BACKGROUND

Germ cell tumors are the most commonplace of the cancers afflicting young men between the ages of 15 and 35 (Motzer and Bosl, 1987). The first goal of treatment is achieving complete response, that is, complete disappearance of the tumor. For disseminated germ cell tumors, multiple-drug chemotherapy, including cisplatin, has been used to achieve a complete response in 70 to 80% of patients, yet approximately 10 to 15% of patients relapse, usually within the first 2 years (Bosl and Geller, 1989). While long-term follow-up of these patients is of interest, there is a strong relationship between cure of this disease and complete response, so that complete response is often taken as the major endpoint in clinical trials. The acute and chronic toxicities of cisplatin-based treatment for germ cell tumors are well recognized and include decreased white blood cell and platelet counts, decreased serum magnesium, decreased renal function, nausea and vomiting, mouth sores, and occasional hearing loss (Bosl et al., 1988). Treatment with less toxic drugs is desirable, but not at the risk of decreasing the number of cures. For this reason, good-risk patients, that is, those likely to achieve complete response, have been identified in prognostic factor studies (e.g., Bosl et al., 1983). In these patients, recent clinical trials have been designed with the goal of decreasing toxicity without compromising efficacy. An interesting discussion on clinical trial design in metastatic germ cell tumors can be found in Freedman et al. (1990).

Standard treatment for metastatic germ cell tumors today consists of two or three drug combinations, with cisplatin as one of the drugs (Bosl et al., 1988). Patients are treated with three or four cycles of chemotherapy, which takes approximately 3 months, and then their response is assessed. The current trial randomized patients to one of two two-drug regimens, where cisplatin was retained in the standard treatment arm and replaced by an analog in the experimental treatment arm. The trial was undertaken because the experimental combination was found successful in patients who had failed cisplatin-based therapy and also was less toxic. The experimental regimen could be given on an outpatient basis, whereas the conventional treatment required some hospitalization during each chemotherapy cycle. Nonetheless, the trial design had to consider the possibility that use of the experimental combination might compromise durable response.

II. PROTOCOL

The objective of this trial was to determine the differences in response, toxicity, time to relapse, and survival between two active chemotherapy regimens in a randomized trial for good-risk patients with germ cell tumors. The major endpoint was complete response to chemotherapy or to chemotherapy plus surgery (complete response). In good-risk patients, the current percent of complete response to the standard treatment arm was approximately 90%. The more easily tolerated experimental treatment arm would be comparable if its percentage of complete response were no lower than 77.5%. Thus the alternative hypothesis was that the complete response to the experimental treatment was lower than the complete response to the standard treatment. The trial was designed as a group sequential trial, so that early stopping, before the maximum number of patients was accrued, was permissible. The sample size was set to detect the stated difference in complete response with overall power of at least 0.85 when hypothesis testing was undertaken to maintain an overall significance level of 0.15. A significance level of 0.15 and power 0.85 were chosen, because concluding that the experimental treatment was comparable to the standard treatment if, in fact, the experimental combination was inferior, was considered important.

After eligibility was established, patients were randomized by the biostatistics office via telephone call. Randomization was by the method of random permuted blocks (Simon, 1979). As this was a multicenter trial, the randomization was stratified for patient institution.

This trial was designed according to the proposals of DeMets and Ware (1982) and Lan and DeMets (1983). As the data accumulated, at most five analyses were planned. Assuming that the five analyses would take place after successive groups of 24 patients per arm were evaluated, the sequence of nominal significance levels to be used were 0.0033, 0.0274, 0.0584, 0.0872, 0.1118. The first hypothesis test (based on 24 patients per arm) would be undertaken at the 0.0033 level, and if the difference in complete response proportions in the two arms was not extreme enough to stop the trial, a second group of 24 patients per arm would be accrued and a second analysis undertaken (based on 48 patients per arm) at the 0.0274 level; and so on. Accrual of the required number of patients was anticipated within 3 years. If the complete response proportion in the experimental treatment arm turned out to be 0.8 and the standard treatment arm had response proportion 0.9 as anticipated, the power of this design to detect this difference was 0.75.

For the interim analyses, a (one-sided) Fisher's exact test would be used to compare the complete response proportions. Balance between the two treatment arms in certain known prognostic factors that were explicitly listed in the protocol were to be checked at each interim analysis. These were the tumor markers beta component of human chorionic gonadatropism, alpha fetoprotein, and lactate dehydrogenase; the number of sites of metastasis; and predicted probability of complete response (Bosl et al., 1983). If any imbalance was found, a stratified Fisher's exact test would be used to compare the proportion of complete responses in each arm (Zelen, 1975). Toxicities were to be tabulated by treatment arm, including nadirs of white blood cells (WBC), platelets, hemoglobin, and serum magnesium and maximum creatinine. Beginning at the third interim analysis, time to relapse would also be monitored.

Although the trial was designed as if the interim analyses would occur after each group of 24 patients per arm was evaluated, the alternative possibility that analyses might be scheduled every 6 or 12 months was considered. It was written into the protocol that the interim analyses might be rescheduled at 6, 12, 18, and 30 months and at the end of the accrual period, and then the sequence of nominal significance levels stated above would be modified (since an unequal number of patients would be accrued between analyses) using the computer program of Lan and DeMets (1983).

The interim analyses were to be reported to a small data monitoring committee consisting of the principal investigator, the statistician, and two clinicians with interests in this disease. After an interim analysis was completed, the data monitoring committee was to decide if the trial should stop. Having an even number of committee members would assure that consensus was reached. Results of the trial were not to be reported at a professional meeting until a decision to stop the trial was made.

For the final analysis, time to relapse, survival time, and "event-free survival" (time to relapse or death, whichever came first) would be estimated using the method of Kaplan and Meier (1958), and comparisons of the two treatment arms would be made using the logrank test, stratified if appropriate (Mantel, 1966). It was recognized that the power of these comparisons would depend on the number of events at the time of the final analysis. Since few events were anticipated, these comparisons would mainly assure that one treatment arm was not much worse than the other.

III. MONITORING AND DATA COLLECTION

Data for this trial were entered into a clinical database at Memorial Sloan–Kettering Cancer Center by a research study assistant. After a patient was registered on the trial, laboratory data from the Memorial Hospital Laboratory Data Management computer would be transmitted electronically into the clinical database. Values for a variable that were outside the normal range of values would be flagged automatically. The research study assistant would check both the unusual values as well as normal values by reinspecting the laboratory report on the patient's medical record. Laboratory values as well as clinical observations that represented substantial toxicity were discussed by the research data manager and the principal investigators at their regular meetings.

Comprehensive clinical data were entered on the patients throughout the trial. When a patient completed treatment, the response to therapy was recorded. The results were reviewed frequently by the research study assistant and the principal investigator.

Because the clinical database contained more detailed information than desired for the interim analyses, data were extracted electronically and moved to the biostatistics computer for statistical analysis. The research study assistant downloaded the requested data to a floppy diskette in a rectangular format and this was easily uploaded to the biostatistics minicomputer.

Data from the outside centers were transmitted on data forms and entered into the clinical database at Memorial Hospital. It was not surprising that certain centers were more prompt in reporting data than others. When delay was noted, oral reminders by telephone as well as written reminders as follow-up were transmitted. Fortunately, this was not too great a problem in this trial.

IV. STATISTICAL ANALYSES

Interim analyses were undertaken essentially as originally planned, after groups of approximately 24 patients per arm were evaluated, and each interim analysis was similar. For example, in the third interim analysis, there were 70 patients in the standard treatment arm and 74 in the experimental treatment arm. Balance in the two arms with respect to the prognostic factors was tabulated, but no hypothesis tests were undertaken. The balance in the two arms was not in question, so Fisher's exact test was used to compare the proportion of complete responses. In the third interim analysis, there were 60/70 (85.7%) complete responses in the conventional treatment arm and 65/74 (87.8%) complete responses in the experimental treatment arm. The one-sided Fisher's exact test gave a p-value of 0.448. The conclusion was that the trial should continue.

Because the clinical investigators noticed that there seemed to be an increased incidence of hospital admissions for patients on the experimental treatment arm, at the third interim analysis, monitoring of toxicity (nadirs of WBC and platelets in four cycles of chemotherapy and number of hospital admissions for granulocytic fever) was begun. It was informally agreed that there would be no stopping rule for these variables. These results were also tabulated, but no formal statistical analysis was undertaken.

There was a notable amount of missing data for the nadirs. The median platelet nadir for the experimental treatment arm appeared to be lower than the platelet nadir for the conventional treatment arm.

V. CONCLUSION

Although this trial was still under way, it could be anticipated that at the end, the two treatments would not be found to differ in complete response proportion. However, it is possible that the increased bone marrow suppression in the experimental treatment arm, which leads to fevers requiring hospitalization, might be considered to offset the advantage of treating patients with this regimen outside the hospital.

VI. DISCUSSION

This trial exemplifies the implementation of the classical group sequential methodology as originally developed (Pocock, 1977). The major endpoint, complete response, was short term and was likely to occur within 2 or 3 months after chemotherapy was begun. In addition, there was minimal hypothesis testing undertaken during the trial. Perhaps if an imbalance in the prognostic factors or in the toxicity profiles appeared, a p-value would have been requested, but as of this writing, the only p-values reported were those for the primary endpoint during the monitoring. At the final analysis, the secondary endpoints would also require hypothesis testing. Nonetheless, the overall number of hypothesis tests, hence the likelihood of false positive results, was well limited.

An unusual feature of this cancer clinical trial was that the major hypothesis was one-sided and the design set $\alpha = 0.15$ and $\beta = 0.15$, in contrast to the more frequent $\alpha = 0.05$ and $\beta = 0.2$. This was because this was a test of equivalence: If the experimental treatment compromised complete response, it was important to detect that, and if the experimental treatment was better than the standard one, that was not considered as important.

In group sequential trials, small imbalances in the number of patients per arm are likely to occur due to the stratification on the institutions that were participating. Such imbalances affect the nominal significance level at which testing should occur, but the effect has been shown to be very slight (Lan, 1985). We undertook the first interim analysis on 24 patients per arm, the second on 46 patients on standard treatment and 50 on experimental treatment, and the third on 70 patients on standard treatment and 74 on experimental treatment. One might analyze an equal number of patients per arm in each stage, but then the possibility of ignoring data on "extra" patients arises. If the trial should stop, this overrun must be considered. In the worst case, including the extra patients could make a "significant" result not significant. We note also that the imbalance tends to grow as the number of strata increases and as the data accumulate. Delayed reporting by certain centers leads to decisions made based on the data received, with the delayed data omitted. In particular, the data may not be analyzed in the order in which patients were accrued to the study.

In cancer clinical trials, often investigators cannot be blinded to treatment assignment, and this can lead to added pressures to stop a trial if a difference in treatment effects is found at an interim analysis, even though this difference is less than that specified by the stopping rule. This did not happen in this trial, since differences were not nearly significant. In fact, the decisions to continue the trial were so clear that the data monitoring committee specified in the protocol never needed to meet.

Group sequential methods have been in rapid theoretical development for over a dozen years. This trial illustrates how they can be implemented, even as originally conceived.

REFERENCES

Bosl, G. J., and Geller, N. L. (1989). The management of nonseminomatous germ cell tumors at Memorial Sloan-Kettering Cancer Center. In *Systemic Therapy for Genitourinary Malignancies* (D. E. Johnson, C. J. Logothetis, and A. von Eschenbach, eds.), Yearbook Publishers, Chicago, pp. 331–337.

Bosl, G. J., Geller, N., Cirrincione, C., Vogelzang, N. J., Kennedy, B. J., Whitmore, W. F., Vugrin, D., Scher, H., Nisselbaum, J., and Golbey, R. B. (1983). Multivariate analysis of prognostic variables in patients with metastatic testicular cancer. *Cancer Res 43*: 3403–3407.

Bosl, G. J., Geller, N. L., Bajorin, D., Leitner, S. P., Yagoda, A., Golbey, R. B., Scher, H., Vogelzang, N. J., Auman, J., Carey, R., Fair, W., Herr, H., Morse, M., Sogani, P., and Whitmore, W., Jr. (1988). A randomized clinical trial of etoposide + cisplatin versus vinblastine + cyclophosphamide + actinomycin D + bleomycin + cisplatin in patients with good prognosis germ cell tumors. *J. Clin. Oncol. 6*: 1231-1238.

DeMets, D. L., and Ware, J. H. (1982). Asymmetric group sequential boundaries for monitoring clinical trials. *Biometrika 69*: 661-663.

Freedman, L., Javadpour, N., Sylvester, R., Aso, Y., Debruyne, F. M. J., Fossa, S. D., Geller, N., Horwich, A., Levine, L., Mostofi, F. K., Murphy, G. P., Simon, R., Stenning, S. P., and Stoter, G. (1990). Basic principles of clinical trials as applied to testicular cancer. In *EORTC Gerintourinary Group Monograph 7: Prostate Cancer and Testicular Cancer*, Wiley-Liss, New York, pp. 255-266.

Kaplan, E. L., and Meier, P. (1958). Nonparametric estimation from incomplete observations. *J. Am. Stat. Assoc. 53*: 457-481.

Lan, K. K. G. (1985). The theory of group sequential methods in clinical trials. *J. Chin. Stat. Assoc. 23*: 171-178.

Lan, K. K. G., and DeMets, D. L. (1983). Discrete sequential boundaries for clinical trials. *Biometrika 70*: 659-663.

Mantel, N. (1966). Evaluation of survival data and two new rank order statistics arising in its consideration. *Cancer Chemother. Rep. 50*: 163-170.

Motzer, R., and Bosl, G. J. (1987). Germ cell tumors of the testis. *Urol. Clin. N. Am. 14*: 389-398.

Pocock, S. J. (1977). Group sequential methods in the design and analysis of clinical trials. *Biometrika 64*: 191-199.

Simon, R. (1979). Restricted randomization designs in clinical trials. *Biometrics 35*: 503-512.

Zelen, M. (1971). The analysis of several two by two contingency tables. *Biometrika 58*: 129-137.

IV

APPLICATIONS IN ANTIVIRAL CLINICAL DRUG DEVELOPMENT

9

Early Termination of a Trial of Azidothymidine for the Treatment of Patients with AIDS and AIDS-Related Complex

Anthony C. Segreti

Burroughs Wellcome Company, Research Triangle Park, North Carolina

I. BACKGROUND

Researchers first defined the acquired immunodeficiency syndrome (AIDS) as a distinct disease entity in 1981. The disease is characterized by a profound immune deficiency, which results in susceptibility to various opportunistic infections and cancers and has subsequent high mortality. The agent responsible is a human retrovirus, human immunodeficiency virus or HIV, which was discovered in 1984.

At the time AIDS was first recognized, Wellcome scientists were studying the usefulness of zidovudine, also known as AZT or by the brand name Retrovir, in other therapeutic areas. This drug was first synthesized as a possible anticancer agent in 1964 by Jerome Horwitz of the Michigan Cancer Research Foundation but was found to be inactive. After being resynthesized by Wellcome chemists, AZT was considered for clinical development as an antibacterial agent. Due to a limited spectrum of activity, Wellcome opted not to develop it in this area.

Soon after the discovery of HIV, Wellcome began to pursue treatments for AIDS. In a preliminary screening process, AZT was identified as possibly having anti-HIV activity by Burroughs Wellcome scientists, who then sent it to the

National Cancer Institute for further testing, specifically against HIV. The anti-HIV activity of AZT in a human cell line was demonstrated by Samuel Broder's laboratory in early 1985.

The pre-IND process was expedited by Wellcome's earlier work performed while the drug was being evaluated as an antibacterial agent, and the IND was submitted in June 1985. The Food and Drug Administration (FDA) approved the IND in 7 days and Burroughs Wellcome Co. began a phase I trial on July 3, 1985. Improvements in disease symptomatology and immune response as well as weight gain were seen in the initial 35 patients studied. Based on these encouraging results, Burroughs Wellcome and the FDA agreed that a controlled trial to assess the efficacy and safety of AZT was warranted.

II. PROTOCOL

When this trial was being planned, there was a widely held belief that no drug would be effective as an antiretroviral agent because of the ability of the virus to mutate readily and to be incorporated into the host cell genome. These facts, as well as a dearth of knowledge of the natural history of the disease and the lack of clinical trial data, made planning this study a challenge.

The objectives of the phase II study were to assess the safety and efficacy of AZT over a 6-month period. Assessment of efficacy had three major components: (1) clinical improvement with primary endpoints of frequency and severity of opportunistic infections and secondary endpoints, including weight gain and Karnofsky score; (2) immune response; and (3) antiviral effect. Patients were required to have a diagnosis of AIDS with a first episode of *Pneumocystis carinii* pneumonia (PCP) within the previous 120 days or to be diagnosed as having advanced AIDS-related complex (ARC) with select symptomatology and a CD4+ lymphocyte cell count of 500 or less. Patients were stratified by study center and by CD4 count (≤ 100, >100) at randomization.

The lack of natural history information and the difficulty in defining a clinically important difference in the absence of previous clinical trials precluded conventional determination of sample size. Instead, the target sample size of 130 patients in each of the AZT and placebo groups was chosen because of the limited availability of drug at the beginning of this study. The possibility of randomizing twice as many placebo patients as AZT patients was considered as a way to increase power without requiring more drug. This option was rejected since it would not allow the Data and Safety Monitoring Board (DSMB) to remain blinded to treatment.

The DSMB was seen from the onset of protocol development as an integral part of this trial. Because of the ethical concerns in a placebo-controlled trial of a disease with high mortality and no therapeutic alternatives, an independent scientific review committee was essential. The role of the DSMB was to assess the accumulating safety and efficacy information and recommend modifications or termination of the trial as appropriate. The committee was formed under the auspices of the National Institute of Allergy and Infectious Diseases (NIAID) and included clinical researchers, a statistician, and an ethicist.

The data to be reviewed were determined jointly by the committee, Burroughs Wellcome, and the FDA. The schedule called for interim analyses at 2, 4, and 6 months after completion of enrollment. The protocol did not specify a statistical procedure for these interim analyses, but the DSMB chose the procedure suggested by O'Brien and Fleming (1979). With this method, the three interim analyses would be performed at p-values of 0.0001, 0.005, and 0.03, respectively.

III. MONITORING AND DATA COLLECTION

The study involved 12 study centers and five primary study monitors. The case report form was designed to be retrieved from the field in discrete parts to simplify the creation of a database for interim analyses. Each monitor visited his or her assigned study sites every 2 to 3 weeks to review and retrieve the data collected since their last visit. After the data were brought in-house, it was edited by the monitor and a data editor before immediate entry into a database. This editing resulted in queries for the investigator and possibly changes to the database. This single-entry database was used for reports to the DSMB. After the study was terminated, a verified database was created through double-entry and comparison to eliminate keystroke errors. This database was quality assured by comparing a random sample of case report forms to the database.

IV. STATISTICAL ANALYSES

The study began in February 1986 and enrollment was completed by June. The DSMB performed the first interim analysis of the data in early August. This involved tabulations of mortality, progression to AIDS (for ARC patients), recurrent *Pneumocystis*, and other opportunistic infections as well as the occurrence of severe or life-threatening toxicities. Results were presented by treatment group, but the identities of the groups remained blinded. Individual patient laboratory listings were also provided. At an initial (telephone) meeting, the DSMB concluded that the trial should continue as planned.

While preparing the database for the second interim analysis, an apparent difference in mortality between the treatment groups was seen. Consequently, a second meeting of the DSMB, scheduled for early October, was moved up to September 10, 1986. This committee reviewed updated versions of the tables seen earlier but also requested a survival analysis using Cox's regression model (1972) to assess the effect of AZT. After reviewing these results, the DSMB felt there was strong evidence of a treatment effect but wanted additional analyses before recommending the irrevocable step of terminating the trial. The board asked for an examination of the baseline comparability of the treatment groups as well as a current update of the survival status of all 281 patients in the trial. These results were supplied quickly and the DSMB recommended on September 19, 1986 that the study be stopped. At this time, there had been 19 deaths in the placebo group and only one in the AZT group.

Because of the extreme time pressure, the analyses sent to the DSMB were very selective and did not address the effect of covariates. The analyses described here were those provided to the FDA for regulatory approval and reported by Fischl et al. (1987). The great majority of time-to-event analyses were done using Cox's regression model. The effect of each factor was assessed using a chi-square statistic, based on the difference in log-likelihoods, after adjusting for all other effects in the model. The only exception occurred when a lack of any deaths in the AZT group in selected subsets of the data precluded the use of this model and an accelerated failure-time model was used instead (Kalbfleisch and Prentice, 1980). For variables such as CD4+ lymphocyte count, the van Elteren (1960) modification of the Wilcoxon rank-sum test was used. This test summarizes across all strata a series of Wilcoxon tests done within individual strata. This procedure was used to compare the changes in CD4+ count over time for the AZT and placebo groups across the four strata (AIDS, ARC; high, low CD4+).

Since little was known about the natural history of AIDS at the start of this study, the analysis explored various subgroups, especially AIDS and ARC patients. This gave information on the effect of prognostic factors as well as the effect of AZT in these subgroups.

The analysis of overall mortality as well as the AIDS and ARC subgroups is presented in Table 1. In each case, the effect of AZT was highly significant. Log CD4+ count is the only covariate that had any effect in this analysis. Surprisingly, AIDS patients did not have higher mortality in this trial than these late-stage ARC patients.

Table 2 provides the analyses of opportunistic infections. The results closely paralleled the earlier mortality analyses. AZT emerges as a highly significant factor for all patients and for AIDS patients. A strong trend is apparent for ARC patients. Relative risks are similar for AIDS and ARC patients. Log CD4+ count was an important factor in the development of opportunistic infections, as it was in mortality.

Finally, change in CD4+ lymphocytes over time is seen in Table 3. AZT patients showed fairly consistent increases over the course of the study, while placebo patients had consistent decreases. The effect of AIDS versus ARC was

Table 1 Analysis of Overall Mortality

Factor	Log-likelihood chi-square	Beta (S.E.)	Relative risk	95% Confidence interval	p-value
		All patients			
AIDS/ARC	0.20	−0.22 (0.49)	0.80	0.31, 2.12	0.655
Log CD4+	3.54	−0.91 (0.46)	0.40	0.16, 1.00	0.060
Treatment	22.17	−3.08 (1.03)	0.05	0.01, 0.34	<0.001
		AIDS patients			
Log CD4+	1.07	−0.68 (0.64)	0.51	0.14, 1.78	0.301
Time from PCP	0.02	−0.001 (0.01)	1.00	0.98, 1.02	0.888
Treatment	13.15	−2.69 (1.04)	0.07	0.01, 0.52	<0.001
		ARC patients			
Log CD4+	2.98	−1.19 (0.67)	0.30	0.08, 1.13	0.084
Treatment	5.84[a]	NA	NA	NA	<0.016

[a] Since no ARC patients treated with AZT died in this trial, Cox's regression model could not be used in this case. Instead, an accelerated failure-time model was used to test for a treatment effect after stratifying for CD4+ lymphocytes at entry.

Table 2 Analysis of Opportunistic Infections

Factor	Log-likelihood chi-square	Beta (S.E.)	Relative risk	95% Confidence interval	p-value
		All patients			
AIDS/ARC	2.33	−0.43 (0.29)	0.65	0.37, 1.15	0.127
Log CD4+	19.21	−1.19 (0.26)	0.30	0.18, 0.51	<0.001
Treatment	12.33	−0.87 (0.26)	0.42	0.25, 0.69	<0.001
		AIDS patients			
Log CD4+	9.96	−1.08 (0.34)	0.34	0.18, 0.66	0.002
Time from PCP	0.52	0.004 (0.01)	1.00	0.99, 1.01	0.471
Treatment	8.35	−0.83 (0.29)	0.42	0.24, 0.78	0.004
		ARC patients			
Log CD4+	8.91	−1.33 (0.43)	0.26	0.11, 0.61	0.084
Treatment	3.37	−0.93 (0.53)	0.40	0.14, 1.12	0.066

Table 3 Changes in CD4+ Lymphocytes Count During the Trial

Diagnosis	Wk.	AZT N	AZT Median	AZT Mean	AZT S.E.	Placebo N	Placebo Median	Placebo Mean	Placebo S.E.	van Elteren p-value
AIDS	4	69	60	83	11	68	−9	−2	6	<0.001
	8	72	40	57	10	60	−9	−17	9	<0.001
	12	67	14	37	11	56	−14	−26	8	<0.001
	16	44	3	10	10	36	−17	−28	12	0.008
ARC	4	54	56	52	15	51	−13	−8	12	<0.001
	8	54	14	22	15	47	−23	−25	16	0.003
	12	46	53	38	19	47	−31	−27	23	<0.001
	16	38	24	41	17	38	−31	−22	15	<0.001
Overall	4	123	60	70	9	119	−11	−5	6	<0.001
	8	126	32	42	8	107	−13	−20	9	<0.001
	12	113	21	37	10	103	−17	−26	11	<0.001
	16	82	10	24	10	74	−18	−25	10	<0.001

Reprinted with permission from the *N. Engl. J. Med. 317*: 189, 1987.

minimal in these analyses. This examination of the data was complicated by the changing patient population over time since patients were entered sequentially and followed until death or study termination.

V. CONCLUSION

Based on the interim analysis, the DSMB recommended termination of the trial. The company agreed and the study ended on Sept. 19, 1986. Both placebo and AZT patients in the trial were given the opportunity to receive open-label AZT at that time. After discussions with FDA, a treatment IND was initiated on October 11, 1986 to allow other AIDS patients with previous PCP infections to begin AZT therapy before approval for marketing. Because of a limited drug supply, entry into the treatment IND was restricted to AIDS patients, who were shown most clearly to benefit.

Burroughs Wellcome began immediate preparation for the new drug application (NDA). An analysis plan for the clinical data was generated and circulated to the FDA Medical and Biometrics reviewers for comment. The NDA was submitted in early December 1986. After expeditious review and a favorable vote by an FDA advisory committee, licensing was granted in March 1987, only 107 days after NDA submission. AZT was initially indicated for use in AIDS patients with a prior PCP episode and advanced ARC patients with CD4+ lymphocytes under 200.

The decision of the FDA to restrict the indication for AZT in ARC patients to those with CD4+ lymphocyte count of less than 200 is an interesting one. The study, as conceived and carried out, stratified patients at randomization on the basis of CD4+ lymphocytes. This was done to ensure an unbiased treatment effect since CD4+ was thought, correctly, to strongly predict subsequent morbidity and mortality. There was no expectation that AZT therapy would have a differential effect based on the patient's CD4+ count. After study completion, an a posteriori data analysis by FDA staff suggested that placebo patients with ARC and CD4 counts over 200 had low mortality; only a modest effect on survival was observed when these patients were compared to similar AZT patients, who had no mortality. The power to detect a treatment effect was limited here because of the low mortality and the small number of patients. Restricting access to AZT, under the label, to those ARC patients with CD4+ count under 200 provided a clearly delineated benefit to this population. At approval, the risks of AZT were unknown to a greater extent than usual, and this restriction was intended to ensure a positive benefit/risk ratio for those patients falling within the labeled indication and to exclude those patients where benefit was less conclusively established. However, patients could have received drug outside this indication if the prescribing physician perceived a likely benefit.

In contrast to a typical NDA including data from 2000 to 3000 patients, this NDA included data from only 281 patients treated in a controlled trial (144 on AZT) for a mean of 4.5 months, of whom about 80% received open-label drug for a mean of 5 additional months as well as data from the 35 phase I patients. As a result of the limited pre-NDA experience, the sponsor agreed to follow these open-label patients after NDA approval and to report their progress periodically to the FDA. Burroughs Wellcome also committed to doing additional studies in patients with less severe disease, including asymptomatic HIV-infected patients, as well as studies to optimize the dosing regimen.

VI. DISCUSSION

The use of interim analyses was crucial to the effective conduct of this study. Without the interim analyses built into the protocol, it would have been difficult or perhaps impossible to conduct this trial. Inevitably, a placebo-controlled trial in a life-threatening disease will engender ethical concerns. Here, the lack of therapeutic alternatives under investigation meant that patients had little recourse to this placebo-controlled trial: this fact heightened concerns. Review of the accumulating data by an independent DSMB gave the assurance that the trial would be terminated as soon as conclusive evidence of drug efficacy was seen. Early termination of this study allowed HIV-infected patients, both within and outside the trial, to benefit from this drug earlier than they otherwise would have, while still providing the substantial evidence of safety and efficacy required for regulatory approval. A large number of other trials of AZT have confirmed these results in other HIV-infected populations. Although the recommended dosing has been modified since this early trial, the essential benefits and risks of AZT were identified here accurately and in a timely manner.

In this trial, the data and safety monitoring board strengthened the study immeasurably by providing interim data review independent of the sponsor and the regulatory agency. The fundamental responsibility of such a committee is to protect the patients of the study while maintaining scientific integrity. At the same time, if a DSMB recommends an action opposed by sponsor or FDA, the drug approval process may be delayed. For example, if a study is terminated early but a regulatory agency does not find compelling evidence of efficacy, the sponsor will not be able to market the product. The decision to terminate a study may preclude the initiation of another similar study because of ethical concerns. To avoid this impasse, the DSMB, sponsor, and FDA must communicate effectively throughout the study. The DSMB must be independent of the other groups in the drug development process, but remain aware of their concerns. This tension ensures that the role of the review committee is both vital and difficult.

Although the interim analyses and early termination of the trial expedited the availability of AZT therapy, there was a significant and unavoidable penalty that resulted from this process. Long-term efficacy and safety of AZT could not be assessed definitively because of the lack of a concurrent control group. This was of concern to the scientific and regulatory communities since innovative therapies for HIV disease would, of necessity, be compared against AZT. The effect of AZT beyond 6 months was analyzed primarily through the open-label experience of the patients in the phase II study after the initial controlled portion was completed.

The follow-up of these patients continued for almost 4 years; long-term benefits and risks of this cohort were determined by comparison to historical controls. Although this follow-up was necessary and informative, establishing the long-term efficacy and safety of AZT was complicated by the absence of a randomized control group as well as the fact that patients originally assigned to placebo had less AZT therapy than the original AZT group. Having pointed out this difficulty, it should not be overemphasized. The ethical advantages of interim analyses clearly outweighed the scientific disadvantages, given this early study of therapy for a life-threatening disease.

REFERENCES

Cox, D. R. (1972). *J. R. Stat. Soc. B 34*: 187.

Fischl, M. A., Richman, D. D., Grieco, M. H., Gottlieb, M. S., Volberding, P. A., Laskin, O. L., Leedom, J. M., Groopman, J. E., Mildvan, D., Schooley, R. T., Jackson, G. G., Durack, D. T., King, D., and the AZT Collaborative Working Group (1987). *N. Engl. J. Med. 317*(4): 185.

Kalbfleisch, J. D., and Prentice, R. L. (1980). *The Statistical Analysis of Failure Time Data*, Wiley, New York, pp. 143–162.

O'Brien, P. C., and Fleming, T. R. (1979). *Biometrics 35*: 549.

van Elteren, P. H. (1960). *Bull. Inst. Int. Stat. 37*: 351.

10

Interim Analysis of a Parallel Comparison Study of Dideoxycytidine Versus Azidothymidine in Patients with AIDS or Advanced AIDS-Related Complex

Amy H. Lin and Samuel V. Givens

Hoffmann–La Roche, Inc., Nutley, New Jersey

I. BACKGROUND

A. AIDS

The acquired immunodeficiency syndrome (AIDS) is a syndrome characterized by profound alterations of immune function. Patients with this syndrome have a significant suppression of the number of T helper-inducer cells (CD4), resulting in an increased incidence of opportunistic infections and unusual malignancies, including Kaposi's sarcoma. The patients also develop systemic symptoms, including weight loss, fever, and sweating. Other patients present with systemic symptoms without having had opportunistic infections or Kaposi's sarcoma and are classified as having AIDS-related complex (ARC). Still others present earlier in the disease syndrome with lymphadenopathy (LAS). Finally, there are others who are asymptomatic but are seropositive for the human immunodeficiency virus (HIV), a human retrovirus that is believed to be the etiologic agent responsible for these illnesses.

B. Dideoxycytidine

In vitro it has been shown that HIV replication can be inhibited by nucleoside analogs. One of the first analogs was azidothymidine (AZT, now referred to as zidovudine or ZDV), which has been shown to be effective in the treatment of AIDS or advanced ARC. Other necleoside analogs have also been studied as antiretroviral agents. One of the most potent of these analogs in vitro is dideoxycytidine (ddC). In the clinical studies by the National Cancer Institute (NCI), the National Institute of Allergy and Infectious Diseases (NIAID), and Roche, ddC exhibited antiviral activity in reducing serum p24 antigen levels. The 0.01 mg/kg q8h dose regimen caused reduction of p24 antigen equivalent to that reported for ZDV. CD4 lymphocyte increases were also observed. Because of the demonstrated antiviral activity, low incidence of mild, reversible peripheral neuropathy and absence of hematologic toxicity with low-dose ddC therapy, a long-term phase II/III study comparing ddC versus ZDV in patients with AIDS or advanced ARC was warranted.

II. PROTOCOL

At the time this chapter was written, the trial was under way but had reached only the halfway point in patient observation. Statistical methods were in place and blinded data were being collected but no analysis has been conducted. We therefore change tenses to show what has and will be done.

This was a randomized, double-blind, comparative study of ddC versus ZDV in outpatients with AIDS or advanced ARC. Patients were stratified by pretreatment CD4 lymphocyte counts (CD4 $\leqslant$ 100 or $>$ 100). A separate randomization list was prepared for each stratum. To ensure the blinding of this study, on entry patients were randomized to receive either active ddC and placebo ZDV or active ZDV and placebo ddC.

The objective of this trial is to demonstrate that ddC monotherapy is at least as efficacious as ZDV monotherapy in the treatment of AIDS or advanced ARC and exhibits a different safety profile. The primary endpoint is patient survival. The secondary endpoints are occurrence and frequency of AIDS-defining opportunistic infections and neoplasms, serum levels of HIV p24 antigen, CD4 cell count, body weight, and neuropsychological test results.

A. Hypotheses and Sample Size Determination in Terms of Survival Rates

The clinicians felt that ddC could be considered to be at least as efficacious as ZDV if the 1-year survival rate of ddC is no worse than that of ZDV by more than 15%. Therefore, the statistical hypotheses of interest to test are:

H_o: true ZDV 1-year survival rate − true ddC 1-year survival rate $\geqslant 0.15$

versus

H_a: true ZDV 1-year survival rate − true ddC 1-year survival rate < 0.15

The sample size was computed based on a method described in Makuch and Simon (1978). To assure with probability $(1 - \beta)$ that the upper 100 $(1 - \alpha)\%$ confidence limit of the difference $(\pi_1 - \pi_2)$ will not exceed δ, the number of patients required for each treatment is

$$N = [\pi_1(1 - \pi_1) + \pi_2(1 - \pi_2)] \left[\frac{Z_{\alpha/2} + Z_\beta}{\delta - (\pi_1 - \pi_2)} \right]^2$$

$$= [0.85(1 - 0.85) + 0.8(1 - 0.8)] \left(\frac{1.96 + 1.28}{0.15 - 0.05} \right)^2$$

$$= 302$$

where $Z_{\alpha/2}$ and Z_β are the upper $\alpha/2$ and β tail points of the standard normal distribution, respectively. π_1 and π_2 are the true 1-year survival rates, and δ is the allowable difference to still claim equivalence. Therefore, approximately 300 patients per treatment group will be required assuming that the true 1-year survival rate for ZDV patients is 85% and for ddC patients is 80%.

The conventional approach for detecting treatment differences uses the following hypotheses:

$$H_o*: \quad \text{true difference} \leqslant 0.05$$

$$H_a*: \quad \text{true difference} > 0.05$$

Failure to reject H_o does not imply equivalence. For a given sample size, testing H_o* versus H_a* is equivalent to testing H_o versus H_a with the type I and II errors reversed. That is, a power of 95% (where power is calculated at a true difference of 0.05) can be achieved in establishing equivalence with a significance level of 20%, assuming that the sample size is adequate to test H_o* versus H_a*, at a significance level of 0.05 with a power of 80% (where power is calculated at a true difference of 0.15).

The sample size required by directly reversing the type I and II errors, that is, using a significance level of 0.1 to reach a power of 0.95 in testing the conventional hypotheses (which will result in testing the hypotheses for establishing equivalence at a significance level of 0.05, with a power of 90%) is

$$N = \frac{[Z_{\alpha/2}(\pi_{1o}(1-\pi_{1o})+\pi_{2o}(1-\pi_{2o}))^{1/2}+Z_\beta(\pi_{1a}(1-\pi_{1a})+\pi_{2a}(1-\pi_{2a}))^{1/2}]^2}{[(\pi_{1a}-\pi_{2a})-(p_{1o}-\pi_{2o})]^2}$$

$$= \frac{[1.645(0.85(1-0.85)+0.8(1-0.8))^{1/2}+1.645(0.85(1-0.85)+0.7(1-0.7))^{1/2}]^2}{[(0.85-0.8)-(0.85-0.7)]^2}$$

$$= 338$$

which is slightly larger than that was calculated based on Makuch and Simon's approach.

B. Interim Analyses and Group Sequential Design

Duration of the study is 2 years from entry for all patients. Three interim analyses and a final analysis were planned. Due to staggered entry and slow accrual, the first interim analysis was scheduled to be conducted when 75% of the patients have completed 6 months, and the second 6 months later, and the third 6 months after the second. The final analysis will be conducted at the end of the study. Since the original O'Brien–Fleming design for serial looks at the data requires an extremely low level of significance at the initial look ($\alpha = 0.0001$), a two-sided group sequential design by Fleming et al. (1984) was adopted. Under this design, the nominal α levels are 0.007, 0.008, 0.010, and 0.040 and the standardized normal deviates are 2.713, 2.641, 2.567, and 2.051 for the first, second, third, and the fourth look at the data, respectively. Notice that the power of the test statistic is essentially maintained at the last look.

The protocol stated that the hypotheses H_o and H_a will be tested using the Kaplan–Meier estimates of the 1-year survival rates and the 100 $(1 - \alpha)\%$ confidence intervals from these estimates. Since the property of the Kaplan–Meier estimates is unknown under the foregoing group sequential design, and a sequentially computed logrank test has been shown to be appropriate for sequential analysis of clinical trials with survival response, the logrank test was chosen to detect treatment differences.

C. Hypotheses in Terms of Relative Risk

Under the proportional hazards model,

$$\begin{aligned}\text{relative risk of ddC to ZDV} &= \text{hazard ratio of ddC to ZDV}\\ &= \exp(-\theta)\\ S_{\text{ddC}}(t) &= [S_{\text{ZDV}}(t)]^{\exp(-\theta)}\end{aligned}$$

and

$$\exp(\theta) = \frac{\log[S_{\text{ZDV}}(t)]}{\log[S_{\text{ddC}}(t)]}$$

where $S(t)$ denotes the survival function. ddC can be considered to be as efficacious as ZDV in patient survival if

$$S_{\text{ZDV}}(1) - S_{\text{ddC}}(1) < 0.15$$

that is,

$$S_{ZDV}(1) - [S_{ZDV}(1)]^{\exp(-\theta)} < 0.15$$

Since the left-hand side of the inequality above is increasing with increasing $\exp(-\theta)$, this implies that

$$\exp(-\theta) < 2.195$$

or

$$\exp(\theta) > 0.45$$

assuming that the true ZDV 1-year survival rate is 85%. Since the relative risk is assumed to be constant across time, the upper bound to be placed on the difference in survival rates at any time t cannot exceed

$$S_{ZDV}(t) - [S_{ZDV}(t)]^{2.195}$$

This function has a bell shape which reaches a maximum value of 0.28 when the survival rate is 52%. It has a value of 0.15 and 0.09 for survival rates of 0.85 and 0.92, respectively. This means that a bound of 9% would have to be placed on the upper confidence limit of the difference of the 36-week survival rates if a bound of 15% were placed at that of the 1-year survival rates, assuming that the ZDV 36-week and 1-year survival rates are 92% and 85%, respectively.

Therefore, the following hypotheses H_o' and H_a', which are equivalent to H_o and H_a under the Cox proportional hazards regression model, will be tested instead.

$$H_o': \text{ hazard ratio of ZDV to ddC} \leqslant 0.45$$

$$H_a': \text{ hazard ratio of ZDV to ddC} > 0.45$$

assuming that the true 1-year survival rate for ZDV patients is 85%. ddC could be considered to be no worse than ZDV if the lower confidence limit of the hazard ratio of ZDV to ddC is above 45%.

D. Sample Size Determination in Terms of Relative Risk

When computed at time t, the logrank test statistic $T(t)$ has an asymptotic normal distribution (Kim and Tsiatis, 1990)

$$T(t) - N(\theta V(t), V(t))$$

The asymptotic variance $V(t)$ is closely related to the expected number d of failures observed by time t by the relation

$$V(t) - d/4$$

provided that the treatment allocation is at random and equal for both treatments, and the treatment difference measured by θ is not too large.

An approximate $100(1-\alpha)\%$ confidence interval for $(d\theta/4)$ is

$$(T(t) - Z_{\alpha/2}(d/4)^{1/2},\ T(t) + Z_{\alpha/2}(d/4)^{1/2})$$

Following similar steps used in Makuch and Simon (1978), the confidence statements can be written

$$\Pr[d\theta/4 < T(t) - Z_{\alpha/2}(d/4)^{1/2}] = \alpha/2$$

$$\Pr[T(t) - Z_{\alpha/2}(d/4)^{1/2} < \delta] = \beta \tag{1}$$

It follows that

$$\Pr\left[\frac{T(t) - d\theta/4}{(d/4)^{1/2}} < \frac{\delta - d\theta/4}{(d/4)^{1/2}} + Z_{\alpha/2}\right] = \beta$$

This implies that

$$\frac{\delta - d\theta/4}{(d/4)^{1/2}} + Z_{\alpha/2} = -Z_\beta$$

$$(Z_{\alpha/2} + Z_\beta)(d/4)^{1/2} + \delta = d\theta/4 \tag{2}$$

To place a lower bound of 0.45 on the hazard ratio of ZDV to ddC [i.e., $\exp(\theta)$] is to place a lower bound of $(d/4)\log(0.45)$ on $d\theta/4$. Substituting $(d/4)\log(0.45)$ for δ in (2) and solving for d yields

$$d = 4\left[\frac{Z_{\alpha/2} + Z_\beta}{\theta - \log(0.45)}\right]^2$$

If the true 1-year survival rate is 85% for ZDV and 80% for ddC, the true hazard ratio of ZDV to ddC is

$$\exp(\theta) = \frac{\log(0.85)}{\log(0.80)} = 0.73$$

or

$$\theta = \log(0.73)$$

Therefore, the total number of deaths required is

$$d = 4\left[\frac{1.96 + 1.28}{\log(0.73) - \log(0.45)}\right]^2$$

$$= 180$$

We need to observe 180 deaths to assure with probability 90% that the lower 95% confidence limit of the hazard ratio of ZDV to ddC will not fall below 0.45.

Assume that failure at time t occurs with hazard rate $\lambda(t)$. Then $\lambda(t) = \lambda$ when survival distribution is exponential. The expected number of failures by time t becomes (Kim and Tsiatis, 1990)

$$E_{\lambda(t)} = C\left[S_a - \frac{e^{-\lambda(t)}}{\lambda}(e^{\lambda S_a} - 1)\right] \qquad \text{if } t > S_a$$

where patient accrual has been assumed to be uniform during the accrual period $(0, S_a)$ with a constant accrual rate C. If S_f is the length of the follow-up period, the expected number of deaths by $S_a + S_f$ is

$$E(S_a + S_f) = \tfrac{1}{2}[E\lambda_{\text{ZDV}}(S_a + S_f) + E\lambda_{\text{ddC}}(S_a + S_f)]$$

Assuming that $S(t) = e^{-\lambda t}$, then $\lambda = -[\log S(t)]/t$. Since $S^{(1)}_{\text{ZDV}} = e^{-\lambda_{\text{ZDV}}(1)} = 0.85$ and $S_{\text{ddC}}(1) = e^{-\lambda_{\text{ddC}}(1)} = 0.8$, we have $\lambda_{\text{ZDV}} = -\log(0.85) = 0.1625$ and $\lambda_{\text{ddC}} = -\log(0.8) = 0.2231$.

$$E(S_a + S_f) = \tfrac{1}{2}C\left\{\left[S_a - \frac{e^{-0.1625(S_a + S_f)}}{0.1625}(e^{0.1625(S_a)} - 1)\right] + \left[S_a - \frac{e^{-0.2231(S_a + S_f)}}{0.2231}(e^{0.2231(S_a)} - 1)\right]\right\}$$

The average patient accrual is about 50 patients per month (i.e., 600 per year). Let $C = 600$ and $S_f = 0.5$ in the formula above, we can solve for S_a so that $E(S_a + S_f) = 180$. It turns out that $S_a = 1.5$. That is, we need a total of 900 patients (18-month accrual) to assure with 90% confidence that the lower 95% confidence limit of the hazard ratio does not fall below 0.45 6 months after the patient accrual has completed.

E. Decision Rules

The evaluation of the first interim analysis of the data will be based on the intent-to-treat analyses of patient survival, opportunistic infectious and neoplasms, and CD4 cell count, in that order of importance, plus the intent-to-treat analyses of key safety parameters. The intent-to-treat population consists of all patients who are randomized and who have at least one follow-up observation.

Although these analyses are interim analysis from the perspective of occurring before the end of the trial, they will *not* lead to an early stop of the trial. They may lead to a submission based on the interim analysis, but unless the drug is unsafe, the trial will continue to completion, which is 2 years from entry for all patients. That is, the intent of the interim analysis is to assure an FDA submission at the earliest possible time, thus providing an effective treatment for public use quickly; in the meantime the trial will continue to collect long-term safety information. These are intense political pressures to approve AIDS drugs as soon as possible.

1. Efficacy Parameters

The primary assessment of efficacy will be patient survival. ddC will be considered to be at least as efficacious as ZDV if it can be shown to be so in terms of patient survival alone. If the results from patient survival do not have the power to demonstrate that ddC is as efficacious as ZDV, the results from AIDS-defining opportunistic infections (OIs) and neoplasms, and CD4 cell counts, will be used together to demonstrate efficacy of ddC. In this case, ddC will be considered to be at least as efficacious as ZDV if (1) it can be considered so in terms of time to first OI, and (2) it cannot be shown that ZDV is significantly better than ddC in terms of both the average area under curve (AUC) of the CD4 cell counts per unit of time in study and the CD4 cell count at week 24. (The blinded observation that there were few fatalities early in the study gives a very small chance that early interim analyses will have the power to detect equivalence in survival rates.)

A committee of ddC investigators who are participating in the ddC–ZDV pivotal trial will meet to review each opportunistic infection, neoplasm, or condition reported in the study and determine if these events meet the CDC definitions of AIDS-defining events (as further detailed by guidelines established by the NIAID Opportunistic Infection Committee. These decisions will be made without breaking the treatment code.

The criteria for claiming ddC to be at least as efficacious as ZDV (i.e., ddC is either superior or equivalent to ZDV) in terms of survival or OIs are given in greater detail below. To achieve this, the upper confidence limit (CL) of the difference of event-free rates (ZDV minus ddC) has to be no more than a prespecified bound. The CLs will be constructed using the standardized normal deviate of 2.713, which is appropriate for the first interim analysis according to the group sequential plan specified in the protocol. The types of analyses and the definitions of superiority and equivalence are as follows:

a. Patient Survival. Patient survival across time (survival curves) will be compared in terms of relative risk of death using the Cox proportional hazards regression model. Under the Cox model, the relative risk of death is assumed to be constant across time. According to the protocol, ddC will be considered to be at least as efficacious as ZDV in terms of patient survival if the upper confidence limit of the difference (ZDV minus ddC) of the 1-year survival rate does not exceed 15%. This 15% bound needs to be reduced when survival rates at a time point less than a year are compared. However, a time-independent lower bound can be placed on the relative risk of death of ZDV to ddC if an upper bound of 15% were placed at the difference of the 1-year survival rates (see Section II.C).

b. Opportunistic Infections. Time to the first OI or neoplasm will be determined for each patient. OI-free rates across time will be compared in terms of relative risk of OIs using the Cox proportional hazards regression model. ddC can be considered to be at least as efficacious as ZDV in terms of OI if the upper confidence limit of the difference (ZDV minus ddC) of the 1-year OI-free rates does not exceed 20%. This is equivalent to a time-independent lower bound of 44% to be placed on the relative risk of OIs of ZDV to ddC (see Section II.C).

c. CD4 Cell Counts. Although CD4 cell counts correlate well with the subsequent clinical course of a patient, CD4 cell counts of patients on ZDV were known to improve, peaking around 8 to 12 weeks, and then to decrease often back to baseline by 24 weeks. Factors such as absolute changes from baseline, lengths of time above or below baseline, and last CD4 counts all provide evidence in evaluating CD4 data. ddC and ZDV will be compared using both the area under the curve of CD4 cell counts and the week 24 CD4 cell count.

A CD4 curve across time is formed by connecting data points, beginning from baseline value and terminating at the last observed data point. Under this curve, any area falling above the baseline CD4 count is considered a positive area, and any area falling below is considered a negative area. For each patient, the net area (sum of positive areas minus sum of negative areas) averaged per unit of time in study is determined. For each patient, the week 24 CD4 cell count is the average of all CD4 counts falling within a window of ±6 weeks (i.e., from weeks 18 through 30).

Both the average area under the curve and the change from baseline in CD4 cell count at week 24 will be analyzed using analysis of covariance (ANCOVA), with baseline CD4 count as a covariate, and effects of center, treatment, and center by treatment interaction. The effect on CD4 cell count will be examined between and within treatments. Since it is difficult to place an upper bound on the difference (ZDV minus ddC) of the AUC of the CD4 cell counts or the difference of the changes from baseline CD4 count at week 24, equivalence will be determined using a very liberal significance level. A two-tailed significance level of 0.20 will be used to test if ZDV is significantly different from ddC (see Section II.A). (Within-treatment effects will also be examined to see if the average AUC is different from zero, and to see if the week 24 CD4 cell count is significantly different from the baseline CD4 cell count. As this is part of the interim analysis, the nominal significance level, 0.007, will be used.)

2. Safety Parameters

Since ddC and ZDV have very different safety profiles, no formal statistical analyses will be performed to compare treatments. Key safety parameters, including hematologic toxicities, peripheral neuropasy, and liver function elevations, will be summarized for AIDS and advanced ARC patients separately, and additionally for those patients with low CD4 cell counts (CD4 $\leqslant$ 100) and high CD4 cell counts (CD4 $>$ 100) separately.

F. Data Safety Monitoring Board and Blinding

A meeting was held with the U.S. Food and Drug Administration (FDA) to discuss the DSMB and the blinding issues. Since this trial will not terminate at interim analyses, the FDA agreed that no data safety monitoring board (DSMB) was required for this trial. Also, since ddC and ZDV have nonoverlapping toxicities, and once the safety parameters are seen, the blind is essentially broken. The FDA therefore agreed that the code could be broken for the interim analyses but that control of dissemination of results should be exercised.

The method that has been used until the interim analysis was to enter only the double-blind bottle code (the randomization code with the study month appended to it) onto the database. A separate file with the mapping of the bottle code to the treatment was stored in a secured file. If there were no interim analysis, then at the end of the study after all corrections and decisions are made about the individual patients, that file will be unlocked and merged into the database. For interim analyses, that file is merged with the data outside the database by the statistician, so that anyone querying the database remains blinded. The results of the interim analyses are kept under tight control internally, and as much as possible, are restricted to results pooled over treatment groups rather than as individual patients. We furthermore attempt to limit who see the summary and also try to limit the information they see by restricting their ability to see each patient's treatment assignment. After interim analysis, the treatment codes will again be locked.

G. Censoring and Follow-up

Legakos et al. (1990) gave a good discussion of the two approaches commonly used for censoring a patient: (1) censoring at the time of treatment termination, and (2) censoring at the last time that a patient is known to be alive (the intent-to-treat analysis). As an example, suppose that a patient stopped taking test medication and left the study at 8 months after treatment began. We later found out that he died at 10 months. Approach 1 will censor him at 8 months, while approach 2 will say that he died at 10 months. If, instead, that patient was followed up until 10 months, and lost to follow-up afterward, approach 1 still censors him at 8 months, but approach 2 will censor him at 10 months. Approach 1 produces inference about the hazard of failing while a patient in the trial is still continuing on treatment; this hazard is in general different from the hazard that would have been experienced had that patient not terminated treatment. These two hazards would be equal only if those patients who terminate treatment do not differ from those who continue on treatment (in most situations, this does not hold). The rationale behind the intent-to-treat approach (approach 2) is that patients in the trial who terminate their treatments do so for the same reasons that would apply were the treatment to become part of routine medical practice. Thus the hazard estimated from the trial would be expected to reflect the benefit from use of the treatment in practice.

In this trial, we plan to take approach 2 in censoring patients. According to the protocol, patients who dropped out early were supposed to return to the study site every month to have a physical exam and lab tests. But most of the time, patients did not return, and follow-up was very difficult.

III. MONITORING AND DATA COLLECTION

A total of 26 centers participated in this trial; the enrollment of each center was limited to 60 patients to avoid overrepresentation of any center. Eligibility is determined by a screening process that takes place within 2 weeks prior to entry. Patients are seen weekly for the first 10 weeks, and biweekly thereafter for the duration of the study. At each visit, a case report form module was completed for a patient. This created a tremendous amount of case report from modules to be collected at the time of the first interim analysis (approximately 14,000 modules). To reduce the amount of information to be collected, visits were rescheduled to be at monthly intervals after the first 6 months, and running logs were used for several key sections of the case report form (e.g., test medication, OIs). Source document of the case report forms was done for about 20% of the patients.

IV. STATISTICAL ANALYSES

Summaries will be performed on all efficacy and safety parameters if an NDA submission is decided. This will include analyses of nonprimary parameters, analyses on patients following the protocol (standard analyses as opposed to more inclusive intent-to-treat analyses), and other subgroup analyses. An additional analysis of the CD4 cell counts, using duration of response, will also be examined. The duration of response for a patient is defined as the first time to four consecutive CD4 recordings that are below the baseline CD4 count. A patient who never had four consecutive CD4 recordings below baseline before dropping out (or by the clinical cutoff date) will have his or her duration of response censored at the time of dropout (or at the clinical cutoff date). In addition to the intent-to-treat analysis that will be performed on all efficacy and safety parameters, standard analyses will be performed on all efficacy parameters. The standard analysis population will include only patients who were not excluded after a strict set of exclusion criteria were applied.

Although confidence intervals are sufficient for establishing superiority and equivalence between the two treatment groups, most AIDS literature reports *p*-values from treatment comparisons. Therefore, comparison between treatment groups will be made in the full analysis in addition to the confidence intervals. Logrank tests stratified by centers will be used to compare the time-to-event distributions. Cox proportional hazards model will be used to estimate relative risks and to relate pretreatment predictors to the time to event. Analysis of covariance with effects of centers, treatment, and center-by-treatment interaction will be used for change from baseline variables. Mantel–Haenszel tests stratified by centers will be used for 2×2 tables. All analyses will be repeated among AIDS patients and advanced ARC patients, and among low- and high-CD4-cell-count patients.

V. CONCLUSION

The first interim analysis was expected to be performed at the beginning of 1991.

VI. DISCUSSION

The determination of sample size was not based on the group sequential design used by the trial. Instead, it was based on fixed-sample-size calculation for establishing equivalence. The group sequential design we chose is appropriate for testing treatment equality, as the null hypothesis is rejected if the confidence interval does not cover zero. It is also appropriate for establishing one treatment to be no worse than the other treatment; that claim is established if the lower confidence limit of the hazard ratio is greater than, say, 0.45, in our trial (in other words, the confidence interval should not contain 0.45). The group sequential design also requires equal increments of information to be collected at each look (i.e., equal number of deaths occurred between successive analyses). [This does not appear to be a serious violation according to the simulations done by DeMets and Gail (1985).] Since the information time (number of deaths by the first interim analysis out of the total expected to die by 2 years) is less than 0.1 (= 29/300), a design with a prespecified α spending function would seem to be more appropriate. The gamma family of α spending functions (Hwang, 1989)

$$\alpha(r,t) = \begin{cases} \alpha \dfrac{1 - e^{-rt}}{1 - e^{-r}} & r \neq 0 \\ \alpha t & r = 0 \end{cases}$$

with $r = -2.8$, produces boundary points 2.940, 2.674, 2.376, and 2.054, with equal number of deaths between interim looks of the data, which are similar in spirit to those of the design used by our protocol (the boundary points are 2.713, 2.641, 2.567, and 2.051 for our protocol). With the very small amount of information collected at the first interim look, say, at the information time of 0.1, the boundary point is 3.2778, larger than that obtained when 25% of the total deaths are observed at the first interim look.

Since it is clear from the relatively low death and OI rates observed prior to the first interim analysis that we will not have enough power to test H_o' versus H_a', a method to combine information from patient survival and OIs, and some of the surrogate markers, such as CD4 and P24, would be of interest. Pocock et al. (1987) derived a global test statistic in which quantitative, binary, and survival endpoints could all be combined. Lin (1990) developed a method using a weighted sum of the logrank statistics in a group sequential setting. Lin's method could be used to compute the combined logrank statistic from patient survival and time to an OI. Yet another way of combining multiple points by classifying each patient as a responder or a nonresponder, depending on whether a patient experienced any OIs, gained weight, had improved CD4 cell counts, or felt better, can also be considered. The clinicians, however, objected to this procedure, as it implies weighing all parameters equally. Although different scores (or weights) can be assigned to various parameters to come up with a summary score for each patient, it was considered to be too arbitrary, and therefore the idea was dropped.

Since both CD4 cell counts and P24 antigen levels are quite variable, a logarithmic transformation of the data to reduce variability seems desirable (one would be added to each count to avoid the problem of taking logs of zero). Either analysis of covariance on these log-transformed data or analysis of variance of the logs of relative changes (defined as log[(posttherapy CD4 + 1)/(baseline CD4 + 1)]) could be performed.

The protocol was amended two times. Two months into the trial, protocol was amended to allow entry of patients with 3 months prior ZDV therapy. Six months into the trial, when a low-dose regimen of ZDV was approved by the

FDA, the protocol was amended to switch all existing patients who were on high-dose ZDV to low-dose ZDV, and to give low-dose ZDV to all new patients (existing patients must have completed at least 28 days of high-dose ZDV, new patients must have 28 days of high-dose ZDV, before switching to the lower dose). Subgroup analyses in patients with, and without prior ZDV therapy, and in patients entered before and after the switching dose policy became effective, were planned to examine the impact of prior ZDV therapy and the switching dose policy. However, none of these amendments were considered in the original sample size calculation. Consequently, any attempt to examine the effect of prior ZDV therapy, or the poolability of high- and low-dose ZDV groups (which is also confounded by time), might fail as a result of inadequate sample size in any of the subgroups compared.

REFERENCES

DeMets, D. L., and Gail, M. H. (1985). Use of logrank tests and group sequential methods at fixed calendar times. *Biometrics 41:* 1039–1044.

Fleming, T. R., Green, S. J., and Harrington, D. P. (1984). Considerations for monitoring and evaluating treatment effects in clinical trials. *Controlled Clin. Trials 5:* 55–66.

Hwang, I. K. (1989). Interim analysis: the flexible approach using a family of alpha spending functions, *11th Annual Spring Symposium*, ASA Northern New Jersey Chapter, Morristown, N.J., May 1.

Kim, K., and Tsiatis, A. A. (1990). Study duration for clinical trials with survival response and early stopping rule. *Biometrics 46:* 81–92.

Lagakos, S. W., Lim, L. L., and Robins, J. M. (1990). Adjusting for early treatment termination in comparative clinical trials. *Stat. Med. 9*: 1417–1424.

Lin, D. Y. (1990). Nonparametric sequential testing in clinical trials with incomplete multivariate observations. To appear in *Biometrika*.

Makuch, R., and Simon, R. (1978). Sample size requirements for evaluating a conservative therapy. *Cancer Treatment Rep. 62*(7): 1037–1040.

Pocock, S. J., Geller, N. L., and Tsiatis, A. A. (1987). The analysis of multiple endpoints in clinical trials. *Biometrics 43:* 487–498.

11

An Application of the Sequential Probability Ratio Test to an Unblinded Clinical Trial of Ganciclovir Versus No Treatment in the Prevention of CMV Pneumonia Following Bone Marrow Transplantation

Charles Du Mond

Syntex Research, Palo Alto, California

I. BACKGROUND

Cytomegalovirus (CMV) interstitial pneumonia is a leading cause of death in patients undergoing allogeneic (matched sibling) bone marrow transplantation for the treatment of hematologic malignancies. Mortality associated with CMV pneumonia can be as high as 90%. Ganciclovir is an antiviral drug active against CMV. Ganciclovir inhibits the viral replication of CMV in infected cells. At the time of this study, ganciclovir had been approved in the United States for the treatment of CMV retinitis (a CMV infection of the retina that occurs in approximately 25% of AIDS patients), but had not yet been approved for the treatment of CMV pneumonia.

In an open-label, compassionate-use trial of ganciclovir in immunocompromised patients with severe CMV disease, there was evidence of antiviral activity and some suggestions of clinical efficacy in treating CMV disease, including CMV pneumonia. It was therefore reasonable to construct a protocol to study the use of ganciclovir as prophylaxis or early treatment of CMV infections in patients at risk of developing CMV pneumonia.

II. PROTOCOL

The objective of this study was to determine the effectiveness of prophylactic ganciclovir by comparing the incidence of CMV pneumonia in patients receiving ganciclovir versus patients receiving no treatment. A goal associated with this objective was that the study design had to permit termination of the study as soon as possible, to minimize the number of patients randomized to no treatment.

This was a two-center, randomized, open-label study. Eligible patients had received an allogeneic bone marrow transplant for hematologic malignancy and had no clinical or radiographic evidence of CMV pneumonia at study entry. A bronchoscopy with bronchoalveolar lavage (BAL) was performed on day 35 posttransplant. Those patients whose BAL showed evidence of CMV by cytology, immunochemical staining, or virus culture were randomized (1:1) to either the ganciclovir group or the control group (no treatment or observation-only patients). The randomization was stratified by age group (25 years or younger versus older than 25 years) and presence or absence of graft-versus-host disease (GVHD) at study entry.

Following randomization, treated patients received intravenous ganciclovir at a dose of 5 mg/kg every 12 h for 14 days, followed by a maintenance dose of 5 mg/kg once daily, 5 days a week, through day 120 posttransplant. This was a randomized, unblinded study. When the study was designed, the investigators believed that a placebo-controlled study was not appropriate, since it might require prolonged hospitalization for placebo administration. Also, the use of an indwelling catheter for the placebo infusions could increase the risk of infection while offering no potential benefit to the patient.

The primary measurement of efficacy was the proportion of patients who achieved a normal protocol completion ("treatment success"), that is, patients who survived to day 120 without developing CMV pneumonia. Treatment failure was defined as the development of CMV pneumonia before day 120 or premature termination due to death. The proportions of patients in the ganciclovir-treated and control groups were compared after each patient had completed the study or reached a decision point (normal protocol completion, development of CMV pneumonia, or death) using a sequential probability ratio test (SPRT) as described in Whitehead (1983). Patients were included in the sequential analysis in the same order in which they were randomized into the study. Patients who terminated from the study prior to day 120 for reasons other than CMV disease or death were evaluated at day 120 and classified as treatment successes or failures depending on the presence or absence of CMV disease through day 120.

III. MONITORING AND DATA COLLECTION

Patients were evaluated daily during hospitalization. Following discharge, they were evaluated twice weekly through day 100 and weekly thereafter through day 120. Study visits were scheduled for days 35 (study entry), 42, 49, 56, 63, 70, 77, 91, 105, and 120 posttransplant. Patients were observed for signs and symptoms of CMV pneumonia. Any patient who developed interstitial pneumonia was terminated from the study and treated as clinically indicated. When possible, if more than a week had elapsed from the previous BAL, a repeat BAL was performed to determine the etiology of the interstitial pneumonia.

Case report forms (CRFs) on each patient were completed from the patient's medical chart by the study center after the patient developed CMV pneumonia, survived 120 days posttransplant, or died. A subset of the CRF questions were identified as necessary for the sequential analysis. These questions received a 100% review by medical personnel. After an individual patient was completed and verified, his or her data was released to statistical analysis.

The algorithm for determining treatment success or failure keyed off two forms: Form T, the termination reason form, and Form PS, the poststudy follow-up form. The algorithm proceeded as follows:

1. If the patient had a normal completion on Form T, the patient was classified as a treatment success.
2. If the patient had death or CMV interstitial pneumonia as a termination reason on Form T, the patient was classified as a treatment failure.
3. If the patient had any other reason (noncompliance, study administration problem, adverse event, etc.) as a termination reason on Form T, Form PS would determine the patient's success or failure.
   a. If Form PS indicated that the patient was alive at day 120 and that the patient had *not* developed CMV interstitial pneumonia, the patient was classified as a treatment success.
   b. If Form PS indicated that the patient had died or developed CMV interstitial pneumonia prior to day 120, the patient was classified as a treatment failure.

As each patient was entered into the analysis, a sequential analysis report was generated which provided the following information: number of completed patients in each group, number of successes in each group, current values of the test statistics, current values of the stopping rule boundaries, and the study management decision (continue or stop study). An example of a sequential analysis report is provided in Table 1. A complete description of the statistical methodology is provided in the next section.

Table 1 Example of Sequential Analysis Report ($n = 24$)

Number of completed patients	
Ganciclovir (m)	10
Control (n)	14
Number of successes[a]	
Ganciclovir (S)	7 (70.0%)
Control (T)	3 (21.4%)
Test statistics	
$Z = \dfrac{nS - mT}{m + n}$	2.83
$V = \dfrac{mn(S + T)[(m - S) + (n - T)]}{(m + n)^3}$	1.42
Critical values for Z	
$U = 2.580 + 0.675V$	3.54
$L = -2.580 + 0.675V$	−1.62
Study management decision[b]	
Continue study	

[a] A patient is considered a treatment success if he or she completes the study (120 days posttransplant) without developing CMV pneumonia.

[b] If $Z > U$, stop the study and conclude that ganciclovir is statistically significantly better than the control (no treatment). If $Z < L$, stop the study and conclude that there is no evidence of a statistical difference between ganciclovir and no treatment. If $L \leqslant Z \leqslant U$, continue the study and recompute the statistics after the next patient completes the study.

IV. STATISTICAL ANALYSES

All statistical analyses were performed using SAS Version 6, Release 6.06 (SAS Institute, 1989). In the sequential, patient-by-patient analysis, the following statistics were computed (see Whitehead, 1983):

$$Z = \frac{(nS) - (mT)}{m + n}$$

$$V = \frac{(mn)(S + T)[(m - S) + (n - T)]}{(m + n)^3}$$

where m is the number of patients in the ganciclovir group, n the number of patients in the control group, S the number of ganciclovir patients who are a treatment success, and T the number of control patients who are a treatment success. The boundaries of the SPRT (or stopping rules) were defined in the following way:

$$U \text{ (upper boundary)} = a + bV$$
$$L \text{ (lower boundary)} = -a + bV$$

where

$$a = \frac{1}{\Theta_R} \log\frac{(1-\alpha)}{\alpha} - 0.583\sqrt{I}$$

$$b = 0.5\Theta_R$$

$$\Theta_R = \log\frac{p_N(1-p_s)}{p_s(1-p_N)}$$

$$I = \frac{1}{4}p_M(1-p_M)$$

$$\alpha = 0.025$$

where p_N and p_s are the assumed probabilities of success under the alternative hypothesis, and p_M is the assumed probability of success under the null hypothesis.

As was specified in the study protocol, the prestudy estimate for the rate of CMV pneumonia in untreated patients was 30%. The alternative hypothesis was that ganciclovir would reduce this rate to 10%. Hence, p_s, the assumed proportion of successes on standard therapy (no treatment—the control group), was 0.7. Similarly, p_N, the assumed proportion of successes on the new therapy (ganciclovir), under the alternative hypothesis, was 0.9. Under the null hypothesis of no treatment effect, the proportion of successes, p_M, is 0.7. To maintain a two-sided test with an overall significance level of 0.05, α was chosen to be 0.025. These assumptions led to the following values determining the boundaries for the SPRT:

$$\Theta_R = 1.350$$
$$I = 0.0525$$
$$a = 2.580$$
$$b = 0.675$$

Hence the stopping rules were as follows:

1. If $Z > 2.580 + 0.675V$, stop the study and conclude that ganciclovir is

statistically significantly better than no treatment, with a two-sided $\alpha = 0.05$.

2. If $Z < -2.580 + 0.675V$, stop the study and conclude that there is no evidence of a statistically significant difference between ganciclovir and no treatment.
3. If Z falls between these two boundaries, continue the study. Recompute the statistics after the next randomized patient reaches an endpoint.

Enrollment in the study was stopped after 31 patients (14 in the ganciclovir group, 17 in the control group) had reached study endpoints and the SPRT revealed a significant difference in the incidence of CMV pneumonia. One control group patient, who had terminated from the study prematurely because of suspected CMV pneumonia, was excluded from the analysis because his illness was later diagnosed as pulmonary aspergillosis. Hence only 30 patients were included in the final SPRT analysis.

Table 2 provides a complete listing of the sequential analysis computations. Figure 1 provides a graphic display of the SPRT as the statistic approaches statistical significance and eventually crosses the boundary, leading to the end of the study. At the time the SPRT analysis was completed and further enrollment was discontinued, nine additional patients had already been enrolled. Four of these patients had completed the study but had not been eligible for inclusion in the SPRT calculation, since patients were entered into the SPRT according to their time of enrollment. Five patients had not yet completed the study. Because these five patients had all been randomized to the ganciclovir group, they were allowed to continue treatment according to the protocol.

V. CONCLUSION

The efficacy analysis of 30 patients (14 in the ganciclovir group, 16 in the control group) demonstrated that ganciclovir was significantly better ($p < 0.05$) than no treatment in preventing the development of CMV pneumonia. In this analysis, 3 of 14 ganciclovir-treated patients (21%) were treatment failures as opposed to 12 of 16 control patients (75%).

VI. DISCUSSION

Since this was an unblinded study, this raises the question of bias in the reporting of CMV pneumonia. Although the protocol stated that all patients would have chest x-rays twice a week, control group patients actually had radiographs taken more frequently. This difference in x-ray frequency may have

Table 2 Listing of Sequential Analysis Computations

Observation	m	n	S	T	Z	V	L	U	Study management decision
1	0	1	0	0	0.00	0.00	−2.58	2.58	Continue study
2	1	1	1	0	0.50	0.12	−2.50	2.66	Continue study
3	1	2	1	0	0.67	0.15	−2.48	2.68	Continue study
4	2	2	1	0	0.50	0.19	−2.45	2.71	Continue study
5	2	3	1	0	0.60	0.19	−2.45	2.71	Continue study
6	2	4	1	0	0.67	0.19	−2.46	2.71	Continue study
7	2	5	1	1	0.43	0.30	−2.38	2.78	Continue study
8	3	5	2	1	0.88	0.44	−2.28	2.88	Continue study
9	4	5	3	2	1.22	0.55	−2.21	2.95	Continue study
10	4	6	3	2	1.40	0.58	−2.19	2.97	Continue study
11	4	7	3	2	1.55	0.59	−2.18	2.98	Continue study
12	4	8	3	2	1.67	0.59	−2.18	2.98	Continue study
13	5	8	4	2	2.08	0.73	−2.09	3.07	Continue study
14	6	8	4	2	1.86	0.79	−2.05	3.11	Continue study
15	6	9	4	2	2.00	0.80	−2.04	3.12	Continue study
16	6	10	4	2	1.75	0.87	−1.99	3.17	Continue study
17	6	11	4	3	1.53	0.93	−1.95	3.21	Continue study
18	6	12	4	3	1.67	0.95	−1.94	3.22	Continue study
19	6	13	4	3	1.79	0.95	−1.94	3.22	Continue study
20	7	13	5	3	2.20	1.10	−1.84	3.32	Continue study
21	8	13	5	3	1.95	1.17	−1.79	3.37	Continue study
22	8	14	5	3	2.09	1.19	−1.78	3.38	Continue study
23	9	14	6	3	2.48	1.30	−1.70	3.46	Continue study
24	10	14	7	3	2.83	1.42	−1.62	3.54	Continue study
25	11	14	8	3	3.16	1.51	−1.56	3.60	Continue study
26	12	14	9	3	3.46	1.60	−1.50	3.66	Continue study
27	12	15	9	4	3.22	1.66	−1.46	3.70	Continue study
28	12	16	9	4	3.43	1.70	−1.43	3.73	Continue study
29	13	16	10	4	3.72	1.79	−1.37	3.79	Continue study
30	14	16	11	4	4.00	1.87	−1.32	3.84	Stop study

Note: m = number of patients receiving ganciclovir; n = number of patients in the control group; S = number of treatment successes in the ganciclovir group; T = number of treatment successes in the control group; Z = test statistic; V = variance/information measure; $L = 2.58 + 0.675V$, the lower boundary for stopping the study; $U = -2.58 + 0.675V$, the upper boundary for stopping the study.

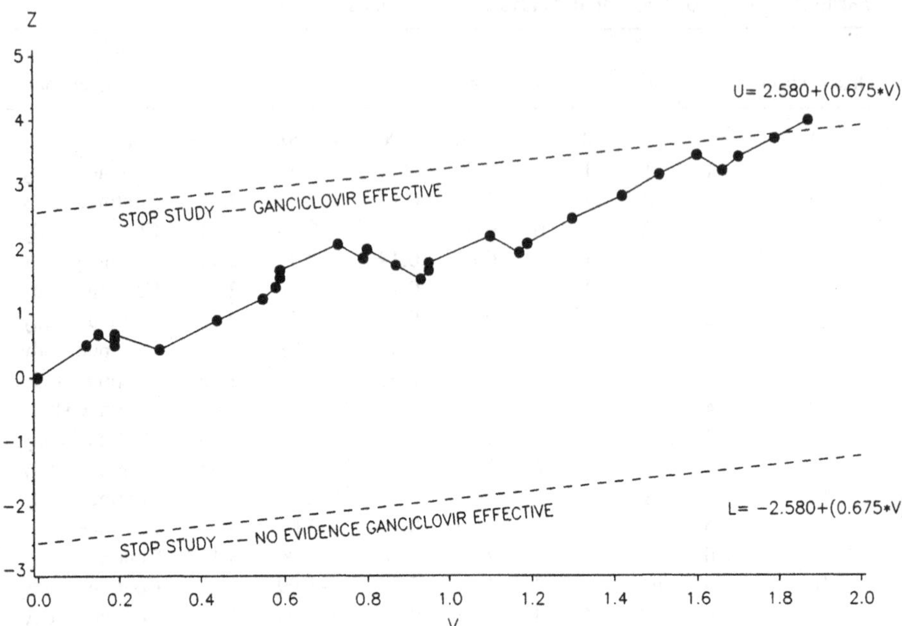

Figure 1 Graphic display of the behavior of the patient-by-patient SPRT, as the statistic approaches statistical significance and eventually crosses the boundary, leading to the end of the study. *Z*, test statistic; *V*, variance/information measure.

been prompted by pulmonary symptoms in the control group or by the investigator's apprehension about disease occurring in patients who were not receiving antiviral therapy. If the primary comparison had been time to development of CMV pneumonia, this difference in x-ray frequency could have biased the results. However, efficacy was based only on the occurrence of interstitial infiltrates, not time to occurrence; therefore, these variations in timing of the x-rays did not affect the results.

It is very important that the patients be included in SPRT calculation in the same order in which they were randomized into the study. This preserves the sequential probability theory associated with the SPRT. Although the SPRT was an effective technique for analyzing and terminating this study, it would not be appropriate for all clinical situations. Several factors contributed to the choice of the SPRT: life-threatening disease, unblinded treatment assignment, and slow patient accrual.

CMV pneumonia has a high mortality rate in bone marrow transplant patients. No FDA-approved therapies exist for the treatment of CMV pneumonia. In this setting, a patient-by-patient SPRT allows the investigator to stop randomizing patients to a nonefficacious treatment (such as observation-only) as soon as a statistically significant difference is identified. If the disease was not life threatening or other efficacious treatments existed, a fixed sample size may be more appropriate.

This study was unblinded. The investigators knew which patients were receiving ganciclovir and which patients were observation only. The SPRT statistic could be computed after each patient reached an endpoint without compromising the study blind. The patient-by-patient SPRT could be used in a blinded study, but the distribution of sequential analysis reports (as in Table 1) would have to be controlled to maintain the overall study blind.

This study had very slow patient accrual. The study started in October 1987, and the 30th patient did not complete the study until February 1990, an accrual rate of approximately one patient per month. At this rate it was reasonable to complete, verify, and analyze each patient's data. If the patients are entering and completing the study faster than the SPRT can be calculated, one of the ethical advantages of the SPRT is lost: the study cannot be stopped soon enough to prevent patients from being randomized to a nonefficacious therapy. In situations where enrollment is too fast for a patient-by-patient SPRT, a group sequential approach [as described in Fleming et al. (1984)] might be more appropriate.

REFERENCES

Fleming, T. R., Harrington, D. P., and O'Brien, P. C. (1984). *Controlled Clin. Trials 5:* 348.

SAS Institute (1989). *SAS/STAT User's Guide, Version 6, 4th ed., Vol. 1 and 2,* SAS Institute, Cary, N.C.

Whitehead, J. (1983). *The Design and Analysis of Sequential Clinical Trials,* Ellis Horwood, Chichester, West Sussex, England.

V

APPLICATIONS IN CARDIOVASCULAR CLINICAL DRUG DEVELOPMENT

12

Bayesian Methods in the Monitoring of Survival in Congestive Heart Failure

Nathan H. Enas, Federico Dies, and Celedon R. Gonzales

Eli Lilly and Company, Indianapolis, Indiana

Donald A. Berry*

University of Minnesota, Minneapolis, Minnesota

I. BACKGROUND

A. Description of Congestive Heart Failure

Congestive heart failure (CHF), a syndrome characterized by dyspnea, fatigue, and edema, is associated with many different forms of heart disease. Although ventricular diastolic dysfunction may be an important contributor to the pathophysiology of CHF, in most patients the clinical manifestations of CHF are usually asociated with decreased myocardial contractility. Functionally, CHF is characterized by decreased cardiac output ("forward failure") and increased left and right ventricular filling pressures with pulmonary congestion and edema ("backward failure"). At first these abnormalities are manifest only during exercise (i.e., failure to increase cardiac output appropriately and excessive increments in left and right ventricular pressures upon exertion), but eventually they become apparent at rest as well. Typically, in patients with CHF the ability to exercise is limited by dyspnea and fatigue. The occurrence

* Current affiliation: Duke University, Durham, North Carolina

of these symptoms at various intensities of exercise is the basis for the frequently used New York Heart Association (NYHA) Functional Classification of CHF (from no limitation of physical activity in class I, to inability to carry on any physical activity without discomfort in class IV).

Maintenance of cardiovascular homeostasis in patients with CHF is mediated by a series of compensatory mechanisms, such as increased neurosympathetic activity, including elevated plasma catecholamines; and increased secretion of renin and angiotensin, aldosterone, vasopressin, and atrial natriuretic factor. These mechanisms cause tachycardia, vasoconstriction, and fluid retention that help maintain cardiac output and arterial pressure. However, marked and/or protracted increments in these compensatory mechanisms may be deleterious to the structure and function of the heart and blood vessels, eventually leading to the establishment of complex vicious cycles. As a result, CHF is a progressive malignant disorder that decreases patient survival. The nature of the disease provides a rationale for using clinical symptoms, measurements of hemodynamic performance and cardiac contractility, estimates of the ability to exercise, and quantification of neurohormonal activity, as well as both duration and quality of life to monitor the magnitude and progression of the disease process and the impact of therapeutic interventions.

B. Congestive Heart Failure as a Health Problem and a Disease

Congestive heart failure is a leading cause of disability and death in most countries. Available statistics in the United States indicate that in the early 1980s the prevalence of CHF was 2.3 million cases and the incidence was 0.4 million cases per year (Smith, 1985). In those years CHF was listed as a diagnosis in 1.5 million hospital discharges and was listed as the principal diagnosis in 0.44 million hospital discharges (Gillum, 1987). Also, CHF was listed as a diagnosis in 4 million outpatient office patient visits and was the first listed or principal diagnosis in 1.8 million visits (Gillum, 1987).

In addition to being a frequent health problem, CHF is a malignant disease. In 1982 heart failure was mentioned nearly 0.2 million times on death certificates, either as the underlying cause (in 30,000 cases) or as a contributing factor (Gillum, 1987). The survival probabilities within 4 years of first diagnosis of CHF were 48% for men and 66% for women, regardless of the underlying cause (Smith, 1985). The survival probabilities of patients with NYHA classes I to III heart failure were 75% at 1 year and 48% at 5 years, and those for patients with NYHA class IV heart failure were 34% at 1 year and 18% at 3 years (Smith, 1985). Clearly, the life prognosis for CHF is similar to or worse than that in most forms of cancer.

Over the period 1970–1983 there was little if any change in the rate of death attributed to CHF (Gillum, 1987), despite substantial reduction in overall mortality from cardiovascular disease (Sytkowski et al., 1990). One possible explanation for this apparent discrepancy is that decreased mortality from acute myocardial infarction and improved survival among patients with angina pectoris and hypertensive heart disease may have led to an increased prevalence of chronic heart disease and CHF in the population, especially in elderly people (65 years of age and over). Whatever the explanation, it is clear that current therapeutic options are not totally effective.

C. Evaluation of New Treatments

The inadequacy of current therapy for a frequent and malignant disease provides the impetus to develop and investigate new forms of treatment for CHF to improve the patient's symptomatology, ability to exercise, quality of life, and survival. However, the choice of appropriate clinical endpoints for evaluating new treatments for CHF has been controversial, partly because of the unexpected lack of correlation between different clinical and functional variables in patients with CHF. Typically, the effect of medications on hemodynamic variables in acute experiments fails to predict their effect on exercise capacity and clinical symptoms. The seemingly more clinically relevant submaximal exercise tests (e.g., the 6- and 12-minute walking distance tests) are more subject to error than is the more objective maximal oxygen uptake test. However, athletic performance may differ in fundamental ways from ordinary daily activities, and thus its estimation by maximal oxygen uptake may not be clinically relevant. Assessment of survival is not technically difficult, but it is not always practical because it usually requires large patient samples and long periods of observation.

There is now general agreement that the best assessment of efficacy of new treatments for CHF is obtained in placebo-controlled, randomized clinical trials in which the new treatment or placebo is added, for ethical reasons, to optimal current standard therapy and in which the effects on multiple endpoints over a period of many weeks to several months is determined (Braunwald and Colucci, 1984; Guyatt, 1985; Packer, 1987). The recommended endpoints include survival, clinical symptoms, exercise capacity, quality of life, cardiac performance (e.g., left ventricular ejection fraction), cardiac size, and concentration of various hormones in plasma (norepinephrine, renin, aldosterone, vasopressin, atrial natriuretic factor) in patients who are well characterized clinically at baseline.

D. Evaluation of Mortality

Early uncontrolled clinical trials with newer positive inotrope vasodilators [see Packer and Leier (1987) for a review] suggested that mortality in patient populations treated with the newer agents was greater than expected. The case was made that constant pharmacologic stimulation of cardiac contractility might, in fact, accelerate the natural downward course of patients with CHF (Katz, 1978; LeJemtel and Sonnenblick, 1984; Packer et al., 1984). Accordingly, clinical trials of a new treatment for CHF should test the hypothesis that the new treatment does not increase mortality (with acceptable α and β error rates), even if the converse hypothesis that the treatment does not prolong survival is not formally tested. The effect of an experimental treatment on mortality is best evaluated by comparing it concurrently with placebo. Other treatments for CHF that improve the patient's well-being, ability to exercise, and even survival (Cohn et al., 1986; Consensus Trial Study Group, 1987) should not be withheld, for obvious ethical reasons. Accordingly, in designing clinical trials to assess mortality, patients should be stabilized on standard therapy and then randomly allocated to receive the experimental agent or placebo in addition to standard therapy.

II. PROTOCOL

A. Objectives and Statistical Hypothesis

The trial was a phase II, multicenter, randomized, placebo-controlled clinical trial of CHF patients who were treated with a new positive inotrope vasodilator called indolidan. The trial was designed to address the following six objectives:

1. Define the relationship between intravenous dose of indolidan and cardiovascular response.
2. Define the relationship between once-a-day oral dosing of indolidan and cardiovascular response.
3. Evaluate the safety of a 2-week, fixed-dose, titration schedule.
4. Determine the pharmacokinetics of indolidan.
5. Compare the efficacy of indolidan to a placebo for the treatment of patients who suffer from CHF.
6. Compare the mortality rates of CHF patients on indolidan and placebo.

To meet these six objectives, we designed a clinical trial consisting of five sequential segments. The initial segment was a screening and baseline examination. In the second segment, approximately 100 patients who met the entry criteria were to be accepted into the clinical trial and hospitalized for hemodynamic evaluation of the intravenous and oral indolidan formulations. Patients who responded and tolerated the medication would be randomized to a combination of standard treatment and either indolidan or placebo. This randomization of the patients began the third segment of the trial. Patients would receive the oral form of the medication once daily for 5 days while remaining in the hospital. In the fourth trial segment, patients who tolerated the oral medication during these 5 days would continue treatment as outpatients for approximately 3 months. During this outpatient treatment, a fixed-titration schedule would be used to adjust the dose of indolidan in order to improve the patients CHF symptoms. The final segment included study drug withdrawal and patient follow-up in which the status of each patient would be assessed approximately 1 month after completion of the trial. Indolidan patients would be given the choice of continuing treatment or not, and placebo patients would be allowed to cross over to indolidan or discontinue the trial.

The following discussion addresses our attempt to accomplish the sixth objective, which was important because of the mortality controversy surrounding use of positive inotrope vasodilators. Historically, the mortality rate for CHF patients under standard treatment has been approximately 10% for a 3-month period. In addition, it was viewed as clinically imperative to detect a 50% increase in mortality rate in a new treatment, such as indolidan. Assessment of the mortality difference between the two groups could have been accomplished by a fixed-sample-size design, given levels of power, α, and expected treatment difference.

However, continual monitoring of data presents a major incompatibility with the classical paradigm. Monitoring of any severe adverse drug reaction is a necessary process. Although monitoring is commonplace, we wanted to use an objective method to aid in the process of deciding if the trial should continue. To accomplish this goal, we chose the Bayesian method developed by Berry (1989), which allows continual monitoring of data without the caveats usually associated with multiple "looks" at the data.

B. Sample Size and Decision Rule

We designed the trial to assure detecting a difference between the two groups with respect to cardiac output and exercise duration. In addition, we designed the trial to test the hypothesis the mortality in the indolidan group would be 20 percentage points greater than in the placebo group, assuming a placebo mortality rate of 10%. The specification of this one-tailed hypothesis with $\alpha = 0.05$ and 80% power required 50 patients per treatment group. A decision rule was chosen to formalize when the mortality rates of the two groups would be considered different. This rule stated that if the probability that indolidan's mortality rate was higher than that of placebo became at least 0.95, a clinical assessment of each death would be reviewed to determine whether to stop the trial. Since the statistician (N.E.) was blinded to treatment group, this rule was interpreted to mean that either 0.95 or 0.05 would be used as critical probabilities to initiate the decision-making process.

III. MONITORING AND DATA COLLECTION

To expedite transfer of data used for study monitoring, a special form was created and sent to each study site (Figure 1). The completed form provided baseline information that was useful in predicting mortality, concomitant to progression of the CHF. The instructions stated that after a patient was randomized to and infused with study treatment, the investigator should complete the form and send it to the Lilly clinical research administrator (CRA). The same data were recorded on clinical report forms and processed as usual, so this duplicate data transmission was used solely for the purpose of keeping monitoring current. If the data were not received by the CRA after a reasonable amount of time (about 2 weeks), she would contact the site and collect the appropriate information by telephone.

Subsequently, the CRA would enter the data into a SAS data base using a data-entry system programmed with SAS/AF (a software system for creating user-friendly "front ends" to information-processing programs). This "intelli-

```
                                  INVESTIGATOR          __________
                                  INVESTIGATOR NO.      __________
                                  PATIENT INITIALS      __________
                                  PATIENT NO.           __________
BASELINE MEASUREMENTS

        |__| lb
_____                             Weight
        |__| kg
_____   ml/min                    VO2 (max)   ETT #1
_____   ml/min                    VO2 (max)   ETT #2
_____   %                         Ejection Fraction
____/____/____                    CHF Date of Onset
Mo.  Day  Year
_____   VT Events/Day             Holter #1
_____   VT Events/Day             Holter #2
_____   1 = No                    Ischemic Heart Disease?
        2 = Yes
_____   cm                        Thoracic Diameter from PA film
_____   cm                        Heart Diameter from PA film
_____   mmol/L                    BUN
_____   mmol/L                    Na

                                  ________________________
                                  Signature

                                  ________________________
                                  Date
```

Figure 1 Case report form for monitoring mortality.

gent" software system bypassed the traditional data-entry process without sacrificing its strengths. For instance, the system was programmed to detect unlikely values and notify the user of the possibility of errors in the data. Any questions concerning data integrity were posed by the CRA to the site administrator before entry into the computer. Figure 2 illustrates the initial menu and the data "browse" screen.

In addition to such quality assurance measures, the system preprocessed the data for analysis. As examples, weight was converted to common units; replicate measurements of the same variable were averaged; cardiothoracic ratio and time since onset of CHF were computed from raw data. Also, since the data-entry and analysis systems were located on the same computer, the data were immediately available for statistical summary and analysis upon entry into the data base. In terms of time to accessibility, this feature is superior to typical processes, which presently require transfer of data between several computers via several software systems before analysis can be performed.

IV. STATISTICAL ANALYSES

For calculating the probability that the mortality rate (per 90-day period) for indolidan plus standard therapy, say λ_I, is greater than that for placebo plus standard therapy, say λ_P, we used the model described by Berry (1989). This model assumes that a patient's mortality rate depends multiplicatively on the treatment and on the patient's prognosis. Suppose that patient k has prognosis x_k and set $w_k = -\log(1 - x_k) \approx x_k$ for small x_k. The mortality rate of patient k is assumed to be

$$\lambda_{ik} = w_k \lambda_i$$

where i = I or P.

That indolidan has a greater mortality rate than does placebo means that $\lambda_I > \lambda_P$. Both rates are unknown. In the Bayesian approach, all unknowns have probability distributions, assessed as described by Spiegelhalter and Freedman (1986), for example. We took λ_I and λ_P to be independent lognormal variables with $\log(\lambda_i)$ having mean 0 and standard deviation $\sigma = 1.5$. This standard deviation corresponds to what was considered to be a noninformative, or open-minded, prior distribution in the sense that even a small amount of data dominates the prior in calculating the posterior probability of $\lambda_I > \lambda_P$. We discuss sensitivity of the conclusion to σ below. Since λ_I and λ_P are exchangeable initially, the initial probability of $\lambda_I > \lambda_P$ is 0.5.

Suppose that t_k is the total number of days patient k is in the study, and let d_I and d_P denote the respective numbers of deaths on indolidan and placebo. For i = I or P, let

$$T_i^* = \sum w_k t_k$$

```
Select Option ===>                              Press END to return

                I N D O L I D A N    E L A G

     M O R T A L I T Y   M O N I T O R I N G   S Y S T E M


     What would you like to do?


                1.  Enter/Change patient information

                2.  Browse patient information

                3.  Print patient information

                4.  Run statistical report
```

(a)

```
                       Browse SAS data set: DATA.DATA                Screen   1
Command ===>                                                          Obs      1

  DATE DATA RECEIVED: ______   (mmddyy)           C O M M A N D S
        INVESTIGATOR:    ___                   *************************
            INITIALS:    ___                   *     CMD 9 - ADD       *
             PATIENT:    ___                   *     CMD 3 - END       *
     DATE RANDOMIZED: ______   (mmddyy)        *     CMD 8 - FORWARD   *
   RANDOMIZATION NO.:   ____                   *     CMD 7 - BACKWARD  *
            END DATE: ______   (mmddyy)        *************************
               DEATH:      _   (1=NO, 2=YES)   * ===> 1 (start at the  *
              WEIGHT:    ___   LBS             *           beginning)  *
                -or-     ___   KGS             * ===> find patient=xxx *
       VO2 (max) #1:    ____   ml/min          * ===> can (cancel chgs)*
       VO2 (max) #2:     ___   ml/min          * ===> del (delete page)*
  EJECTION FRACTION:      __   %               *************************
   CHF DATE OF ONSET: ______   (mmddyy)
    VT Events/Day #1:     __
    VT Events/Day #2:     __
           ISCHEMIC:       _   (1=NO, 2=YES)
   THORACIC DIAMETER:    ___   cm
      HEART DIAMETER:    ___   cm
                 BUN:    ___   mmol/L
                  NA:    ___   mmol/L
```

(b)

Figure 2 (a) Initial menu for mortality monitoring system; (b) "browse" screen in mortality monitoring system.

where the sum is over the patients assigned to treatment i. At any given time, the likelihood function of λ_i is

$$\lambda_i^{d_i} \exp(-\lambda_i T_i^*)$$

for $i = \text{I}$ and P. Thus the sufficient statistics are $(d_\text{I}, T_\text{I}^*, d_\text{P}, T_\text{P}^*)$.

Considering patients' prognoses serves to adjust for treatment assignments that are not balanced with respect to prognosis. Suppose that patient 1 is assigned to treatment I, patients 2 and 3 are assigned to treatment P, and that w_1 is twice as large as $w_2 = w_3$. Then if all three patients have been in the study for the same amount of time ($t_1 = t_2 = t_3$) and none of the three patients have died, patients 2 and 3 combined make the same contribution to the likelihood function of λ_P that patient 1 alone makes to that of λ_I.

The current probability of $\lambda_I > \lambda_P$ is as follows [Berry, 1989, eq. (12)]:

$$P(\lambda_I > \lambda_P | \text{current data}) = \frac{\int_0^\infty g(v; d_P, T_P^*) \int_v^\infty g(u; d_I, T_I^*)\, du\, dv}{\int_0^\infty g(v; d_P, T_P^*) \int_0^\infty g(u; d_I, T_I^*)\, du\, dv}$$

where

$$g(x;d,T) = e^{-Tx}x^{d-1(\log x/2\sigma^2)}$$

We evaluated this probability numerically after each death to help decide whether the trial should be stopped because of increased mortality among patients on indolidan. Figure 3 shows an example of the density with $T_I^* = 10$, $T_P^* = 15$, $d_I = 1$, $d_P = 2$, $\sigma = 1.5$. In this example, $P(\lambda_I > \lambda_P \mid \text{these data}) = 0.613$. The SAS code used to perform this analysis is included in the appendix and is based on an algorithm developed by one of the authors (D.B.).

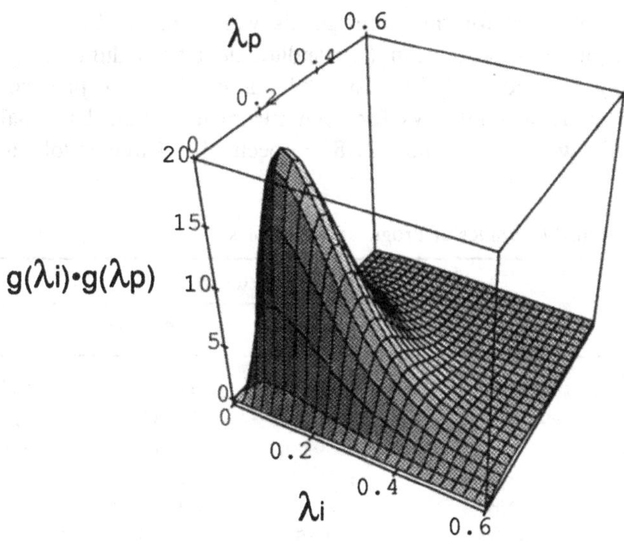

Figure 3 Example of density integrated numerically.

A. Covariate Information

As described above, we incorporated each patient's baseline or initial prognosis as a covariate in the analysis. This was interpreted as the patient's estimated probability of death during the 3-month randomized phase of the study, assuming standard therapy. This probability was computed as follows. Based on the literature and on previous Lilly clinical trials (Cohn et al., 1986; Dargie et al., 1987; Lee and Packer, 1984; Likoff et al., 1987; Pfeffer and Pfeffer, 1987; Szlachcic et al., 1985), we selected eight predictors of mortality. For each predictor we assigned relative weights to values or ranges of values corresponding to their predictive worth, greater weight indicating worse prognosis (Table 1). For simplicity, we chose to define prognosis as a function of total score (i.e., the sum of the eight weights). One of us (F.D.) chose a variety of patient types and assessed his subjective probabilities that such patients would die within 3 months. Then we fit a linear function as follows:

$$\text{initial prognosis} = \frac{0.4(\text{total score} - 3)}{100}$$

Since possible total scores range between 8 and 52, the initial prognoses are between 0.02 and 0.196. Thus initial prognosis was estimated quite conservatively over a relatively small range of possible values.

B. Results

Forty and 41 patients were randomized to indolidan and placebo, respectively. The treatment group medians for initial prognosis were similar: 0.100 for indolidan, 0.108 for placebo. The mean (±standard deviation) duration on study was 81 (±28) days for indolidan and 89 (±14) days for placebo. Median duration on study was 89 days for each treatment group. The final values for T_I^* and T_P^* were 353.3 and 429.8, respectively. Three indolidan

Table 1 Weights Assigned to Values of Prognostic Variables

	Assigned weight			
Predictor	1	3	5	9
VO_2 max. (mL/min)	>14		12–14	<12
Ejection fraction (%)	>35		25–35	<25
CHF duration (years)	<2		2–4	>4
VT events/day	⩽3	4–10	⩾11	
Ischemic?	No		Yes	
Cardiothoracic ratio	⩽0.5	0.5–0.55	>0.55	
BUN (mmol/L)	<11	11–14	>14	
Na (mmol/L)	>132	128–132	<128	

patients died during the randomized phase of the study, as did two placebo patients. Table 2 displays the study results for each patient.

The data analysis was integrated into the same SAS/AF system used for data entry and management. This meant that the data could be analyzed with ease immediately upon entry into the data base or at any other time. As stated in the protocol, the data were analyzed after each death was reported and the patient's data entered into the data base. Figure 4 summarizes the analysis by showing how T_I^* and T_P^* changed over time, indicating when the deaths occurred on I and P, and displaying weekly posterior probabilities. The final probability that $\lambda_I > \lambda_P$ was 0.738.

Using the data from placebo patients and the maximum likelihood estimate discussed by Berry (1989), we updated the initial prognostic algorithm used at the outset (Figure 5). Evidently, our prognostic algorithm overestimated the probability of death. For example, a patient with an initial prognosis of 0.20 has an estimated probability of death of only 0.09. This new algorithm can be used in future studies of similar patients.

C. Sensitivity Analysis

We posed a question concerning the influence of our choice of prior mortality rate distribution on the results: How did $\sigma = 1.5$ affect both early and final probabilities. To answer this question, we performed two sets of probability computations, allowing σ to vary from 0.1 to 10.0 in increments of 0.1: one

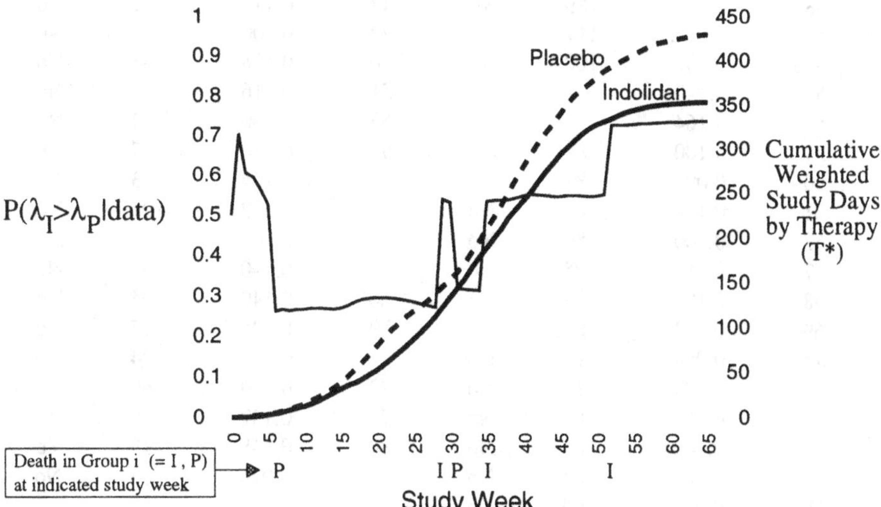

Figure 4 Sufficient statistics by study week. I and P, death in group at indicated study week.

Table 2 Study Results by Patient

Placebo				Indolidan			
Patient number	Initial prognosis	Days on study	Death	Patient number	Initial prognosis	Days on study	Death
1	0.036	90	No	2	0.060	92	No
3	0.092	87	No	4	0.132	89	No
5	0.156	26	Yes	6	0.052	90	No
8	0.124	90	No	7	0.060	59	No
9	0.100	87	No	11	0.036	89	No
10	0.076	85	No	13	0.100	88	No
12	0.124	94	No	14	0.060	89	No
15	0.084	89	No	16	0.108	89	No
17	0.164	87	No	21	0.100	85	No
18	0.132	91	No	23	0.116	94	No
19	0.148	89	No	25	0.148	85	No
20	0.116	86	No	26	0.100	97	No
22	0.060	90	No	28	0.108	87	No
24	0.052	90	No	30	0.156	102	No
27	0.084	89	No	31	0.116	87	No
29	0.084	90	No	32	0.100	82	No
34	0.116	91	No	33	0.092	88	No
35	0.124	88	No	36	0.084	88	No
38	0.100	54	No	37	0.100	263	No
40	0.148	100	No	39	0.068	90	No
41	0.132	102	No	43	0.060	45	Yes
42	0.148	93	No	44	0.100	104	No
46	0.108	69	Yes	45	0.052	88	No
48	0.092	89	No	47	0.116	12	No
52	0.084	111	No	49	0.100	−8	No
53	0.132	108	No	50	0.108	93	No
54	0.140	101	No	51	0.116	96	No
56	0.164	96	No	55	0.100	92	No
59	0.100	89	No	57	0.148	7	No
60	0.092	87	No	58	0.124	93	No
61	0.108	85	No	62	0.132	101	Yes
63	0.100	89	No	64	0.100	85	No
67	0.156	95	No	65	0.140	91	No
68	0.100	88	No	66	0.140	94	No
69	0.124	88	No	70	0.124	117	No
73	0.084	90	No	71	0.124	124	No
75	0.124	111	No	72	0.100	60	No
76	0.084	87	No	74	0.132	89	No
77	0.148	89	No	80	0.148	19	Yes
78	0.164	103	No	81	0.076	54	No
79	0.060	90	No				

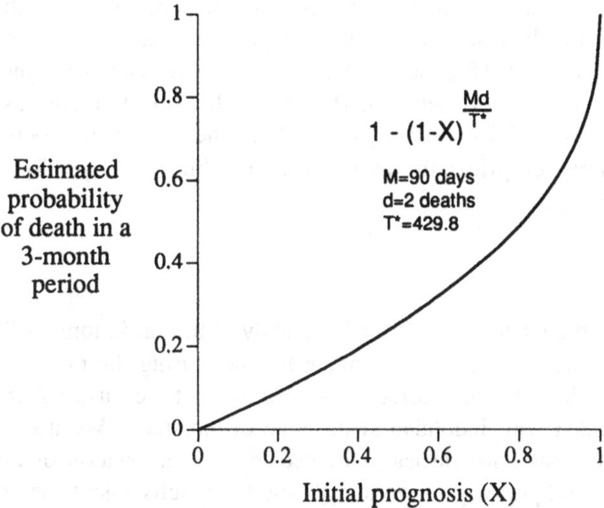

Figure 5 Updated prognostic algorithm using placebo patients.

for all patients enrolled within approximately 3 months of the beginning of the study (to include at least one death), and the other of the entire patient sample. Figure 6 shows the results of these computations for the 15 patients who enrolled within 3 months. Early calculations are not severely affected by the choice of σ.

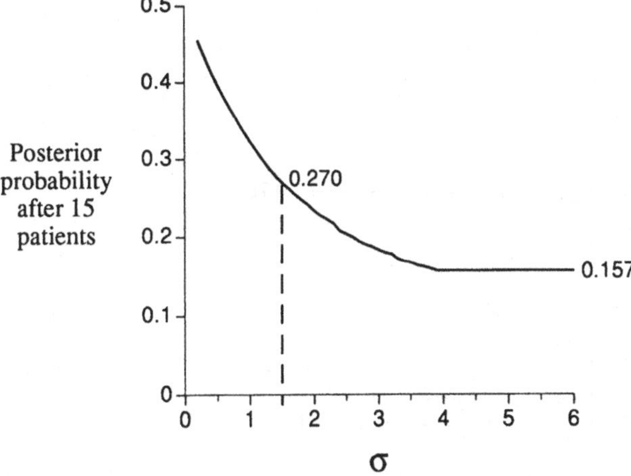

Figure 6 Effect of varying σ on early ($N = 15$) posterior probability of $\lambda_I > \lambda_P$.

Figure 7 shows the results for all 81 patients. As would be expected, the final probability is relatively insensitive to the choice of σ since it uses data from 81 patients compared to 15 patients early in the study. As is true generally, the probability of $\lambda_I > \lambda_P$ tends to 0.5 as $\sigma \to 0$. This limiting case corresponds to known λ_I and λ_P, with $\lambda_I = \lambda_P$. The other extreme, $\sigma \to \infty$, corresponds to an improper prior; the asymptotic probability of $\lambda_I > \lambda_P$ is achieved by about $\sigma = 4$.

V. CONCLUSION

In an elaborate, placebo-controlled, multisegment study of the cardiotonic drug indolidan, we incorporated a Bayesian technique for monitoring the mortality rates in each group. Monitoring mortality was important because of the unknown risks associated with indolidan at the time of the study. We used a method that provided a basis for decisions related to the continuation of the trial. We found the technique easy to work with and the results easy to interpret. A bonus was that we avoided the problems of multiplicity of interim analyses associated with classical statistical techniques.

VI. DISCUSSION

Continuously monitoring data in a clinical trial with the possibility of stopping the trial early—or otherwise altering its design—can affect classical statistical inferential tools, such as p values. This is so even if the trial is not actually

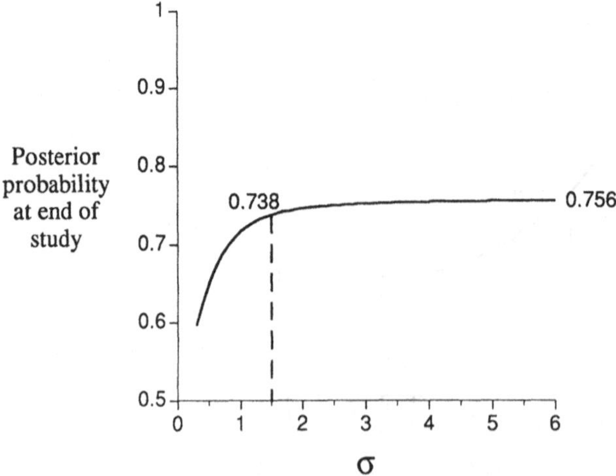

Figure 7 Effect of varying σ on final ($N = 81$) posterior probability of $\lambda_I > \lambda_P$.

stopped early and its design is not altered. In the present study we felt it unethical not to monitor death as a safety variable. Classical inferences are affected only if death is correlated with the measurements in question. We do not know whether such correlations exist, so we do not know whether and how classical inferences should be adjusted. But we felt it necessary to sacrifice the ability to adjust appropriately because we regarded safety to be of paramount importance. We did not plan to make adjustments in any classical inferences had the study not terminated early, but the matter became moot when the study was stopped because the drug lacked sufficient efficacy. (This lack of efficacy was determined by an interim analysis of the data, which included about 80% of the planned patient enrollment.)

Stopping a clinical trial is a complicated decision problem. A drug may increase the mortality rate somewhat, yet improve quality of life sufficiently for most patients that it will still constitute an appropriate treatment. Or the drug may decrease the mortality rate substantially, yet be worthless because it causes intolerable side effects. Therefore, we do not propose that stopping a clinical trial should be based on the probability that an experimental drug's mortality rate is greater than that of standard therapy. However, this probability is an important consideration and can serve as a guide for deciding whether and when to stop.

APPENDIX: SAS CODE FOR COMPUTING POSTERIOR PROBABILITIES

```
TITLE1 'BAYESIAN MONITORING OF MORTALITY IN CLINICAL TRIALS';

*  THE FOLLOWING SAS MACRO INPUTS THE SUFFICIENT STATISTICS (T1, D1, T2,
   D2) AND THE PRIOR STANDARD DEVIATION (S) AND OUTPUTS THE POSTERIOR
   PROBABILITY (I1);

%MACRO SEQBAYES(T1,D1,T2,D2,S);
  DATA INITIAL;
    TA=&T1; T1=&T1; DA=&D1;
    TB=&T2; T2=&T2; DB=&D2;
    IF TA>TB THEN DO;
      TB=TB/TA;
      TA=1;
    END;
    ELSE DO;
     TA=TA/TB;
     TB=1;
    END;
    H=0.2; * H IS THE WIDTH OF THE "DELTA" RECTANGLE FOR INTEGRATION;
    L=1/(2*&S*&S);
    V =LOG((DB+0.01)/(TB+0.01));
    VV=LOG((DA+0.01)/(TA+0.01));
    XY=4 * MAX(V,VV) + 1;
    KK=1;
```

```
RUN;

DATA FINAL;
  SET INITIAL;
  ARRAY PA{500} PA1 - PA500;
  ARRAY PB{500} PB1 - PB500;

  I2 = 0;

INIT:  KK=1; N=0; A1=0; A2=0; A3=0; D1=0; D2=0; VZ=0.005;


SUMS:  IF KK>1.2 THEN N=N-1;
       U=(N+0.5)*H;
       U1=LOG(U);
       UU=U**(-U1*L);
       PB{N+1}=EXP((DB-1)*U1-U*TB)*UU;
       PA{N+1}=EXP((DA-1)*U1-U*TA)*UU;
       Q1=0; Q2=0;
       DO N = 1 TO KK;
         Q1=Q1+PB{N};
         Q2=Q2+PA{N};
       END;
       Q1=PA{KK}*(Q1-PB{KK}/2);
       Q2=PB{KK}*(Q2-PA{KK}/2);
       SS+Q2;
       WW+Q1+Q2;
       IF NOT(WW=0) THEN DO;
            A1=SS/WW;
            A4=A3;
            A3=A2;
            A2=A1;
       END;
       KK=KK+1;

       IF U<XY OR MOD(KK,10) THEN GO TO SUMS;

       Z1=A4-A3;
       Z2=A3-A2;
       Z3=Z1-Z2;
       AD=Z2*Z2/Z3;
       D1=A1-AD;

       IF ABS(D1-D2)>VZ THEN DO;
         D2=D1;
         GO TO SUMS;
       END;
       I1=D1;

       IF ABS(I1-I2)>VZ THEN DO;
         I2=I1;
         H=H/2;
         GO TO INIT;
       END;
```

```
          ELSE PROB = ROUND(I1,.001);

LABEL DA = 'DEATHS GROUP A'
      DB = 'DEATHS GROUP B'
      T1 = 'TOTAL WEIGHTED STUDY TIME A'
      T2 = 'TOTAL WEIGHTED STUDY TIME B';

PROC PRINT DATA=FINAL LABEL;

      VAR DA T1 DB T2 PROB;
    RUN;
  %MEND SEQBAYES;

  %SEQBAYES(429.8, 2, 353.3, 3, 1.5);
```

REFERENCES

Berry, D. A. (1989). *Biometrics 45*: 1197–1211.

Braunwald, E., and Colucci, W. S. (1984). *J. Am. Coll. Cardiol. 3*: 1570.

Cohn, J. N., Archibald, D. G., Ziesche, S., Franciosa, J. A., Harston, W. E., Tristani, F. E., Dunkman, W. B., Jacobs, W., Francis, G. S., Flohr, K. H., Goldman, S., Cobb, F. R., Shah, P. M., Saunders, R., Fletcher, R. D., Loeb, H. S., Hughes, V. C., and Baker, B. (1986). *N. Eng. J. Mdd. 314*: 1547.

Consensus Trial Study Group (1987). *N. Engl. J. Med. 316*: 1429.

Dargie, J. H., Cleland, J. G. F., Leckie, B. J., Inglis, C. G., East, B. W., and Ford, I. (1987). *Circulation 75*: IV–93.

Gillum, R. F. (1987). *Am. Heart J. 113*: 1043.

Guyatt, G. H. (1985). *J. Chronic Dis. 38*: 353.

Katz, A. M. (1978). *N. Engl. J. Med. 299*: 1409.

Lee, W. H., and Packer, M. (1984). *Circulation 70*: II–113.

LeJemtel, T. H., and Sonnenblick, E. H. (1984). *N. Engl. J. Med. 310*: 1384.

Likoff, M. J., Chandler, S. L., and Kay, H. R. (1987). *Am. Cardiol. 59*: 634.

Packer, M. (1987). *J. Am. Coll. Cardiol. 9*: 433.

Packer, M., and Leier, C. V. (1987). *Circulation 75*: IV–55.

Packer, M., Medina, N., and Uyshak, M. (1984). *Circulation 70*: 1038.

Pfeffer, M. A., and Pfeffer, J. M. (1987). *Circulation 75*: IV–93.

Smith, W. M. (1985). *Am. J. Cardiol. 55*: 3A.

Spiegelhalter, D. J., and Freedman, L. S. (1986). *Stat. Med. 5*: 1–13.

Sytkowski, P. A., Kannel, W. B., and D'Agostino, R. B. (1990). *N. Engl. J. Med. 322*: 1635.

Szlachcic, J., Massie, B. M., Kramer, B. L., Topic, N., and Tubau, J. (1985). *Am. J. Cardiol. 55*: 1037.

13

Interim Analysis in the Norwegian Multicenter Study

Irving K. Hwang

Merck Sharp & Dohme Research Laboratories, Rahway, New Jersey

Bruce E. Rodda

Bristol-Myers Squibb Company, Princeton, New Jersey

I. INTRODUCTION

Recent developments in group sequential methods have had a great impact on the design and analysis of randomized clinical trials. This is especially true for those trials that are of "pivotal" or "confirmatory" nature in support of a new drug application (NDA). The pros and cons of performing interim analyses on accumulating data in these trials have been discussed in numerous papers in the literature (e.g., Rodda et al., 1988; Pocock and Hughes, 1989; Davis and Hwang, 1992), and its use for the determination of efficacy and safety is a frequent and necessary practice.

To illustrate the application of group sequential methods (e.g., Pocock, 1977; O'Brien and Fleming, 1979; Lan and DeMets, 1983; Hwang et al., 1990) in performing interim analyses and to demonstrate the use of group sequential testing for a general class of linear rank tests (Chatterjee and Sen, 1973; Tarone and Ware, 1977; Prentice, 1978; Harrington and Fleming, 1982; Tsiatis, 1982), we use the results of a long-term clinical trial in survivors of an acute myocardial infarction conducted by the Norwegian Multicenter Study Group (1981). In particular, demonstrations are given for the use of a general and flexible family (i.e., γ-family) of α spending functions proposed by

Hwang et al. The trial design and results were reported by the Norwegian Multicenter Study Group and are reviewed in Section II [see also Pedersen (1982) and Rodda (1983)].

In Section III we briefly display the one-parameter γ-family of α spending functions, and in Section IV we demonstrate with three different approaches: the fixed-event, fixed-time, and actual-event analyses for performing retrospective interim analyses using the total mortality data from the Norwegian Multicenter Study.

II. THE NORWEGIAN MULTICENTER STUDY

The Norwegian Multicenter Study, also known as the Blocadren Myocardial Infarction Study (BMIS), was a long-term, randomized, double-blind, multicenter clinical trial to assess the efficacy and safety of Blocadren (timolol maleate) 10 mg twice daily versus placebo in secondary prevention of mortality and reinfarction in survivors of a confirmed acute myocardial infarction. Twenty county, municipal, and university hospital centers in Norway participated in this multicenter study. A total of 11,182 hospital admissions were screened and 3583 patients who survived the acute phase of a myocardial infarction were evaluated for trial eligibility. Fifty-two percent, a total of 1884 patients, satisfied the inclusion and exclusion criteria and were randomized to treatment with either Blocadren or placebo between 7 and 28 days after their infarction. The first patient entered and began treatment on January 14, 1978 and patient recruitment was completed on October 20, 1979. The trial was officially terminated on October 20, 1980, after the last randomized patient had completed 1 year of follow-up. Of the total 1884 patients who entered the trial, 945 were randomized to the Blocadren treatment group and 939 to the placebo group. The patients were stratified into three risk groups (high, reinfarction, and low) according to protocol definitions; 1091, 352, and 441 patients, respectively, were entered into the high, reinfarction, and low-risk groups. The mean age was 61 years and there were 1484 males and 400 females. The average patient experience was 17 months and all patients were treated for at least 1 year, except those who died or dropped out during the course of the trial. Maximum exposure to study therapy was 34 months.

The total mortality from all causes (intention to treat) at trial conclusion (October 20, 1980) for the 1884 randomized patients was 250 deaths, 98 occurring in the Blocadren group and 152 in the placebo group. The cumulative mortality rates based on the Kaplan–Meier product-limit estimator (Kaplan and Meier, 1958) were, respectively, 13.3% for Blocadren and 21.9% for placebo, representing an overall 39.3% reduction in total mortality for the Blocadren-treated patients relative to those treated with placebo. The normalized logrank test statistic (Mantel, 1966) calculated under the null hypothesis of equal survival distributions was $z = 3.71$, which gives a p-value of approximately 0.0003 (two-sided). Table 1 tabulates the total mortality data by time-interval grouping (1 month = 30 days) for the 34 months of study. The corresponding Kaplan–Meier life-table curves and their standard errors (Greenwood, 1926) are summarized in Table 2. The mortality curves for both the Blocadren and placebo groups are shown in Figure 1. These two curves diverge early and remain separated for the duration of the trial. A proportional hazards regression model (Cox, 1972) was used to analyze the total mortality data.

III. THE γ-FAMILY OF α SPENDING FUNCTIONS

Hwang et al. (1990) proposed a general γ-family of α spending functions to provide a range of options in group sequential designs. Briefly, the family is in the form of the following one-parameter truncated exponential distributions:

$$\alpha(\gamma,t) = \begin{cases} \alpha \dfrac{1 - e^{-\gamma t}}{1 - e^{-\gamma}} & \gamma \neq 0 \\ \alpha t & \gamma = 0 \end{cases} \qquad \text{for } 0 \leqslant t \leqslant 1$$

so that $\alpha(\gamma,0) = 0$ and $\alpha(\gamma,1) = \alpha$, for all γ. The parameter γ specifies the α spending rate, which, in turn, determines the shape of the group sequential

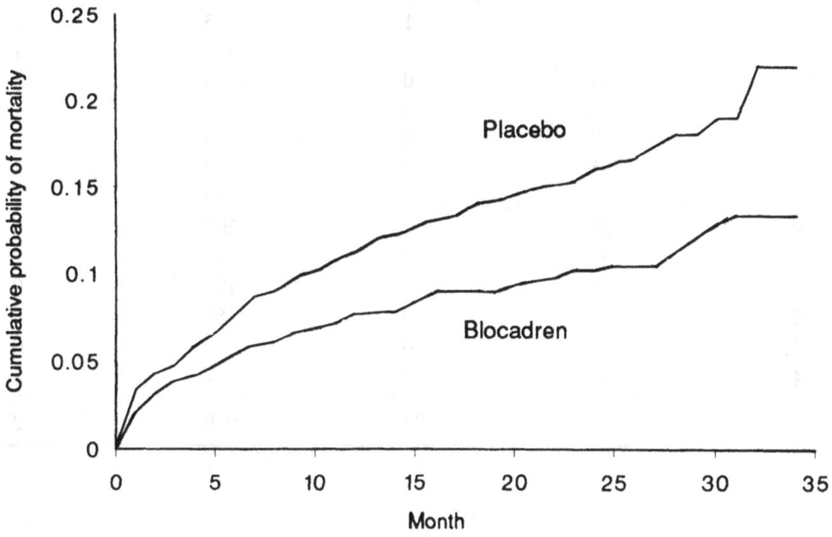

Figure 1 Life-table for total mortality: the Norwegian Multicenter Study.

Table 1 Thirty-four-Month Total Mortality Data: the Norwegian Multicenter Study

	Blocadren		Placebo	
Month	At risk	Death	At risk	Death
1	945	19	939	31
2	926	10	908	9
3	916	7	899	4
4	909	3	895	10
5	906	5	885	7
6	901	6	878	10
7	895	5	868	10
8	890	2	858	3
9	888	5	855	7
10	883	2	848	4
11	881	3	844	6
12	878	5	838	5
13	873	1	833	6
14	836	0	801	2
15	806	5	764	5
16	767	5	737	3
17	722	0	702	3
18	672	0	649	4
19	631	0	599	1
20	592	2	558	3
21	542	2	523	2
22	507	1	483	1
23	463	2	442	1
24	419	0	393	3
25	375	1	352	2
26	337	0	315	1
27	295	0	278	2
28	267	2	242	2
29	237	2	207	0
30	197	2	172	2
31	145	1	126	0
32	100	0	81	3
33	50	0	39	0
34	12	0	7	0
	945	98	939	152

Table 2 Thirty-four-Month Life-Tables on Total Mortality: the Norwegian Multicenter Study[a]

	Blocadren		Placebo	
Month	KM mortality	S.E.	KM mortality	S.E.
1	0.0201	0.0046	0.0330	0.0058
2	0.0307	0.0056	0.0426	0.0066
3	0.0381	0.0062	0.0469	0.0069
4	0.0413	0.0065	0.0575	0.0076
5	0.0466	0.0069	0.0650	0.0080
6	0.0529	0.0073	0.0756	0.0086
7	0.0582	0.0076	0.0863	0.0092
8	0.0603	0.0077	0.0895	0.0093
9	0.0656	0.0081	0.0969	0.0097
10	0.0677	0.0082	0.1012	0.0098
11	0.0709	0.0083	0.1076	0.0101
12	0.0762	0.0086	0.1129	0.0103
13	0.0772	0.0087	0.1193	0.0106
14	0.0772	0.0087	0.1215	0.0107
15	0.0830	0.0090	0.1272	0.0109
16	0.0890	0.0093	0.1308	0.0110
17	0.0890	0.0093	0.1345	0.0112
18	0.0890	0.0093	0.1398	0.0114
19	0.0890	0.0093	0.1413	0.0115
20	0.0920	0.0095	0.1459	0.0118
21	0.0954	0.0098	0.1491	0.0119
22	0.0972	0.0099	0.1509	0.0120
23	0.1011	0.0103	0.1528	0.0122
24	0.1011	0.0103	0.1593	0.0126
25	0.1035	0.0105	0.1641	0.0130
26	0.1035	0.0105	0.1667	0.0132
27	0.1035	0.0105	0.1727	0.0138
28	0.1102	0.0115	0.1796	0.0145
29	0.1177	0.0125	0.1796	0.0145
30	0.1266	0.0139	0.1891	0.0158
31	0.1327	0.0151	0.1891	0.0158
32	0.1327	0.0151	0.2191	0.0228
33	0.1327	0.0151	0.2191	0.0228
34	0.1327	0.0151	0.2191	0.0228

[a] KM, Kaplan–Meier product-limit estimate (Kaplan and Meier, 1958); S.E., standard error estimate (Greenwood, 1926).

boundary generated. In this formulation, t represents the proportion of the total information accumulated up to the time of the interim analysis. The information is usually measured in terms of the number of patients or endpoint events in a trial (Lan et al., 1984), but interim analyses may often be scheduled at specified calendar times, although theoretically, they should occur in terms of information times (Lan and DeMets, 1989). Applying the standard Brownian motion process to $\alpha(\gamma,t)$ functions (Lan and DeMets, 1983), one can compute discrete group sequential boundaries c_i, with respect to t_i and various γ values, consecutively spending the available type I error probability. For a theoretical development of the γ-family of α spending functions, refer to Hwang (1988).

IV. RETROSPECTIVE ANALYSES USING THE GROUP SEQUENTIAL APPROACH

The Norwegian Multicenter Study was designed as a fixed-sample trial without incorporating any group sequential design because many methods had not yet been fully developed. Despite this, there were three interim analyses and one final analysis performed during the course of the trial. In all the analyses, the primary endpoint (i.e., total mortality) and secondary endpoints (e.g., sudden deaths, nonfatal reinfarctions, and rehospitalizations) as well as many subgroups were evaluated, and the p-values were reported without any adjustments for repeated testing. The first interim analysis of April 20, 1979 was done at the request of the independent Ethical Review Committee (ERC) of the trial. The purpose was to evaluate whether a treatment effect or trend would exist 1 year postrandomization of the first patient. Because the interim results on total mortality was approaching statistical significance (logrank $z = 1.79$, $p \cong 0.07$), the ERC recommended a second analysis to be done 3 months later for determination of patient enrollment. The second analysis of July 20, 1979 showed a significant treatment difference between the Blocadren and placebo groups (logrank $z = 2.17$, $p \cong 0.03$). The ERC decided to extend patient enrollment an additional 3 months. The last patient was randomized on October 20, 1979, and the trial was finally terminated on October 20, 1980, based on the overwhelming results of the third analysis of March 20, 1980 (logrank $z = 3.328$, $p \cong 0.0009$). The decision to terminate the trial was based on a combination of many factors, with strong statistical evidence playing a crucial part.

As stated previously, group sequential methods were not used to determine early stopping of the trial. To ascertain whether the outcome would have been different had these methods been employed, we analyze the total mortality data retrospectively using the discrete group sequential boundaries constructed by the γ-family of α spending functions. To simplify the problem, we restrict our attention to the primary endpoint, total mortality of all causes, based on the intention-to-treat approach. Although the trial was designed as a fixed-sample multicenter study, the total sample size, $n \cong 1800$ to 2000 (actual $n = 1884$) patients, was not estimated in a straightforward manner, nor was there an estimate given for the total information (i.e., total number of deaths). Hence, to simplify the problem further, and for convenience in demonstrating the use of group sequential methods, we assume the total number of deaths (250) was the total information planned for this trial.

The assumption above turns out to be quite reasonable. If patients who suffer an acute myocardial infarction have a 2-year cumulative mortality rate of 15% on placebo and Blocadren reduces it by one-third during this period, the total sample size required would be approximately 2000 patients, to provide a 90% power at $\alpha = 0.05$, two-sided, and the estimated total information for the trial would be exactly 250 deaths.

We consider a Cox proportional hazards regression model and test the hypotheses

$$\mathbf{H}_0\colon \zeta = 1 (\Leftrightarrow \beta = 0) \quad \text{versus} \quad \mathbf{H}_1\colon \zeta \neq 1 (\Leftrightarrow \beta \neq 0)$$

where ζ denotes the relative hazard ratio and β the regression coefficient for the proportional hazards model. We follow the recommendation of Pocock (1982) and restrict the maximum number of repeated analyses to $N \leqslant 5$ and proceed with three different approaches in analyzing the total mortality data of the Norwegian Multicenter Study.

A. The Fixed-Event Approach

One simple approach is to divide the trial into five equally spaced analyses in terms of total number of deaths and perform a group sequential significance test after every 50 deaths. Since the time parameter t, which represents the process or information time, is rescaled in terms of the total information (i.e., total number of deaths) in the sample, the general class of sequentially computed linear rank statistics, S_i, $i = 1, \ldots, 5$ form a partial-sum process of independent, identically distributed normal random variables. The process is multivariate normal with independent and equal increments in variance; that is, $t_i = i/5$, $i = 1, \ldots, 5$ or $t = \{0.20, 0.40, 0.60, 0.80, 1.00\}$ as shown in Table 3. Hence we can simply compute the linear rank test statistics sequentially after every 50 deaths and compare the resulting normalized z scores against the chosen group sequential boundary, c_i, $i = 1, \ldots, 5$. Instead of prespecifying a single boundary, we choose a number of boundaries to demonstrate the use of the γ-family of α spending functions, as well as the well-known Pocock and O'Brien–Fleming boundaries. The boundaries chosen among the γ-family are those of $\alpha(-4, t)$, $\alpha(-1, t)$, and $\alpha(1, t)$, where the boundaries of

Table 3 Results of Retrospective Group Sequential Analyses Based on the Fixed-Event Approach: the Norwegian Multicenter Study

	Analysis i				
	1	2	3	4	5
Rescaled time, t_i	0.20	0.40	0.60	0.80	1.00
Number of deaths, D_i	50	100	150	200	250
Blocadren	18	41	62	77	98
Placebo	32	59	88	123	152
Hazard ratio, ζ	0.56	0.69	0.69	0.61	0.62
Calendar date	Nov. 14, 1978	May 6, 1979	Oct. 10, 1979	Apr. 14, 1980	Oct. 20, 1980
Study days	305	478	635	822	1,011
Standard z score (two-sided)[a]					
Logrank	2.013	1.851	2.218	3.507	3.711
P-P Wilcoxon	1.990	1.837	2.187	3.455	3.664
T-W	1.878	1.775	2.057	3.332	3.601
Two-sided group sequential boundary, $\|c_i\|$[a]					
(i) $\alpha = 0.05$					
$\alpha(-4, t)$	3.259	2.987	2.694	2.375	2.027
$\alpha(-1, t)$	2.729	2.590	2.453	2.315	2.182
$\alpha(1, t)$	2.455	2.419	2.400	2.392	2.395
O'B-F	4.555	3.221	2.630	2.277	2.037
P	2.413	2.413	2.413	2.413	2.413
(ii) $\alpha = 0.01$					
$\alpha(-4, t)$	3.694	3.457	3.206	2.938	2.652
$\alpha(-1, t)$	3.227	3.121	3.013	2.908	2.802
$\alpha(1, t)$	2.989	2.981	2.984	2.988	3.000
O'B-F	5.847	4.135	3.376	2.924	2.615
P	2.986	2.986	2.986	2.986	2.986

[a] P-P, Peto–Prentice; T-W, Tarone–Ware; O'B-F, O'Brien–Fleming; P, Pocock.

$\alpha(-4,t)$ and $\alpha(1,t)$ generate boundaries similar to the O'Brien–Fleming and Pocock boundaries, respectively, and $\alpha(-1,t)$ generates boundaries intermediate of the two. In addition, throughout the exercise of analyzing the mortality data, we sequentially calculate the linear rank test statistics, namely, the logrank (Mantel, 1966; Peto and Peto, 1972; Cox, 1972), Peto–Prentice Wilcoxon (Prentice, 1978), and Tarone–Ware (Tarone and Ware, 1977) statistics, under the null hypothesis H_0. The results for the fixed 50-death analysis are summarized in Table 3. A modified version of the SAS macros developed by Hwang and Bolognese (1980) is used for performing all the calculations of the linear rank tests and life tables.

Table 3 shows that all boundaries, including those at $\alpha = 0.01$ level, are crossed at the fourth analysis with a total of 200 deaths observed. The cumulative distribution of deaths is 77 and 123, respectively, in the Blocadren and placebo groups, with a relative hazard ratio $\zeta = 0.61$. The z scores calculated for the logrank, Peto–Prentice Wilcoxon, and Tarone–Ware tests at the fourth analysis are, respectively, 3.507, 3.455, and 3.332, which are all greater than the largest boundary value, $c_4 = 2.988$, corresponding to $\alpha(1, t_4)$ at $\alpha = 0.01$. Hence, based on the fixed-event analysis, we reject H_0 and conclude that Blocadren is superior to placebo in secondary prevention of mortality at the fourth interim analysis with 200 deaths observed. The results are highly significant at $\alpha = 0.01$ level, regardless of the boundaries chosen or the linear rank statistics used. Therefore, the trial would be recommended for early termination after the fourth analysis as of April 14, 1980 (on study day 822).

B. The Fixed-Time Approach

Another approach is to divide the study into approximately five equally spaced periods and perform a group sequential test after approximately every 6-month interval. To restrict the maximum number of analyses to $N = 5$, the time interval between the fourth and fifth analyses is not 6 months, but approximately 9 months. Nevertheless, the first four analyses are indeed equally spaced 6 months apart, and as will be discussed later, this deviation from the fixed-time definition does not affect the outcome of the retrospective group sequential tests. Unlike that in the fixed-event approach, the rescaled time parameter $t = \{0.112, 0.284, 0.476, 0.704, 1.000\}$, in terms of the total 250 deaths (see Table 4), is no longer equally spaced. That is, $t_i \neq i/5$, $i \leqslant 5$, and hence the condition requiring a partial-sum process or the sequentially computed linear rank statistics to have equal increments in variance is no longer satisfied. Accordingly, the group sequential boundaries of Pocock and O'Brien–Fleming, based on the assumption of equal variance increments, are no longer appropriate. This problem is addressed by constructing discrete group sequential boun-

Table 4 Results of Retrospective Group Sequential Analyses Based on the Fixed-Time Approach: the Norwegian Multicenter Study

	Analysis i				
	1	2	3	4	5
Rescaled time, t_i	0.112	0.284	0.476	0.704	1.000
Number of deaths, D_i	28	71	119	176	250
Blocadren	9	29	50	69	98
Placebo	19	42	69	107	152
Hazard ratio, ζ	0.47	0.69	0.72	0.63	0.62
Calendar date	July 20, 1978	Jan. 20, 1979	July 20, 1979	Jan. 20, 1980	Oct. 20, 1980
Study days	188	372	553	737	1,011
Standard z score (two-sided)[a]					
Logrank	1.948	1.547	1.798	3.011	3.711
P-P Wilcoxon	1.959	1.327	1.767	2.967	3.664
T-W	1.949	1.517	1.631	2.836	3.601
Two-sided group sequential boundary, $\lvert c_i \rvert$					
(i) $\alpha = 0.05$					
$\alpha(-4, t)$	3.481	3.172	2.885	2.523	2.008
$\alpha(-1, t)$	2.993	2.711	2.549	2.369	2.145
$\alpha(1, t)$	2.645	2.487	2.427	2.379	2.342
$\alpha_1^*(t)$	>5.0	4.058	3.051	2.450	2.004
$\alpha_2^*(t)$	2.626	2.489	2.439	2.389	2.337
(ii) $\alpha = 0.01$					
$\alpha(-4, t)$	3.897	3.618	3.371	3.060	2.631
$\alpha(-1, t)$	3.407	3.218	3.090	2.944	2.763
$\alpha(1, t)$	3.157	3.029	2.995	2.968	2.944
$\alpha_1^*(t)$	>5.0	>5.0	3.910	3.156	2.596
$\alpha_2^*(t)$	3.143	3.031	3.006	2.976	2.939

[a] P-P, Peto-Prentice; T-W, Tarone-Ware.

daries using the γ-family of α spending functions. Again, the boundaries chosen among the γ-family are $\alpha(-4,t)$, $\alpha(-1,t)$, and $\alpha(1,t)$. Also included are boundaries corresponding to $\alpha_1^*(t)$ and $\alpha_2^*(t)$ of Lan and DeMets (1983). As seen in Table 4, $\alpha(-4,t)$ and $\alpha_1^*(t)$ can be used to generate the O'Brien–Fleming-like boundaries, in situations where information time is not equally spaced, with $\alpha(-4,t)$ providing less stringent boundaries values for $t \leqslant 0.5$. The Pocock-like boundaries can be constructed equally well by using either $\alpha(1,t)$ or $\alpha_2^*(t)$.

The results of sequential analyses in Table 4 demonstrate that all boundaries are crossed at the fourth analysis, with a total of 176 deaths observed. The cumulative deaths are 69 and 107, respectively, in the Blocadren and placebo groups with a hazard ratio $\zeta = 0.63$. The corresponding z scores for the logrank, Peto–Prentice Wilcoxon, and Tarone–Ware tests at the fourth analysis are, respectively, 3.061, 2.967, and 2.836, which exceed all boundaries values at $\alpha = 0.05$ level. Note that the logrank z score also exceeds all boundary values at $\alpha = 0.01$. Therefore, based on the fixed-time analysis, the trial would be again recommended for termination at the fourth analysis as of January 20, 1980 (on day 737 of the trial).

C. The Actual-Event Approach

As mentioned earlier, the trial was designed as a fixed-sample study and there were actually four formal analyses carried out during the course of the trial. The recommendation by the Ethical Review Committee to stop the trial somewhat before schedule was based on the unadjusted p-value ($p \cong 0.0009$) at the third interim analysis of March 20, 1980. The data are reanalyzed using the group sequential methods with $N = 4$, based on the interim analyses that actually took place. Table 5 summarizes the results based on this actual-event analysis.

Once again, the rescaled time parameter $t = \{0.388, 0.536, 0.785, 1.000\}$ is not equally spaced, and hence we avoid the problem of unequal variance increments by using the γ-family to construct discrete group sequential boundaries for $\alpha(-4,t)$, $\alpha(-1,t)$, and $\alpha(1,t)$. Similarly, the boundaries corresponding to $\alpha_1^*(t)$ and $\alpha_2^*(t)$ are also included. Table 5 shows that all boundaries are crossed at the third analysis with a total mortality of 76 and 120 in the Blocadren and placebo groups, respectively. The hazard ratio of Blocadren relative to placebo at analysis 3 is $\zeta = 0.62$. The calculated linear rank test z scores are, respectively, 3.328, 3.285, and 3.186 for the logrank, Peto–Prentice Wilcoxon, and Tarone–Ware tests, respectively; each exceeds all the boundary values at the $\alpha = 0.01$ level.

The retrospective early stopping decision rule is in accord with what had actually happened, and it recommends termination of the trial after the third

Table 5 Results of Retrospective Group Sequential Analyses Based on the Actual-Event Approach: the Norwegian Multicenter Study

	Analysis i			
	1	2	3	4
Rescaled time, t_i	0.388	0.536	0.785	1.000
Number of deaths, D_i	97	134	196	250
Blocadren	40	55	76	98
Placebo	57	79	120	152
Hazard ratio, ζ	0.69	0.68	0.62	0.62
Calendar date	Apr. 20, 1979	July 20, 1979	Mar. 20, 1980	Oct. 20, 1980
Study days	462	553	797	1,011
Standard z score (two-sided)[a]				
Logrank	1.790	2.173	3.328	3.711
P-P Wilcoxon	1.769	2.138	3.285	3.664
T-W	1.703	1.954	3.186	3.601
Two-sided group sequential boundary, $\lvert c_i \rvert$				
(i) $\alpha = 0.05$				
$\alpha(-4, t)$	2.926	2.802	2.384	2.021
$\alpha(-1, t)$	2.464	2.502	2.296	2.168
$\alpha(1, t)$	2.237	2.400	2.345	2.372
$\alpha_1^*(t)$	3.418	2.866	2.303	2.026
$\alpha_2^*(t)$	2.235	2.410	2.351	2.363
(ii) $\alpha = 0.01$				
$\alpha(-4, t)$	3.397	3.304	2.943	2.646
$\alpha(-1, t)$	2.997	3.057	2.886	2.791
$\alpha(1, t)$	2.805	2.985	2.945	2.981
$\alpha_1^*(t)$	4.369	3.668	2.972	2.612
$\alpha_2^*(t)$	2.803	2.993	2.950	2.973

[a] P-P, Peto–Prentice; T-W, Tarone–Ware.

interim analysis as of March 20, 1980 (on study day 797), based on the group sequential testing approach.

V. DISCUSSION

Interim analyses are scientifically, ethically, and administratively essential in large clinical trials conducted over extensive periods of time. They must be planned and done in a logical manner; their consequences must be considered carefully when selecting a specific decision rule. We have used the total mortality data from the Norwegian Multicenter Study to demonstrate the use of a general class of linear rank statistics for group sequential significance testing in survival analysis. Three different approaches have been examined—the fixed-event, fixed-time, and actual-event analyses—for cases where the information time is both equally spaced and unequally spaced, so that the overall type I error probability is maintained at the prespecified α level. In particular, we have shown that the boundaries constructed by the γ-family of α spending functions are flexible and useful. As demonstrated in the fixed-time and actual-event analyses, it is very difficult to schedule interim analyses at calendar times that satisfy the requirement of equal increments in information time. However, this problem can be avoided by constructing group sequential boundaries based on the $\alpha(\gamma, t)$ function with respect to t_i and γ value chosen consecutively by spending the available α, regardless of the disposition of the time parameter t_i.

In the design of a group sequential trial using the γ-family of α spending functions, one single member of the γ-family, which characterizes the spending rate of the overall type I error probability α, should be selected at the design stage. Instead, we have included a few members of the γ-family along with the well-known boundaries (e.g., Pocock, O'Brien–Fleming, and similarly α_2^* and α_1^* of Lan and DeMets) to illustrate the use of the α spending functions in performing group sequential analysis. In addition, among the class of linear rank statistics, the calculated logrank test statistics have uniformly exhibited the largest z scores among its class for all the analyses performed. The finding further supports the validity of fitting a proportional hazards regression model under the family of Lehmann alternatives to the total mortality data. Furthermore, the exercise of analyzing the total mortality data of the fixed-sample Norwegian study retrospectively confirms that the recommendation by the Ethical Review Committee of the Norwegian Multicenter Study Group was indeed a correct one (see the summary results in Table 6), even though a group sequential design with an early stopping decision rule was never incorporated, simply because appropriate group sequential methods were not available at that time.

Nevertheless, since statistical methodology is now sufficiently well developed, proper utilization of the methods for interim analysis is essential for all trials with long-term follow-up. To satisfy the ethical, statistical, and regulatory concerns, we ought to plan ahead for the inevitable. That is, group sequential methods should be used and incorporated in the study protocol as an integrated part of the study design. Details such as the nature of the sequential boundary, references to methodology, and early stopping decision rules should

Table 6 Boundary Crossing Based on the Two-Sided Logrank Test for the Retrospective Group Sequential Analyses: the Norwegian Multicenter Study

	Group sequential analytic approach		
	Fixed-event	Fixed-time	Actual-event
Number of analyses, N	5	5	4
Equally spaced in rescaled information time	Yes	No	No
Boundary crossing observed at:[a]			
N^*	4	4	3
τ^*	0.800	0.704	0.785
Overall significance level	<0.01	<0.01	<0.01
Number of deaths observed	200	176	196
Calendar date	Apr. 14, 1980	Jan. 20, 1980	Mar. 20, 1980
Study days	822	737	797

[a] τ^*, boundary crossing time or early stopping time in terms of total information.

be provided. In addition, there should be adequate documentation to indicate when interim analyses were done and what the consequences were.

REFERENCES

Chatterjee, S. K., and Sen, P. K. (1973). Nonparametric testing under progressive censorship. *Calcutta Stat. Assoc. Bull. 22*: 13.

Cox, D. R. (1972). Regression models and life tables (with discussion). *J. R. Stat. Soc. B 34*: 187.

Davis, R. L., and Hwang, I. K. (1992). Interim analysis in clinical trials. In *Statistics in the Pharmaceutical Industry,* 2nd ed. (C. R. Buncher and J. Y. Tsay, eds.), Marcel Dekker, New York.

Greenwood, N. (1926). The natural duration of cancer. In *Report of Public Health and Medical Subjects,* H.M.S.O., London, Vol. 33, p. 1.

Harrington, D. P., and Fleming, T. R. (1982). A class of rank tests procedures for censored survival data. *Biometrika 69*: 553.

Hwang, I. K. (1988). Group sequential significance tests for clinical trials, Ph.D. dissertation, Department of Statistics, The Wharton School, University of Pennsylvania.

Hwang, I. K., and Bolognese, J. B. (1980). SAS macros for survival analysis, *5th SAS Users Group International Conference Proceedings*, pp. 417–422.

Hwang, I. K., Shih, W. J., and deCani, J. S. (1990). Group sequential designs using a family of type I error probability spending functions. *Stat. Med. 9*: 1439.

Kaplan, E. L., and Meier, P. (1958). Nonparametric estimation from incomplete observations. *J. Am. Stat. Assoc. 53*: 457.

Lan, K. K. G., and DeMets, D. L. (1983). Discrete sequential boundaries for clinical trials. *Biometrika 70*: 659.

Lan, K. K. G., and DeMets, D. L. (1989). Group sequential procedures: calendar versus information time. *Stat. Med. 8*: 1191.

Lan, K. K. G., DeMets, D. L., and Halperin, M. (1984). More flexible sequential and nonsequential designs in long-term clinical trials. *Commun. Stat. Theory Methods 13*: 2339.

Mantel, N. (1966). Evaluation of survival data and two new rank order statistics arising in its consideration. *Cancer Chemother. Rep. 50*: 163.

Norwegian Multicenter Study Group (1981). Timolol-induced reduction in mortality and reinfarction in patients surviving acute myocardial infarction. *N. Engl. J. Med. 304*: 801.

O'Brien, P. C., and Fleming, T. R. (1979). A multiple testing procedure for clinical trials. *Biometrics 35*: 549.

Pedersen, T. R. (1982). Timolol-induced reduction in mortality and reinfarction: a multicenter study on timolol in secondary prevention after infarction. *ACTA Med. Scand.* (Suppl.).

Peto, R., and Peto, J. (1972). Asymptotically efficient rank invariant test procedures. *J. R. Stat. Soc. A 135*: 185.

Pocock, S. J. (1977). Group sequential methods in the design and analysis of clinical trials. *Biometrika 64*: 191.

Pocock, S. J. (1982). Interim analysis for randomized clinical trials: the group sequential approach. *Biometrics 38*: 153.

Pocock, S. J., and Hughes, M. D. (1989). Practical problems in interim analysis, with particular regard to estimation. *Controlled Clin. Trials 10*: 209S.

Prentice, R. L. (1978). Linear rank tests with right-censored data. *Biometrika 65*: 167.

Rodda, B. E. (1983). The timolol myocardial infarction study: an evaluation of selected variables. *Circulation 67*: I101.

Rodda, B. E., Tsianco, M. C., Bolognese, J. A., and Kersten, M. K. (1988). Clinical development. In *Biopharmaceutical Statistics for Drug Development* (K. E. Peace, ed.), Marcel Dekker, New York, p. 273.

Tarone, R. E., and Ware, J. (1977). On distribution-free tests for equality of survival distributions. *Biometrika 64*: 156.

Tsiatis, A. A. (1982). Repeated significance testing for a general class of statistics used in censored survival analysis. *J. Am. Stat. Assoc. 77*: 855.

14

Interim Analysis of the Helsinki Heart Study Primary Prevention Trial

Harry Haber
Warner-Lambert/Parke-Davis Pharmaceutical Research Division, Ann Arbor, Michigan

I. BACKGROUND

Despite recent declines in mortality from coronary heart disease (CHD), CHD remains the major cause of death and disability in industrialized countries of the world. The mortality rate from CHD per 100,000 population in the United States was 250 in 1980 and 236 in 1983 (NCHS, 1983). About 800,000 new myocardial infarctions and 600,000 recurrences are reported each year in the United States (National Heart, Lung, and Blood Institute, 1982). Coronary heart disease is the leading cause of premature permanent disability among American workers, is the third most frequent cause of short-term hospitalization, and is the highest in per admission hospital cost (Kannel and Thom, 1986). The enormous toll of death and disability due to CHD focused concern on its possible prevention by various interventions, particularly through regulating serum cholesterol levels by means of diet and drug therapy.

Epidemiologic and clinical studies left little doubt regarding the role of serum cholesterol in the pathogenesis of CHD (Brown and Goldstein, 1986; Steinberg, 1985; Kannel et al., 1979). In particular, two large, placebo-controlled primary prevention trials, the WHO Clofibrate Trial (Committee of Principal Investigators, 1978) and the Lipid Research Clinics Coronary Primary Prevention Trial (LRC-CPPT) with cholestyramine (Lipids Research Clinics Program, 1984) both demonstrated marked reduction of nonfatal myocardial infarction following drug-induced reduction of serum cholesterol. The serum concentration of HDL-cholesterol appeared to be a strong inverse predictor of the incidence of CHD. Follow-up results of the LRC-CPPT study indicated that for each 1 mg/dL increase in HDL-C, there was a 5.5% decrease in the risk of CHD. Evidence from these and a number of other clinical trials seemed to indicate that lowering elevated serum cholesterol and increasing HDL-cholesterol would have a beneficial effect on the incidence of CHD.

Optimum therapy for the prevention of CHD appeared to be treatment that increased HDL-C while lowering LDL-C. Extensive clinical experience with gemfibrozil had shown it to be a safe and effective lipid-regulating agent that consistently did both. Accordingly, a large-scale, prospective, double-blind epidemiologic study (the Helsinki Heart Study) was undertaken in otherwise healthy, dyslipidemic men in Finland to compare gemfibrozil with placebo in the primary prevention of CHD.

II. PROTOCOL

The objective of the Helsinki Heart Study primary prevential trial was (1) to test the hypothesis that reducing serum total cholesterol and LDL-cholesterol and increasing HDL-cholesterol by the use of gemfibrozil would reduce the incidence of coronary heart disease in an asymptomatic, dyslipidemic, middle-aged male population at high risk of developing CHD, and (2) to record adverse events and evaluate the long-term safety of gemfibrozil. The statistical null hypothesis was that there was no difference in the incidence rates for CHD between the gemfibrozil group and the placebo group. The alternative hypothesis was that the incidence of CHD would be lower in the gemfibrozil group than in the placebo group. The incidence of CHD in the gemfibrozil group was taken to be 10.0 per 1000, a clinical reduction of 33%.

In computing the appropriate sample size for the Helsinki Heart Study, the projected rate of fatal and nonfatal myocardial infarction among placebo subjects was estimated to be 15.0 per 1000, based on Finnish statistics. The sample size was calculated using the normal approximation to the binomial distribution. A two-sided 5% level of significance and power of 90% to detect a reduction of 33% in the treated group was chosen, with an anticipated 20% withdrawal rate. Using these criteria, the sample size was estimated to be 4000.

Efficacy of treatment was determined by comparing the incidence of cardiovascular endpoints. The endpoints were definite fatal and nonfatal myocardial infarction (MI), sudden cardiac death, and unwitnessed cardiac death.

Detailed definitions of these endpoints were described in the protocol and a thorough system of verifying all potential endpoints was established.

The protocol provided for interim analyses with a possible first evaluation after 1 year of follow-up. After 1 year of study experience, the total number of myocardial infarctions and coronary deaths were well below the projected totals. Therefore, the code was not broken and interim statistical analysis was not performed. The first code break occurred in June 1985 when all study participants had completed 3 years of follow-up (two-thirds of the population had completed 4 years, due to staggered entry).

As is common in long-term clinical trials, a group of scientists from various backgrounds was formed to act as an independent decision-making body. Four scientists not involved in the Helsinki Heart Study formed the Ad Hoc Committee for the purpose of providing advice on early termination to the Helsinki Heart Council. Plans for subsequent code breaks and interim analyses after the break at 3 years were not specifically laid out in the protocol. The number of analyses and the timing of them were not defined. For this reason the sequential procedure of Lan and DeMets (1983) was adopted to deal with repeated significance testing and decision making in the Helsinki Heart Study.

III. MONITORING AND DATA COLLECTION

The Helsinki Heart Study began in November 1980 and was completed in March 1987. The study was conducted under the management of the International Advisory Council (IAC), consisting of experts in metabolic disease, cardiology, epidemiology, biostatistics, and clinical toxicology as well as the principal medical officers of the participating institutions and representatives from Warner-Lambert Clinical Research (United Kingdom and United States). The IAC reviewed and approved the study design and protocol and met, in full, twice a year. The daily management of the Helsinki Heart Study was controlled by the Executive Committee of the IAC. The Ethics Committee consisted of all Finnish members of the IAC and met at least once a year. This committee was responsible for the ethical and safety aspects of the study and was the final arbiter for determining termination or continuation of the trial based on recommendations from the Ad Hoc Committee.

All day-to-day aspects of the trial were monitored by the Executive Committee operational staff at the Helsinki Heart Council's Central Office located in Helsinki. The 37 major centers (clinics) were further divided into 77 subclinics where the actual field work was carried out. About 90 nurses worked at these clinics under the supervision of the central office.

A common protocol using identical case reporting forms was strictly adhered to in all clinics to ensure comparability of data. Case reporting forms of all subjects were forwarded to the Parke-Davis Research Division in Ann

Arbor, Michigan for processing and data base entry and subsequent conversion to microfiche.

An SAS (SAS Institute, 1985) data base was created to facilitate analysis and reporting of the data. A 100% check of the data was performed using computerized data listings and comparisons with case report forms. Quality assurance programs were written to double-check critical data based on ranges and exploratory data techniques. All statistical analysis programs were done in SAS or BMDP and were checked for accuracy by programmers and biostatisticians.

IV. STATISTICAL ANALYSIS

The sequential method of O'Brien and Fleming (1979) and the method of Pocock (1977) require that the total number of statistical decision times, k, be specified in advance and that these k times be equally spaced. Lan and DeMets (1983) proposed a sequential procedure that does not require these two assumptions and yields boundaries similar to those of O'Brien–Fleming and Pocock as special cases. The Lan–DeMets procedure is summarized and its use in long-term clinical trials, such as the Helsinki Heart Study, is described in Lan et al. (1984). The basic ideas are as follows.

First, consider a nonsequential trial for which there is one test of significance at the scheduled end of the trial, with no provision for rejecting the null hypothesis and stopping the trial prior to the scheduled conclusion. Thus the alpha error level (e.g., 0.05) is "spent" once and for all at the end of the trial. In contrast, the Lan–DeMets procedure can be described as spending the alpha error level over a period of time, say from 0 to 1 (i.e., time 0 is the start of the study and time 1 is the scheduled end). This is done by specifying, in advance, a function, $\alpha^*(t)$, which characterizes the rate at which the alpha error level is spent.

In a nonsequential trial, the critical value, or boundary, for a two-sided test of a random variable at $\alpha = 0.05$ is 1.96 at time $t = 1$. Since it is not possible to reject earlier, the boundary can be considered to be infinite for $0 \leqslant t \leqslant 1$. In contrast, for the Lan–DeMets procedure, there is a boundary $[b(t), 0 \leqslant t \leqslant 1]$ for the test statistic $(S(t),\ 0 \leqslant t \leqslant 1)$, such that $\alpha^*(t)$ is the probability that the boundary is crossed by time t:

$$\alpha^*(t) = \Pr[S(u) \geqslant b(u) \text{ for some } u,\ 0 \leqslant u \leqslant t]$$

Thus the function $\alpha^*(t)$ characterizes the rate at which the alpha error level is spent during the trial. More specifically, $\alpha^*(t)$ can be interpreted as the probability of type I error spent by time t.

The specification of a boundary, $b(t)$, implies a particular function, $\alpha^*(t)$. Conversely, any function $\alpha^*(t)$ that is chosen to satisfy the three conditions

(1) $\alpha^*(0) = 0$, (2) $\alpha^*(t)$ is nondecreasing, and (3) $\alpha^*(1) = \alpha$ implies a particular boundary, $b(t)$.

In practice, the data are not analyzed continuously, so there are only a finite number of decision times. If the first analysis is done at time t, then by definition of $\alpha^*(t)$, we can spend a probability of $\alpha^*(t_1)$ at t_1 and a corresponding boundary value of b_1 can be computed. If the statistic is at least as large as b_1, the null hypothesis is rejected and the trial stops. Otherwise, the trial continues until a second analysis at time t_2. Since the amount of $\alpha^*(t_1)$ was spent at t_1, there is an amount $\alpha^*(t_2) - \alpha^*(t_1)$ to spend at t_2, and a boundary value, b_2, can be computed to spend this portion of the overall alpha level. This process continues until the end of the trial. It is important to note that at time t_i the boundary b_i can be calculated without knowing k, the total number of decision times, or t, $j = i + 1, \ldots, k$, the future decision times.

Subject only to the three conditions noted above, $\alpha^*(t)$ can be chosen to meet the needs of the study. Three possibilities are noted in Figure 1. The three possibilities are $\alpha_1^*(t)$, $\alpha_2^*(t)$, and $\alpha_3^*(t)$. Each represents a different accounting of the alpha error "spending."

In a study such as the Helsinki Heart Study where long-term effects were of interest, the function $\alpha_1^*(t)$ was chosen because it makes it more difficult to stop the study very early. On the other hand, the boundary values later in the study are closer to the nonsequential boundary (i.e., 1.96 for $\alpha = 0.05$). This was a desirable feature. In addition, the other functions are not strictly convex, and such functions have been observed to generate nondecreasing boundaries. Such boundaries allow the embarrassing possibility of a nonsignificant result at

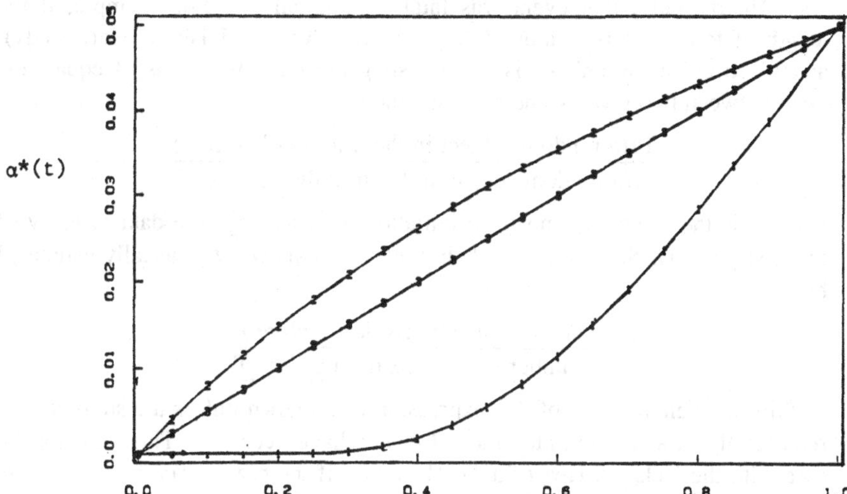

Figure 1 Mode of spending type I error probability for α_i^* $(i = 1, 2, 3)$ when $\alpha = 0.05$.

one analysis when, for some reason, a decision to stop the trial with a significant result at the previous analysis was deferred. The function $\alpha_1^*(t)$ is more robust than $\alpha_2^*(t)$ with respect to the specification of the time parameter (DeMets, personal communication). This was particularly an issue in the Helsinki Heart Study, for which the parameter of interest was time to cardiac events.

The time parameter, t, is not precisely defined except that it has the value 0 at the beginning of the study and the value 1 at the scheduled end of the trial. Loosely speaking, the time parameter, t, represents the proportion of statistical information that has been accumulated when the data are monitored. More precisely, t is the time parameter for a standard Brownian motion process $[B(t),\ 0 \leqslant t \leqslant 1]$. This process time parameter, t, is a monotone function of calendar time, but the functional relationship may not be the identity [i.e., $B(t) = t$]. The functional relationship may have different definitions for different applications.

For example, for an acute study where the response is observed immediately after a patient enters the study, if we monitor at calendar time, t, the corresponding process time is simply

$$\frac{\text{number of patients entered by } t}{\text{target sample size of the trial}}$$

With this definition, the application of the Lan–DeMets procedure is immediate.

However, the situation is more complex for a study where the response variable is survival time, or more generally, the time to an event. In the Helsinki Heart Study, that event was fatal or nonfatal MI. For example, if the length of follow-up is at most T (e.g., 5 years for the Helsinki Heart Study), and if we use a logrank statistic for testing the null hypothesis of equal survival between two groups, the process time is

$$\frac{\Pr(\text{a random subject in the trial dies before } t)}{\Pr(\text{a random subject in the trial dies before } T)}$$

where t is the calendar time from initiation of recruiting (the data of entry of the first patient). Since these probabilities are unknown, t is usually estimated by

$$\frac{\text{number of subjects dead before } t}{\text{number of subjects dead before } T}$$

Still, the denominator of this expression is unknown unless the study design requires the trial to continue until D events have occurred. This was not the case with the Helsinki Heart Study. However, if the hazard rate becomes quite stable after a short period of time (which appeared to be the case with the Helsinki Heart Study), the value of D that will be attained by the designed end of the follow-up, T, can be estimated. An overestimate of D will result in an underestimate of t and thus be conservative in the expenditure of type I error.

DeMets had indicated in personal communication that the Lan–DeMets procedure is quite robust if calendar time is used in lieu of the actual process time. The use of calendar time avoids the problem of estimating D, the number of events at the end of the study. Estimating D in the Helsinki Heart Study was complicated by the fact that subjects were in the trial for varying lengths of time. Although it was straightforward to estimate the probability of having an event by 5 years, it did not appear as straightforward to estimate the total number of events as of a given date. Calendar time also made no difference in the use of O'Brien–Fleming boundaries as long as time was set at 5 years.

Consequently, in determining the Lan–DeMets critical value, process time was approximated by calendar time. The one interim analysis that occurred at the 3-year point actually occurred 72.7% into the study time. The results were not significant. Using the function $\alpha^*(t)$ and the computer program provided by Lan and DeMets, the O'Brien–Fleming critical value at the final analysis was 4.02. The logrank statistic yielded a chi-square value of 5.8 (Frick, 1988).

V. CONCLUSION

The decision reached by the Ad Hoc Committee of the Helsinki Heart Council was to continue the trial until its scheduled completion. The results of the interim analysis were sufficiently positive to imply that the results after 5 years of study time would satisfy the objectives of the trial and reject the null hypothesis of equal treatment effect. In a joint press release, both the company and the Helsinki Heart Council expressed the optimistic results of the interim look at the data and indicated that the trial would continue without further looks until the scheduled endpoint.

VI. DISCUSSION

The most interesting aspect of the interim analysis of the Helsinki Heart Study was the fact that the type of sequential analysis was not described in the original protocol nor was the exact timing of interim looks indicated. All of the statistical details of the interim analysis had to be dealt with at the point that the decision was made to break the code and "peek" at the results. In March 1985 the temporary Ad Hoc Committee of the Helsinki Heart Council was formed. Its purpose was to "evaluate the progress of the HHS after the code break this summer and to make a recommendation to the Ethical Committee as to the future progress of" the study (company memorandum). The Ad Hoc Committee was provided with a blinded list of all definite and possible cardiovascular endpoints, cancer cases, and deaths up to a final date. The committee met to break the code for patients with these conditions. After applying the statistical analysis to the data, a simple chi-square test, the codes were resealed and the results were presented to the Ethical Committee. The Ethical Committee subsequently met to review the results and recommendations of the Ad Hoc Committee and suggest a plan for future action. As an additional safety measure to ensure an accurate decision with minimal bias, an outside committee reviewed all ECG recordings from a random sample of 100 patients with special emphasis on detecting false negative readings. This committee also reviewed the ECG readings of all patients with definite and possible endpoints. These reviews were done in a blinded fashion.

Following this rather careful and detailed interim analysis and the recommendation of continuing the trial without further looks to its scheduled completion, the task of adjusting for this one look was started. Biostatisticians from Helsinki and Parke-Davis investigated all possible methods of adjustment and consulted with various statisticians and clinical trials experts. We were limited, however, to few options because of the prior lack of planning for the interim looks. The Lan–DeMets procedure provided the most appropriate solution. The procedure applied well to our situation and was well accepted by both the scientific and regulatory communities. We were able to apply the Lan–DeMets analysis quite easily to the HHS data, and the result was a rejection of the null hypothesis with proper adjustment for an interim look at the data.

The interim analysis of the Helsinki Heart Study provides a vivid example of the nuances of clinical trials management. Adjustments for analyses not planned for in the original protocol were made and the very positive results of a landmark prospective trial were protected.

REFERENCES

Brown, M. S., and Goldstein, J. L. (1986). A receptor-mediated pathway for cholesterol homeostasis. *Science 232*(4746): 34–47.

Committee of Principal Investigators, W.H.O. Clofibrate Trial (1978). W.H.O. cooperative trial on primary prevention of ischemic heart disease using clofibrate to lower serum cholesterol: mortality follow-up report. *Br. Heart J. 40*: 1069–1118.

DeMets, D. L. (1984). Stopping guidelines vs. stopping rules: a practitioner's point of view. *Commun. Stat. Theory Methods 13*: 2395–2417.

Dixon, W. J. (1981). *BMDP Statistical Software Manual*, University of California Press, Berkeley, Calif.

Frick, M. H., et al. (1987). Helsinki Heart Study: primary prevention trial with gemfibrozil in middle-aged men with dyslipidemia. Safety of treatment, changes in risk factors, and incidence of coronary heart disease. *N. Engl. J. Med. 317*: 1237–1245.

Kannel, W. B., and Thom, T. J. (1986). In *The Heart* (J. W. Hurst, ed.), McGraw-Hill, New York, pp. 557–565.

Kannel, W. B., Castelli, W. P., and Gordon, T. (1979). Cholesterol in the prediction of atherosclerotic disease: new perspectives based on the Framingham study. *Ann. Intern. Med. 90*: 85–91.

Kim, K., and DeMets, D. L. (1985). Group sequential monitoring in clinical trials. *Technical Report 31,* University of Wisconsin–Madison, Madison, Wisc.

Lan, K. K. G., and DeMets, D. L. (1983). Discrete sequential boundaries for clinical trials. *Biometrika 70*: 659–663.

Lan, K. K. G., DeMets, D. L., and Halperin, M. (1984). More flexible sequential and non-sequential designs in long-term clinical trials. *Commun. Stat. Theory Methods 13*: 2339–2353.

Lipid Research Clinics Program (1984). The lipid research clinics coronary primary prevention trial results: I and II. *J. Am. Med. Assoc. 251*: 351–374.

National Heart, Lung, and Blood Institute (1982). Tenth report of the director, National Heart, Lung, and Blood Institute, Vol. 2, *Heart and Vascular Diseases.* 2. Magnitude of the Problem, NIH Publication 84-2357, U.S. Department of Health and Human Services, Washington, D.C., pp. 37–40.

O'Brien, P. C., and Fleming, T. R. (1979). A multiple testing procedure for clinical trials. *Biometrics 35*: 549–556.

Pocock, S. J. (1977). Group sequential methods in the design and analysis of clinical trials. *Biometrika 64*: 191–199.

Public Health Service (1983). *Vital Statistics of the United States, U.S. PHS., Hyattsville, Md., p. 7.*

SAS Institute (1985). *SAS Users Guide: Statistics,* Version 5 ed. SAS Institute, Inc., Cary, N.C.

Steinberg, D. (1987). Lipoproteins and the pathogenesis of atherosclerosis. *Circulation 76*(3): 508–514.

15

Plans for the Enalapril Post-MI Trial (CONSENSUS II)

Steven M. Snapinn

Merck Sharp & Dohme Research Laboratories, West Point, Pennsylvania

I. BACKGROUND

CONSENSUS II (the Cooperative New Scandinavian Enalapril Survival Study) is a trial comparing enalapril (an angiotensin converting enzyme inhibitor) and placebo in the treatment of acute myocardial infarction. The trial was designed and planned during 1989 and early 1990 and is currently (late 1990) recruiting toward a goal of 9000 patients. Although no results are yet available, in this section we describe the various procedural aspects of the trial and plans for statistical analysis, emphasizing the sequential stopping rule.

Angiotensin-converting enzyme (ACE) inhibitors act on the renin-angiotensin system, a hormonal regulatory system that helps maintain the body's blood pressure. One step in the process is the conversion of angiotensin I to angiotensin II, an extremely potent vasoconstrictor. By inhibiting the enzyme that facilitates this conversion, treatment with an ACE inhibitor results in vasodilation and reduction in blood pressure. Enalapril, marketed by Merck Sharp & Dohme (MSD), has Food and Drug Administration (FDA) approval for the treatment of hypertension.

Enalapril, given orally, also has approval as adjunctive therapy in the management of heart failure in patients who are not responding adequately to diuretics and digitalis, based largely on the results of the CONSENSUS trial (CONSENSUS Trial Study Group, 1987). Congestive heart failure is a condition in which the heart fails to perform adequately as a pump, resulting in symptoms which include shortness of breath and fatigue with low levels of activity. In its most severe form (New York Heart Association Class IV) these symptoms are present even at rest, and the patient's prognosis is extremely poor. In the CONSENSUS trial, enalapril or placebo was added to each patient's optimal therapy, and 6-month mortality from all causes was 44% with placebo compared to only 26% with enalapril ($p = 0.002$).

In CONSENSUS II enalapril is now being studied in a new condition: acute myocardial infarction. It is hypothesized that enalapril therapy will limit the amount of damage to heart tissue that occurs during a myocardial infarction, which will result in reduced mortailty, less likelihood of development of congestive heart failure, and fewer reinfarctions.

II. PROTOCOL

All patients admitted to a participating coronary care unit experiencing an acute myocardial infarction are screened for eligibility in the trial. The myocardial infarction must be documented by chest pain lasting more than 20 minutes and confirmed by either electrocardiographic evidence or elevated cardiac enzyme levels. Exclusion criterion include patients with blood pressure below 100 mmHg systolic or 60 mmHg diastolic, patients in cardiogenic shock, and patients with a clear indication for ACE inhibitors. Randomization and initial study treatment must be within 24 hours of the onset of chest pain.

Patients enrolled in the trial continue to receive any necessary medication to treat their myocardial infarction or any other condition, with the exception that ACE inhibitors are not permitted. The initial dose of the study drug (enalapril or placebo) is an intravenous formulation, administered by an infusion lasting 2 hours. The reason for this is the possibility that the first dose of an ACE inhibitor in patients with compromised heart function may cause the patient's blood pressure to drop dangerously low; a slow infusion gives the clinician much greater control over the patient's blood pressure than would an oral dose. After the initial intravenous infusion patients switch to oral study drug and remain on this for the 6-month duration of the trial. Following discharge from the hospital (approximately 10 to 14 days after randomization) patients return for follow-up visits at 1 month, 3 months, and 6 months after randomization. Patients are not followed within the study context beyond their 6-month visit.

The primary objective of this trial is to demonstrate a reduction in all-cause 6-month mortality due to enalapril. Based on prior studies in acute myocardial infarction the 6-month mortality rate in the placebo group was predicted to be

12%. A reduction due to enanalpril of 20% (to 9.6%) was deemed to be both clinically important and reasonable to expect. However, due to the uncertainty in both the placebo-group mortality and the reduction due to enalapril, as well as to the importance of this trial and the difficulty in replicating it, it was decided to plan the trial with relatively high power. The sample size of 9000 patients (4500 per group) is based on 95% power to detect a difference in 6-month mortality of 12% in the placebo group compared to 9.6% in the enalapril with a two-sided chi-square test at the 5% significance level.

Although the power is based on a chi-square test, the major statistical analysis will be based on survival analysis procedures. In particular, the Kaplan–Meier mortality curves will be presented and the difference between the groups assessed with the logrank statistic. There will be analyses of the primary endpoint (all-cause 6-month mortality) as well as many secondary analyses, including 1-month mortality, mortality for specific causes of death, time to first reinfarction, and time to first hospitalization for congestive heart failure. Major subgroups of interest include patients who had had one or more prior infarcts, patients who experienced an anterior infarction, and patients 70 years of age or older. All analyses will be based on an intent-to-treat approach, which includes all randomized patients regardless of adherence to the protocol. Based on past experience with the CONSENSUS trial, in which all 253 randomized patients were followed without a single lost to follow-up, the number of patients lost to follow-up in CONSENSUS II is expected to be small.

III. MONITORING AND DATA COLLECTION

CONSENSUS II is being run under the auspices of two independent committees: the Steering Committee and the Safety Monitoring Committee. The Steering Committee is responsible for the scientific integrity of the trial, including development and approval of the protocol, monitoring adherence to the protocol, decisions on all scientific questions arising during the trial, and publication of the results. This group consists of three clinicians from each of the four participating Scandinavian countries (Denmark, Finland, Norway, Sweden), one statistician, and one representative from the sponsor (Merck Sharp & Dohme).

The Safety Monitoring Committee is responsible for the safety of the patients participating in the trial. This committee, which consists of three clinicians and a statistician, meets periodically to review unblinded statistical analyses of the data prepared by an MSD statistician. During the course of the trial this statistician and the Safety Monitoring Committee are the only ones unblinded to the results. In case of a safety concern or of convincing drug efficacy, the Safety Monitoring Committee is charged with making an appropriate recommendation to the Steering Committee. The recommendation might be to stop the trial or it might be a protocol amendment, but in either case the ultimate decision is made by the Steering Committee.

With over 80 centers in four countries recruiting 9000 patients, the rate of data flow in this trial is enormous. The data are stored initially in our ORACLE databases, one in each of the four countries. The procedures in place to collect, enter, and verify the data are an attempt to obtain clean data as quickly as possible, for the purposes of study monitoring and safety analysis.

Copies of the work booklets are picked up by MSD personnel or mailed from the investigator to that country's Merck subsidiary immediately after a patient has visited the clinic. Prior to entry into the computer, the work booklets are reviewed by a medical monitor in order to identify and correct errors made by the investigator when filling out the form. The data-entry screens themselves are a second line of defense against errors. Logic built into the screens can check for various types of errors: for example, comparing values to normal ranges and checking dates for consistency. The data-entry system also encodes all relevant textual terms (such as adverse experiences and concomitant therapies) using the dictionaries developed by MSD. In addition, a set of computerized screening queries is run against the data to identify more complicated types of errors. After the data have been entered and verified, case report forms (CRFs) are printed sent to the investigator for signature; these become the official study documents.

Special provision is made for entering all key endpoint information. When the patient experiences a major endpoint (reinfarction, hospitalization, or death), the investigator immediately fills out a special form and sends it to the subsidiary. These forms are given the highest priority by MSD, and as a result the endpoint information in the database is usually out of date by no more than a few days. The data are eventually migrated to a consolidated ORACLE database in the United States, where they are subject to further medical review and data verification. Special procedures are in place for making "postsignature" corrections, which ensure that the subsidiary databases remain in agreement with the consolidated database. While the consolidated database will be the one used for the final analysis and filing with regulatory agencies, the subsidiary databases, which are more current, are used for interim analysis.

IV. SEQUENTIAL ANALYSIS PLANS

Given the large number of expected deaths in this trial (approximately 1000), the Safety Monitoring Committee felt strongly that they would need to review the data very frequently. The tentative procedure was for a first analysis after the first 50 deaths and approximately monthly analyses thereafter. Because of the frequency and possibly irregular schedule of the interim analyses, the primary consideration in planning the sequential analysis procedure was flexibility. Accordingly, the procedure that will be used is one based on conditional probabilities, in the spirit of the procedures proposed by Lan et al. (1982).

The basic idea behind this type of procedure is the following. If the data collected at an interim analysis determine the outcome at the planned conclusion of the trial with very high probability, the trial is stopped early. The advantage of this type of procedure is extreme flexibility; since the procedure does not involve repeated significance tests, the frequency and scheduling of the interim analyses is relatively unimportant. The major disadvantage depends on the assumptions made about the distribution of the future, unobserved data. If the conservative assumption is made that the future data will follow the null hypothesis (as in stochastic curtailment), the procedure will rarely stop the trial early. On the other hand, if a less conservative assumption is made, the expected sample size will be reduced, but the effect of the procedure on the overall significance level is difficult to assess. In CONSENSUS II a less conservative assumption about the future data is made, but special measures are taken to assure that the overall significance level is not adversely affected. This procedure is described in detail by Snapinn (1990) and summarized below.

Let p_A and p_B represent the hypothesized event rates in groups A and B upon which the power calculations are based, and let p_{null} represent the common event rate in the two groups under the null hypothesis. Now suppose that an interim analysis has been performed after n_1 patients out of a planned total of n ($n_1/2$ in each group), and the observed event rates in the two groups are q_A and q_B. Also suppose that the one-sided alternative hypothesis is that $p_A > p_B$. For the purpose of calculating the probability of eventual rejection of the null hypothesis, the future event rates in the two groups, r_A and r_B, are predicted to be weighted averages of the observed rates and the null rates, with the weights based on the observed and future sample sizes:

$$r_A = \frac{n_1 q_A + n_2 p_{null}}{n} \qquad (1)$$

$$r_B = \frac{n_1 q_B + n_2 p_{null}}{n}$$

where $n_2 = n - n_1$. Notice that early in the trial the predicted future rates are nearly equal to the null rate in both groups, but that later in the trial the predicted future rate in each group becomes closer to that group's observed rate.

Using the observed data and the predictions above for the future event rates, and making normal-theory assumptions, the predicted probability of rejecting the null hypothesis at the end of the trial can be calculated as

$$\Phi\left(\frac{n_1(q_A - q_B)/2 + n_2(r_A - r_B)/2 + z_{1-\alpha}[n_1 q(1-q) + n_2 r(1-r)]^{1/2}}{[n_2 r(1-r)]^{1/2}}\right) \qquad (2)$$

where $q = (q_A + q_B)/2$ and $r = (r_A + r_B)/2$. The value in (2) is compared to a prespecified cutpoint, p_{rej}, and if greater than p_{rej} the trial is stopped early with the conclusion that the event rate in group A is greater than that in group B. Clearly, the possibility of early rejection of the null hypothesis tends to inflate the significance level of the test, since some trials that will eventually end in acceptance will have very positive early results. Conversely, if early acceptance of the null hypothesis were also possible, this would tend to deflate the significance level, due to the possibility of false early acceptances. The goal of the procedure to be used in CONSENSUS II is to balance the probabilities of false early rejection and false early acceptance, thereby maintaining the overall significance level of the test.

The future event rates in the two groups for the purpose of calculating the probability of early acceptance are

$$r_A = \frac{n_1 q_A + n_2 p_A}{n} \qquad (3)$$

$$r_B = \frac{n_1 q_B + n_2 p_B}{n}$$

Notice that early in the trial these predicted future rates are nearly equal to the rates under the alternative hypothesis, but that later in the trial the predicted future rate in each group becomes closer to that group's observed rate. These predicted future rates are used in (2) to determine the probability of eventual acceptance of the null hypothesis, and this value is compared to a predetermined cutoff point, p_{acc}, to determine whether or not to stop the trial for early acceptance.

The significance level of the overall procedure is maintained by an appropriate choice of p_{rej} and p_{acc}. Based on simulation results, the values $p_{rej} = 0.95$ and $p_{acc} = 0.90$ appear to work well and are the values that will be used in CONSENSUS II. Simulation studies show that with these constants the effect on the significance level of the procedure is negligible, and in addition, the cost in terms of reduction in power is small.

While a valid statistical stopping rule is essential, in practice this will be used only as a guideline by the Safety Monitoring Committee. The committee will have to consider many issues besides the primary efficacy analysis when making their decision, including analyses of secondary endpoints, especially safety issues. Another advantage of the procedure used here is that the predicted probabilities of future rejection and acceptance can be used by the committee as a valuable monitoring tool when weighing all the evidence to make their difficult decision.

V. CONCLUSION

In a trial with a large number of expected deaths, the issue of safety takes on a tremendous importance, and both the data-handling procedures and the sequential stopping rule for CONSENSUS II have been designed to address this issue. The database design and data-handling procedures allow quick access to a clean and up-to-date database. And the sequential analysis procedure gives the Safety Monitoring Committee a valid statistical stopping rule as a guideline while allowing them to monitor the trial as they see fit.

REFERENCES

CONSENSUS Trial Study Group (1987). Effects of enalapril on mortality in severe congestive heart failure: results of the cooperative North Scandinavian enalapril survival study (CONSENSUS). *N. Engl. J. Med. 316:* 23, 1429–1435.

Lan, K. K. G., Simon, R., and Halperin, M. (1982). Stochastically curtailed tests in long-term clinical trials. *Commun. Stat. C1:* 207–219.

Snapinn, S. M. (1992). Monitoring clinical trials with a conditional probability sequential stopping rule. *Stat. Med.* (in preparation).

VI

APPLICATIONS IN GASTROINTESTINAL CLINICAL DRUG DEVELOPMENT

16

Early Termination of Two Trials of Misoprostol in the Prevention of NSAID-Induced Gastric Ulceration

Karl E. Peace

Biopharmaceutical Research Consultants, Inc., Ann Arbor, Michigan

I. BACKGROUND

A few years ago, I had the responsibility of running a large-scale clinical research program of the synthetic prostaglandin (PGE_2) analog, misoprostol. Clinical and statistical evidence from the program formed the primary basis for NDA approval in the United States of misoprostol in the prevention of nonsteroidal anti-inflammatory drug (NSAID)-induced gastric ulcers in osteoarthritic patients requiring NSAIDs in the management of their arthritic symptoms. Statistical aspects of the program, particularly with regard to interim analyses, are presented in this chapter. The program consisted of two identical protocols. A rationale for the program is presented in Section II. The protocols are reviewed in Section III. Monitoring and data management considerations are presented in Section IV. Meeting with the U.S. Regulatory agency is addressed in Section V. Interim analysis plans are outlined in Section VI. Conclusions and final remarks appear in Section VII.

II. RATIONALE

It is important for the reader to understand the rationale for conducting the clinical research. No one conducts a clinical trial merely to show statistical significance. Clinical trials should be conducted to answer a medically and/or scientifically relevant question, when the answer cannot be determined from available information (Peace, 1991). Gastric ulceration, induced by the chronic administration of NSAIDs, represents potentially a major health problem. Some factors to consider are (1) the socioeconomic impact, (2) pathophysiological aspects, (3) clinical management dilemmas, (4) the effect of NSAIDs on the gastroduodenal mucosa of arthritic patients, and (5) the mucosal protective potential of misoprostol against injury by NSAIDs. In discussing these factors in sequence, the views of some of the world's leading researchers in ulcer disease are summarized. These include: Langman (1987), Collins (1987), Roth (1987), Lanza (1987), and Cohen (1987).

Many clinicians believe that NSAIDs cause dyspepsia, ulcers to develop in the stomach and duodenum, and complications of perforation and bleeding. It has, however, been difficult to obtain confirmatory evidence that supports these views. In clinical trials of NSAIDs, although dyspepsia has been noted, ulcer and ulcer complications due to NSAIDs have been rare, and they have been generally well tolerated. Similarly, surveillance studies in both the United Kingdom and the United States have failed to suggest any significant hazard of NSAIDs (Langman, 1987).

In contrast, adverse effects due to the use of NSAIDs account for approximately 20 to 25% of all adverse events reported in the United Kingdom and the United States. Retrospective case-control studies have indicated that the likelihood of ulcer complications among NSAID users may be as high as five times greater than that among nonusers. Based on data from the United Kingdom, ulcer mortality rates may be increasing in the elderly population. This increase has occurred concurrently with an increase in NSAID prescriptions. Although younger persons may be prone to suffer only from dyspepsia following NSAID use, serious adverse events may be prevalent among the elderly (Langman, 1987).

The first NSAID, aspirin—acetylsalicylic acid—was synthesized in 1883 and was widely used to treat arthritic conditions by the last decade of the nineteenth century. Within 15 years of the introduction of aspirin, the medical literature described aspirin-associated symptoms and damage to the upper gastrointestinal (GI) tract that are being recognized and described today. Subsequently, the synthesis of nonaspirin NSAIDs produced drugs with therapeutic profiles and patterns of GI toxicity similar to those of aspirin. In 1971, Sir John Vane proposed that aspirin exerts its anti-inflammatory and antipyretic effects through the inhibition of the synthesis of prostaglandins (PGs). It was found to inhibit PG cyclooxygenase, the enzyme that converts arachidonic acid to all active prostanoids. Subsequently, it was shown that all NSAIDs inhibit this enzyme and therefore decrease the synthesis of active PGs, including

PGE_2. It is widely accepted that PGs (particularly PGE_2 and PGF_2) modulate inflammatory response. They improve the pain and inflammatory properties of other mediators and directly affect the cellular component of the response. Biochemically, all nonaspirin NSAIDs are more potent than aspirin in inhibiting PG cyclooxygenase in vitro. However, this additional potency is not directly reflected in either their anti-inflammatory or toxic effects (Collins, 1987).

The question arises then as to why NSAIDs are associated with damage to the upper GI tract, even when these drugs are given in suppository form. The story that has emerged appears to implicate their ability to decrease PG synthesis, by a mechanism identical to that by which they exert their anti-inflammatory and antipyretic activity (Collins, 1987). NSAIDs appear to cause peptic damage by two mechanisms. One is by *local* physiochemical disruption of the gastric cytoprotective barrier. The other is through *systemic* inhibition of the cytoprotective mechanism, probably due to their effect on cytoprotective PGs. The conventional view of the cytoprotective mechanism is that several components are involved: (1) a mucus layer that is adherent to the gastric epithelium, (2) the production of bicarbonate ions by the underlying mucosal cell, (3) a rapid reproductive property of the cells of the gastric and intestinal mucosa, and (4) submucosal blood flow which is sufficient to support these factors and to remove hydrogen ions that have diffused back from the intestinal lumen (Collins, 1987).

Prostanoids (particularly PGE_1 and PGE_2) have been shown to enhance these components. Thus, by inhibiting these prostanoids, either by the local or systemic action of NSAIDs, cytoprotection is reduced, thus creating a situation in which a breach in the gastric mucosa may occur. The barrier-breaking effect of aspirin can be observed directly by endoscopy, whereas the systemic effect is evident when these drugs are given by routes other than the oral route. This condition can be induced in animals by intravenous or intraperitoneal injection and in humans by rectal administration. In a real clinical therapeutic situation, the gastric damage associated with NSAIDs is likely to be due to a combination of these two effects, although it is unclear how they contribute to damage caused by particular NSAIDs (Collins, 1987).

The primary gastric cytoprotective mechanism may well be breached locally and systemically by NSAIDs, which allows gastric acid and pepsin to attack the underlying mucosa. In peptic ulcer disease not associated with NSAIDs, it has been shown that reducing the hydrogen ion concentration of the luminal content with H_2-receptor blocking drugs contributes to ulcer healing and to a reduction of gastritis. The H_2-receptor blocker cimetidine has been shown not to influence the healing of peptic ulcers associated with NSAID use when the NSAID continues to be taken. It may therefore be assumed that such ulcers are not due primarily to gastric acid assault. Rather, they appear to be NSAID-caused biochemical lesions that persist as long as the NSAID is ingested (Collins, 1987).

Some patients develop peptic ulcers within weeks of ingesting NSAIDs, whereas others appear not to develop such lesions until after years of treatment. The reasons for such heterogeneity are not known (Collins, 1987). The osteoarthritic patient who must stop taking anti-inflammatory medications because of serious gastropathy (gastromucosal damage), with or without symptoms (as many as half the patients have no symptoms) faces compromised control. But to continue such NSAID therapy puts these patients at risk of progressing or recurring gastric lesions (Roth, 1987).

Injury to the gastric mucosal seen with NSAIDs represents the major drawback in the treatment of inflammatory musculoskeletal disorders with these agents. Clinically, the injury is manifested primarily by mucosal erosion and hemorrhage, occasionally by ulcer, and rarely with perforation. Several techniques have been used to study these effects. These include (1) fecal blood loss studies, (2) retrospective reviews of hospital admissions for gastrointestinal bleeding ulcer and perforation, (3) prospective studies of patients taking NSAIDs, and (4) endoscopic studies of normal volunteers. Extensive reviews of hospital admissions in the United Kingdom and the United States have shown an increased relative risk of bleeding, hemorrhage, and perforation in patients being treated with NSAIDs. A large number of short-term, double-blind, controlled studies in normal volunteers have demonstrated these toxic effects on the gastric and duodenal mucosa (Lanza, 1987).

All NSAIDs injure the gastric and duodenal mucosa to some degree. As Collins (1987) points out, at least two mechanisms have been implicated in such injury: (1) direct local irritation, and (2) inhibition of cyclooxygenase activity. The relative importance of these mechanisms depends on the drug. Gastric acid appears to be a prerequisite for injury. Acid plays two key roles: (1) it facilitates absorption of the NSAID; and (2) it causes injury when its back-diffusion exceeds the buffering capacity of the mucosa (Cohen, 1987).

Two double-blind, placebo-controlled, endoscopic studies examined the ability of misoprostol to protect against NSAID injury. Both studies used misoprostol in 200-μg doses (acid inhibitory) concurrently with NSAIDs for approximately 1 week. Lanza (1986) used 500 mg q.i.d. of tolmetin and 200 μg q.i.d. of misoprostol in 60 subjects for 6 days. He found a significant reduction in both gastric and duodenal injury compared to placebo. Aadland et al. (1986) used 500 mg b.i.d. of naproxen and 200 μg b.i.d. of misoprostol for 7 days in 32 volunteers. They found a significant reduction in gastric lesions compared with placebo. No troublesome side effects were reported in either study (Cohen, 1987).

These two studies indicate that misoprostol may prevent gastric mucosal injury due to NSAID use, as assessed by endoscopy. They do not prove that misoprostol is effective in the prevention or treatment of NSAID-induced symptoms, bleeding, ulceration, or perforation, nor can they be adduced as evidence supporting prostaglandin therapy for peptic ulcer disease (Cohen, 1987). However, since misoprostol is known to increase mucus production and to have gastric antisecretory properties, through increasing the production of bicarbonate, the data clearly point to the need for controlled clinical trials of misoprostol in osteoarthritic patients requiring NSAIDs.

III. PROTOCOLS

The clinical research program consisted of two identical protocols in osteoarthritic patients requiring any of three NSAIDs in the management of their symptoms. Each protocol had two strata. Stratum 1 represented patients who at entry had endoscopically confirmed upper gastrointestinal (UGI) or gastric ulcers. Stratum 2 represented patients who at entry were without gastric ulcers as confirmed by endoscopy. Within the treatment stratum, patients were randomized in balanced, double-blind fashion to either a placebo group, or a 200-μg misoprostol q.i.d. group. Within the prophylaxis stratum, patients were randomized in balanced, double-blind fashion to either a placebo group, a 100-μg misoprostol q.i.d. group, or a 200-μg misoprostol q.i.d. group. All patients were to return for follow-up endoscopy and other clinical evaluations after 4 and 8 weeks of study medication administration. Patients in the prophylaxis stratum were also to return for evaluation at the end of their 12-week study medication administration period.

A. Objectives

The objectives were (1) to evaluate the efficacy of misoprostol in treating NSAID-induced UGI symptoms and ulcers; and (2) to demonstrate the effectiveness of misoprostol on UGI symptom relief and in the prevention of gastric ulcers.

B. Admission Criteria

The criteria for inclusion were: (1) the patient must be of legal age of consent or older; (2) males, or females of non-childbearing potential (postmenopausal or surgically sterilized) or practicing an acceptable method of birth control; (3) currently taking either ibuprofen, piroxicam, or naproxen as NSAID therapy for osteoarthritis; (4) currently, the patient has abdominal pain; (5) to enter the treatment stratum, the patient must have an endoscopically identified gastric ulcer which, in the opinion of the investigator, is due to NSAID therapy and is anticipated to require NSAID therapy for at least 8 consecutive weeks after the first dose of study medication; (6) to enter the prophylaxis stratum, the patient must have no gastric ulcers on endoscopy and require at least 3 months of NSAID therapy for their arthritic condition; and (7) the patient (or next of kin) has given informed consent for participation in the study.

C. Efficacy Parameters

The efficacy parameters for the treatment stratum were: (1) ulcers healed at 4 or 8 weeks, as confirmed by endoscopy; (2) UGI pain relief as derived from pain ratings recorded by the patient in a daily diary; and (3) relief of other UGI symptoms. Of these, ulcer healing was primary. The efficacy parameters for the prophylaxis stratum were: (1) ulcer development, as confirmed by endoscopy at weeks 4, 8, or 12; (2) UGI pain relief as derived from pain ratings recorded by the patient in a daily diary; and (3) relief of other UGI symptoms. Of these, the prevention of ulcer development was primary. UGI pain was rated by the patient according to the following scales:

UGI day pain rating scale:

0	None	I had no abdominal pain.
1	Mild	I had some abdominal pain, but it did not interrupt my normal activities.
2	Moderate	I had some abdominal pain sufficient to interrupt my normal activity.
3	Severe	I had severe disabling abdominal pain.

UGI night pain rating scale:

0	None	I had no abdominal pain
1	Mild	I had some abdominal pain, but I was able to go back to sleep.
2	Moderate	I had abdominal pain sufficient to keep me awake for long periods.
3	Severe	I had severe abdominal pain that kept me awake most of the night.

The ratings were recorded on a diary provided by the sponsor as part of the case report forms. The diaries were collected at each follow-up visit.

D. Sample Size Determination

Per protocol sample size determinations revealed that 200 evaluatable patients would be needed to address the primary treatment objective, and 450 evaluatable patients would be needed to address the primary prophylaxis objective.

The numbers for the treatment stratum were determined on the basis of a 5% one-sided (Peace, 1989) type I error rate and a 95% power to detect a 22% difference in healing rates, given an expected healing rate of 50% in the placebo group. The numbers for the prophylaxis stratum were determined on the basis of a 5% one-sided type I error rate and a 95% power to detect a 15% difference in ulcer development rates, given an expected ulcer rate of 25% in the placebo group.

E. Efficacy Endpoints

The primary efficacy endpoints in the treatment stratum was the proportion of patients with healed (complete reepithelization of the ulcer crater) ulcers by 8 weeks. The primary efficacy endpoint in the prophylaxis stratum was the proportion of patients with ulcers by 12 weeks. The secondary endpoint in both strata was the proportion of patients without daytime or nighttime pain. The Mantel–Haenszel (1959) or Fisher's exact test was (to be) used for *statistical analyses* of the endpoints. No plans were provided in the protocol for formal statistical interim analyses of the efficacy endpoints. However, the safety data were to be carefully monitored.

IV. MONITORING AND DATA MANAGEMENT

Successful clinical development programs require good clinical trial management. An important aspect of clinical trial management is staying current with enrollment, dropout, and completion rates of each clinical trial. This allows taking corrective action early, if needed. Beyond an interest in the progress of clinical trials, there is usually strong interest in knowing safety and efficacy outcomes prior to study completion. These interests are genuine and may represent a concern for patient safety, a need to plan future studies, or a desire to stop the study early to permit earlier filing of the registrational dossier (Peace, 1987).

All studies should be *monitored* for *safety*. Ideally, this should be done on a per patient basis without knowledge of the treatment to which the patient was assigned. Monitoring by treatment group can be done if this is important to make a clinical decision as to whether the study should be stopped for safety reasons. In this case it is usually sufficient to separate the safety data into treatment groups without revealing group identity (Peace, 1987). Since the design of studies of a new drug is almost always based on efficacy considerations, it is not likely that monitoring for safety while a study is ongoing will in itself compromise (efficacy) study objectives. However, it is good practice to indicate in the protocol what procedures will be used to monitor safety (Peace, 1989).

As indicated previously, most studies of new drugs are designed to provide answers to questions of efficacy. Therefore, *monitoring* for *efficacy* while the study is in progress, particularly in an unplanned, ad hoc manner, will almost always be seen to compromise the answers. If it is anticipated that the efficacy data will be looked at prior to study termination, for whatever reason, it is wise to include in the protocol an appropriate plan for doing this. The plan should address type I error penalty considerations, what steps will be taken to minimize bias, and permit *early termination.*

The early termination procedure of O'Brien and Fleming (1979) is usually reasonable. It allows periodic interim analyses of the data while the study is in progress, while preserving most nominal type I error for the final analysis upon scheduled study completion—provided that there was insufficient evidence to terminate the study after an interim analysis. The recent paper by the PMA (1991) working group addressing the topic of interim analyses provides a good summary of the concerns about, and procedures for, interim analyses.

As indicated previously, we did not plan to perform interim analyses of the two misoprostol studies at the time we developed the protocols. The primary reason for this was due to the uncertainty associated with our estimate of the placebo ulcer development rate. Although we used 25%, the literature reflected wide variability, and no studies had followed osteoarthritic patients who were on the three NSAIDs required by the protocols for 3 months with monthly endoscopic examination for ulcer development. We did, however, monitor the studies closely and computerized the data aggressively. We knew on a weekly basis the status of the studies as to entry, completion, and ulcer development, without splitting the data into the three treatment groups. Table 1 summarizes such data at about the halfway point during conduct of the studies. Ignoring study and treatment group and based on patient information in the computerized data base, we noticed that the incidence of ulcer development

Table 1 Enrollment/Completion Status of Misoprostol Studies at Approximately Study Midpoint

Protocol	Stratum[a]	Patients entered	Patients completed
1	Tx	87	66
	Px	275	132
2	Tx	120	84
	Px	253	130
1/2	Tx	207	150
	Px	528	262

[a] Tx, treatment; Px, prophylaxis.

Table 2 Ulcer Status of Completed Prophylaxis Patients in Computerized Data Base

Patients	No ulcer	Ulcer	Unknown	% Ulcer
215	156	18	41	8.4[a]
215	156	18	41	10.3[b]
215	156	18	41	27.4[c]

[a] Crude or best-case estimate (an underestimate).
[b] Reduced estimate.
[c] Worst-case estimate (an overestimate).

in the prophylaxis stratum may range from a crude rate of 8.4% to a worst-case rate of 27.4% (Table 2). Parenthetically, comparable rates were also observed among prophylaxis patients whose case report form data had not yet been computerized (Table 3). However, all the ulcers could have been in one of the treatment groups. If this were the case, the incidence within that group could have been three times as high, or anywhere from 25.2 to 82.2%. We therefore felt compelled, on ethical grounds, to meet with the Food and Drug Administration (FDA) to discuss plans for performing an interim analysis of the studies, with the possibility of stopping the studies early.

V. FDA MEETING

We met with the FDA around mid-October 1987. We discussed the data and our procedures for stopping the trials, collecting any remaining data, and statistical analyses. Some of the information presented at the meeting is contained in Tables 1, 2, and 3 in addition to that contained in Tables 4 and 5. Table 4 reflects 215 patients with 18 ulcers being split in a reasonably balanced way

Table 3 Ulcer Status of Completed Prophylaxis Patients Not in Computerized Data Base

Patients	No ulcer	Ulcer	Unknown	% Ulcer
43	34	5	4	11.6[a]
43	34	5	4	12.8[b]
43	34	5	4	20.9[c]

[a] Crude or best-case estimate (an underestimate).
[b] Reduced estimate.
[c] Worst-case estimate (an overestimate).

Table 4 Ulcer Status of Completed Prophylaxis Patients in Computerized Data Base: Possible Grouping Reflecting Dose Proportionality

Group	Patients	No ulcer	Ulcer	Unknown	% Ulcer[a]
A	70	58	0	12	0[b]
B	71	53	6	12	8.5[c]
C	74	45	12	17	16.2[d]
	215	156	18	41	8.4[a]

[a] Crude or best-case estimate (an underestimate).
[b] Worst case = 17.1%; reduced estimate = 0%.
[c] Worst case = 25.4%; reduced estimate = 10.2%.
[d] Worst case = 39.2%; reduced estimate = 21.1%.

across the three treatment groups, with numbers of ulcers per group reflecting a reasonable but perhaps conservative dose-response relationship. Table 5 reflects comparative analyses of the data in Table 4 using confidence intervals and Fisher's exact test (expected to be more conservative than the Mantel-Haenszel test). It should be stressed that Table 4 represents a reasonable distribution of the total number (18) of ulcers under an assumption of dose proportionality. At the time of our meeting with the FDA, the blind had not been broken, nor had we separated the data according to blinded group labels. Since we had not planned to do a formal interim analysis at the protocol development stage, we wanted to make the case to the FDA that we should perform an

Table 5 Ulcer Status of Completed Prophylaxis Patients in Computerized Data Base: Possible Grouping Reflecting Dose Proportionality—*p*-Values and Confidence Intervals

Comparison[a]	% Difference	Standard error	90% CI[b]	*p*-value[c]
B–A (B.C.)	8.5	0.033	(3.1%;13.9%)	0.015/0.028
C–A (B.C.)	16.2	0.043	(9.2%;23.2%)	0.000/0.000
B–A (W.C.)	8.3	0.069	(−2.9%;19.6%)	0.162/0.304
C–A (W.C.)	13.8	0.064	(3.2%;24.4%)	0.003/0.005
B–A (R)	10.2	0.039	(3.7%;16.7%)	0.014/0.027
C–A (R)	21.1	0.054	(12.2%;30.0%)	0.000/0.000

[a] B.C., best case; W.C., worst case; R, reduced.
[b] Normal approximation.
[c] Fisher's exact test (one-sided/two-sided).

interim analysis on ethical grounds, and that if dose-response was observed, we be able to stop the studies early based on a demonstration of prophylaxis efficacy. We wanted to be convincing that if an interim analysis was done, it would be performed in a statistically valid, bona fide manner.

There were three issues that received considerable discussion at the meeting with the agency: (1) When should the trials be terminated? (2) To what extent should blinding be maintained during the interim analysis? (3) At what type I error level should we conduct the interim analysis?

Concerning when to terminate, three possibilities were considered: We could terminate immediately; we could terminate based upon enrollment after 4 additional weeks; or we could continue entry until completion of the interim analysis and then decide on the basis of that analysis. The first two of these possibilities exact no penalty on the type I error, provided that we were prepared to live with the results. The third would, however, and is consistent with the philosophy for performing interim analyses.

Blinding considerations consisted of to what extent investigators, patients, and company personnel should be blinded as to the results of the interim analysis. The primary concern was that if we failed to terminate the studies on the basis of the interim analysis results, the study objectives would not be compromised by having performed the interim analysis.

As to the size of the type I error for the interim analysis, we could take the O'Brien–Fleming approach and use 0.005, and if there was insufficient evidence to stop, allow the studies to continue to completion and conduct the final analysis at the 0.048 level. Another possibility was to use a two-stage Pocock (1977) procedure, which would allocate a type I error of 0.031 to each stage. Yet another possibility was to conduct the interim analysis at the 0.01 level, with the final analysis being conducted at a level determined as per Lan and DeMets (1983) or Peace and Schriver (1987) if insufficient evidence existed for termination at the interim analysis.

The agency was receptive to us performing an interim analysis subject to providing them with written plans. Such plans would address the three issues noted above, as well as any others that would reflect positively on the scientific and statistical validity of the exercise.

VI. INTERIM ANALYSIS PLANS

The interim analysis plans that were submitted to the FDA are summarized below:

1. The interim analysis will be based on all patients who will complete the prophylaxis stratum by October 26, 1987. Completed patients are those who actually completed 12 weeks of treatment and those who terminated prematurely.

2. The interim analysis will focus on the intent-to-treat population:
   a. All patients who entered the studies according to the inclusion/exclusion criteria and who took at least one dose of study medication will be included in the analysis.
   b. All patients who failed to have at least one follow-up endoscopy will be handled in two ways:
      (1) As not having an ulcer—this provides the "crude rate" estimate of ulcer development. It is also the best-case estimate.
      (2) As having an ulcer—this provides the worst-case estimate.

   The best case is the preferred analysis.

Although life-table estimates could be computed, they are not likely to prove fruitful, as there are only two intermediate points of outcome assessment between entry and completion of treatment.

3. The primary efficacy endpoint and the one upon which termination decisions will be based is ulcer development at anytime during the 3-month prophylaxis treatment phase.

4. Symptomatic relief, in particular the proportions of patients without daytime or nighttime pain, are secondary efficacy endpoints. These will be displayed and analyzed but will not contribute to the termination decision nor will they invoke a type I error penalty.

5. Completed case report forms on patients from the studies will undergo blinded review by clinical data editors in the company's data processing department prior to being sent to an outside third-party consulting firm, where the data will be entered into a computerized data base without breaking the blind.

6. Once entry has been completed and the database has been quality assured by the third-party group, they will break the seal containing the randomization schedule and enter patient numbers and treatment group assignment into a separate file that will be quality assured. The treatment groups—placebo q.i.d., misoprostol 100 μg q.i.d., and misoprostol 200 μg q.i.d.—will be relabeled in a randomized manner as A, B, and C. The data file containing patient number and the group labels A, B, and C will then be merged with the data base.

7. Initial analyses will consist of the three pairwise comparisons A versus B, B versus C, and A versus C in terms of the proportions of patients developing ulcers by the end of 3 months of treatment. These analyses are to facilitate the decision as to study termination and will be carried out using Fisher's exact test. The analyses will be performed by the third-party group, who will also compare the treatment groups at baseline in terms of factors such as prior NSAID use in an attempt to identify whether there are factors other than the prospective treatments received that may explain ulcer development. Any such factor identified will necessitate performing adjusted analyses such as Mantel–

Haenszel. Any display reflecting analysis results, until such time as the decision is made to terminate the studies, will reflect the group labels A, B, and C.

8. Once the initial analyses are completed, the third-party group will report to Karl E. Peace the *p*-value corresponding to a comparison of the top-dose misoprostol group with the placebo group. If this *p*-value is less than or equal to 0.01, the studies will be terminated immediately. Full analyses of all study data will then proceed for the purpose of making a submission to the FDA for an NSAID-induced ulcer prevention claim. Data on patients who had not completed the studies at the time of the interim analysis will be appended.

VII. CONCLUSION AND FINAL REMARKS

Several facets of the misoprostol treatment and prevention of NSAID-induced gastric ulceration program deserve comment. First, the study population consisted of osteoarthritic patients who required NSAIDs in the management of their arthritic symptoms. Such patients were being treated for their arthritic condition by a rheumatologist. However, the condition being studied with respect to the effectiveness of misoprostol was gastric ulceration believed to be caused by NSAID administration. Therefore, for the purpose of the clinical research program, the rheumatologist was not the primary investigator. The endoscopist was. At each center, a board-certified gastroenterologist was identified who assessed the degree of ulceration and the presence of UGI symptoms.

Second, two identical protocols comprised the program, yet for the purpose of the interim analysis, they were treated as one multicenter protocol. Concerning this point, it is important to realize that since the protocols were identical and patients were randomized to treatment groups within centers, in actuality the two protocols were equivalent to just one multicenter study. In addition, the primary reason for performing the interim analysis was due to the ethical dilemma of whether to continue to enroll and treat patients in the studies when more than a quarter of the patients may be developing frank ulceration. As mentioned in Section II, NSAID-induced ulcers with continued administration of NSAIDs may lead to perforation and bleeding, particularly in an elderly population. To have conducted interim analyses of each study individually and failed to stop either or both of the studies because of lower power from the reduced sample size would not have been tenable. Since the interim analysis was conducted at about the halfway point of both studies, treating the two studies as one gave us the same statistical power that we had for an individual study at the time of protocol development. For the prophylaxis stratum, this represented 95% power to detect a 15% difference with a one-sided type I error rate of 5%.

Third, attention was paid only to the prophylaxis stratum with respect to the interim analysis stopping rule. The reason for this was that prophylaxis was seen to be the primary indication at the protocol development stage. Prior to the NSAID clinical research program, the company had conducted several phase III clinical trials that established the efficacy of misoprostol in healing peptic ulcers. In fact, the company had submitted a new drug application (NDA) for misoprostol in the treatment of duodenal ulcers which was recommended for approval by an FDA gastrointestinal advisory committee. The FDA failed to approve the drug for that indication due to the fact that it had not been shown to be significantly superior to the already marketed H_2-receptor antagonists and a concern about the abortifacient capacity of misoprostol. The feeling was that if it could be demonstrated that misoprostol was effective for some indication for which the H_2-receptor antagonists were not, this would warrant approval. Since the H_2-receptor antagonists had not been shown to be effective in the prevention of NSAID-induced damage, and the body of evidence suggested (Section II) that misoprostol could be, the company decided to develop the drug for this indication. At screening for the NSAID protocols, patients had to have UGI pain. Only after baseline endoscopy could it be determined whether a patient already had a gastric ulcer. If not, the patient went into the prophylaxis stratum. If so, it was felt more appropriate to offer the patient entry into the treatment stratum rather than just to exclude the patient from further study. Data from the treatment stratum of the NSAID protocols were analyzed and presented in the final clinical study reports.

Fourth, the interim analysis stopping rule was formulated in terms of the single pairwise comparison: 200 μg of misoprostol q.i.d. versus placebo. The other two pairwise comparisons were constructed for interest but did not affect the statistical decision stopping rule. The reason for this was to try to economize with respect to the overall type I error by avoiding a multiple comparison issue. At the protocol development stage, the 200-μg q.i.d. dose of misoprostol was seen as the target dose. The 100-μg q.i.d. dose of misoprostol was included in the prophylaxis stratum for dose-response reasons. One may note that only the acid-inhibitory 200-μg dose was included in the treatment stratum. In addition, the dose comparison trial was making its way into the federal regulations in the mid-1980s through the IND/NDA Rewrite. If the 200-μg dose was statistically significant compared to placebo at the 0.01 level, dose response would have been implied by Williams' (1971, 1972) procedure.

Fifth, the interim analysis was based on Fisher's exact test of the 2 $\times$ 2 table reflecting 200 μg of misoprostol q.i.d. and placebo as the rows and the numbers of patients with ulcers or no ulcers as the columns. That is, the data were lumped across centers for the interim analysis stopping rule. Generally, since randomization was to treatment within centers, an analysis such as Mantel–Haenszel, which blocked on centers, would be seen to be more appropriate. The reason for not using the Mantel–Haenszel procedure directly was that due to small, no, or equal numbers of patients with ulcers (consistent with a large number of investigational centers), the effective sample size was expected to be less than the actual sample size. After stopping the trials, the Mantel–Haenszel procedure was used to address the robustness of the conclusion by collapsing some centers into "pseudocenters."

Finally, as has been acknowledged previously, the interim analysis that was performed was not included in the protocol. This is not to say that it was not planned. The bottom line is that through attentive monitoring, taking the proactive approach to clinical trial/data management, statistical analyses planning, and report development, and working prospectively with the U.S. regulatory agency, a bona fide interim analysis was made. This led to earlier termination of the program. Consequently, the submission was made and approved earlier than it might otherwise have been.

REFERENCES

Aadland, E., Fausa, O., and Vatn, M. (1986). Misoprostol protection against naproxen-induced gastric damage. *Symposium: Advances in Prostaglandins and Gastroenterology,* World Congresses of Gastroenterology, Sao Paulo, Brazil, September 8.

Cohen, M. M. (1987). Mucosal protection by misoprostol against injury by nonsteroidal anti-inflammatory agents excluding aspirin. *Symposium: Clinical Developments on Misoprostol—Peptic Ulcer Disease and NSAID-Induced Gastropathy, Digestive Disease Week,* Chicago, May 8.

Collins, A. J. (1987). Pathophysiologic aspects of NSAID-induced gastropathies. *Symposium: Clinical Developments on Misoprostol—Peptic Ulcer Disease and NSAID-Induced Gastropathy, Digestive Disease Week,* Chicago, May 8.

Lan, K. K. G., and DeMets, D. L. (1983). Discrete sequential boundaries for clinical trials. *Biometrika 70:* 659–670.

Langman, M. J. S. (1987). Nonsteroidal anti-inflammatory drugs: socioeconomic impact of associated gastropathies. *Symposium: Clinical Developments on Misoprostol—Peptic Ulcer Disease and NSAID-Induced Gastropathy, Digestive Disease Week,* Chicago, May 8.

Lanza, F. L. (1986). A double-blind study of prophylactic effect of misoprostol on lesions of gastric and duodenal mucosa induced by oral administration of tolmetin in healthy subjects. *Digest. Dis. Sci. 31*(Suppl.): 131S–136S.

Lanza, F. L. (1987). The effect of NSAIDs on the gastroduodenal mucosa of arthritic patients and normal volunteers. *Symposium: Cytoprotection, NSAIDs, and the Arthritic Patient,* Carlsbad, Calif., May 29–30.

Mantel, N., and Haenszel, W. (1959). Statistical aspects of the analysis of data from retrospective studies of disease. *J. Natl. Cancer Inst. 22:* 719–748.

O'Brien, P., and Fleming, T. (1979). A multiple testing procedure for clinical trials. *Biometrics 35:* 549–556.

Peace, K. E. (1987). Design, monitoring and analysis issues relative to adverse events. *Drug Inf. J. 21*(1): 21–28.

Peace, K. E. (1989). The alternative hypothesis: one-sided or two-sided? *J. Clin. Epidemiol. 42:* 473–476.

Peace, K. E. (1991). Shortening the time for clinical drug development. *Regul. Affairs 3:* 3–22.

Peace, K. E., and Schriver, R. S. (1987). *P*-values and power computation in multiple-look trials. *J. Chronic Dis. 40:* 23–30.

PMA (1991). Pharmaceutical Manufacturers Association Biostatistics and Medical Ad Hoc Committee on Interim Analysis, *Issues in Data Monitoring and Interim Analysis in the Pharmaceutical Industry,* PMA, Washington, D.C.

Pocock, S. (1977). Group sequential methods in the design and analysis of clinical trials. *Biometrika 64:* 191–199.

Roth, S. H. (1987). Nsaid gastropathy: a rheumatologist's perspective. *Symposium: Cytoprotection, NSAIDs, and the Arthritic Patient,* Carlsbad, Calif., May 29–30.

Williams, D. A. (1971). A test for differences between treatment means when several dose levels are compared with a zero dose control. *Biometrics 27:* 103–117.

Williams, D. A. (1972). The comparison of several dose levels with a zero dose control. *Biometrics 28:* 519–531.

17

Famotidine in Upper Gastrointestinal Hemorrhage

Karen L. Walton-Bowen

Merck Sharp & Dohme Research Laboratories, West Point, Pennsylvania

I. BACKGROUND

A high proportion of people admitted to hospitals every year with acute upper gastrointestinal (GI) hemorrhage will have bled from a peptic ulcer (Vellacott et al., 1982). Further hemorrhage after admission (i.e., continued bleeding or rebleeding) is associated with a relatively poor prognosis (Jones et al., 1973), and medical treatment is directed at preventing this complication and reducing the corresponding high mortality and surgical intervention in these patients.

In the markedly acidic environment of the stomach it is likely that hemostasis is severely impaired. This would explain the continuous oozing and tendency to rebleed that characterizes hemorrhage from peptic ulcers. Platelet aggregation and plasma coagulation are both very sensitive to changes in hydrogen ion concentration in vitro. In addition, previously formed platelet aggregates disaggregate at slightly acid pH values, and these effects are enhanced by the presence of pepsin, which is activated at low pH (Green et al., 1978).

It has been suggested that by virtue of their ability to raise gastric pH, H_2-receptor antagonists might be useful agents in preventing continued or recurrent bleeding by allowing platelet and plasma hemostatic mechanisms to operate normally. Pepsin output and activation would also be reduced by these drugs. If this rationale is correct, treatment with H_2 antagonists should be aimed at maintaining the highest possible pH in the stomach. Ostro et al. (1985) demonstrated that gastric pH in severely ill patients could be better controlled by primed syringe pump infusions of cimetidine than by conventional bolus dosage regimens. In all therapeutic trials of H_2-receptor antagonists in acute hemorrhage to date, bolus intravenous (IV) doses, oral doses, or a combination of both have been used. In view of the practical difficulties involved, titration of dosage against pH has not been undertaken in published studies in these patients. Many studies have failed to demonstrate efficacy of H_2 blockers in upper gastrointestinal (GI) hemorrhage; potential underdosage is one possible explanation, but other studies have been flawed in one or more of the following ways: (1) failure to include an adequate number of patients to avoid a type II error, (2) failure to exclude patients with a low risk of further hemorrhage, or (3) failure to include a placebo group, so that absolute efficacy cannot be demonstrated. Nonetheless, Collins and Langman (1985), reviewing 27 randomized controlled trials of H_2-receptor antagonists, reached the conclusion that overall they appeared to be "moderately promising." They, in common with others, urged that a large randomized placebo-controlled study was necessary.

Famotidine (Pepcid, Merck Sharp & Dohme) is a potent H_2-receptor antagonist [on a milligram-per-milligram basis it is approximately 9 times as potent as Ranitidine (Zantac, Glaxo Pharmaceuticals) and 32 times as potent as Cimetidine (Tagamet, SmithKline Beecham)]. In addition, it has a dose-related duration of action; a 40-mg oral dose produces consistent antisecretory activity for 10 to 12 hours. Famotidine does not interfere with the mixed-function oxidase system of the liver and thus does not share the potential of Cimetidine to interact with other drugs at this level; it does not have antiandrogenic properties and in large clinical studies adverse effects have been rare and nonserious. Doses of up to 800 mg daily have been administered for periods of up to 1 year in patients with Zollinger–Ellison syndrome without the identification of any dose-related adverse effects. As a potent and long-acting antisecretory agent, Famotidine may be ideally suited for use in producing a pronounced and prolonged rise in gastric pH at relatively low doses intravenously.

II. PROTOCOL

A. Objectives

The objectives of the study were as follows:

1. To assess the efficacy of intravenous Famotidine in reducing mortality, rebleed, and need for surgical intervention up to the time of discharge from the hospital in patients presenting with bleeding from a peptic ulcer

2. To assess the safety of intravenous Famotidine in such patients

These objectives lead to the following hypotheses:

1. To demonstrate a halving of mortality from the level of around 20% as seen in this high-risk group, as described by Jones et al. (1973). This was latter amended to a halving from the 10% level.
2. To detect clinically important changes in the rate of rebleed, which in this population is approximately 40% (Jones et al., 1973; MacLeod and Mills, 1982)

B. Study Design

The study was designed as a double-blind randomized placebo-controlled multicenter study to be conducted in the United Kingdom and Ireland in patients identified by endoscopy to have bled from a peptic ulcer. Patients were identified by the following set of guidelines:

Criteria for inclusion:

1. Adults over 18 years of age willing to participate in the study
2. The presence of a recent (within 24 hours) clinical history suggesting significant upper gastrointestinal blood loss (i.e., bright red hematemesis and/or typical melena stools ± symptoms of hypovolemic shock)
3. On endoscopy within 24 hours of admission, the presence of an endoscopically identified peptic ulcer with the stigmata of active or recent hemorrhage [i.e., continued oozing and/or fresh or altered clot (including black slough) adhering to ulcer base ± visible vessel in the ulcer base]

Criteria for exclusion:

1. Severe continuous bleeding requiring immediate surgical intervention
2. Bleeding from stress ulcers (e.g., in postoperative multiple trauma or severely ill patients)
3. Presence of an alternative possible source of bleeding (e.g., esophageal varices, Mallory–Weiss tear, hemorrhagic gastritis)
4. Known hypersensitivity to H_2-receptor antagonists
5. Known significant cardiac, pulmonary, blood, liver, pancreatic, or renal ulcer disease, which is considered likely to interfere with the conduct of the trial
6. Uncontrolled diabetes mellitus; active malignant disease; pregnancy or a patient in whom pregnancy is a practical possibility

Such a patient population is at a high risk of rebleeding and exhibits high mortality, as described by Green et al. (1978) and Storey et al. (1981). Patients with a high likelihood of a spontaneously good outcome were excluded in the hope that real differences between active and placebo treatment would not be diluted or masked. Since the majority of episodes of further hemorrhage occur within 48 hours of admission of the initial rebleed (Jones et al., 1973), patients received intravenous therapy for 3 days in a double-blind fashion. This consisted of an initial 10-mg (2.5-mL) bolus dose of either Famotidine or placebo administered intravenously over 2 to 3 minutes followed immediately by a syringe pump infusion of 3.2 mg of Famotidine or placebo per hour for 72 hours (i.e., approximately 80 mg/24 hours). Active oral Famotidine 40 mg nocte was provided for all patients after the 72-hour double-blind study period.

C. Endpoints and Sample Size

During the double-blind study period and at any time prior to discharge, the clinical endpoints of importance—death from any cause—surgery (GI) and rebleeds were recorded. The study was designed with a 1% significance level and a power of 95% to detect an anticipated halving of mortality from the 20% level in the control group to the 10% level in the active group. This implied a sample size of 450 patients per group, which also gave considerable power to detect clinically important changes in the rate of rebleeding (rate of rebleed anticipated at approximately 40% in such a patient population). The study was therefore planned for 1000 patients in total: 500 patients on active Famotidine treatment and 500 patients on placebo for the 3-day double-blind period. It was anticipated that 50 clinics would participate and enter 20 patients per clinic over an 18-month period. The study was later amended to reflect differences from the 10% level in the control group to the 5% level in the active group, with 80% power at a 5% significance level.

D. The Decision Rule and Plans for Analysis

A straightforward group sequential procedure, as described by Pocock (1977), was to be applied to the frequency of mortality from any cause during admission, with an interim analysis after 500 patients had completed the study, to permit termination of the study on ethical grounds if there was early evidence of a benefit with active treatment. A final analysis was planned for when 1000 patients had completed the study if the decision at the interim stage was to continue the trial. This procedure was based on anticipated mortality rates of 10% and 20%, respectively, and a required overall significance level of 1%.

As the trial progressed, a review of the mortality among the first 200 patients to complete the study (without consideration of treatment allocation) indicated an overall mortality rate of 7%. Consequently, a slightly different fundamental approach as proposed by Peto [see Pocock (1982)], which would preserve the nominal significance level of the final test, was adopted. This made the criterion for stopping the trial early more stringent, but this was consistent with the original objective of the analysis.

This procedure was, however, adjusted to allow the study to terminate if there was reasonable evidence of increased mortality in the active treatment arm. If the interim analysis did not conclude that the study should terminate because of overwhelming benefit of active treatment, a less stringent test would be applied to check that the results did not suggest an opposite effect. The calculation of the characteristics of the proposed procedure was based on revised estimates of mortality of 5% and 10%, respectively, on active and placebo treatments. (See Section IV for details and properties of the procedure.)

III. MONITORING AND DATA COLLECTION

Study administration, data collection, data management, and the interim analysis were the responsibility of the clinical research and biostatistics sections at Merck Sharp & Dohme, Hoddesdon, United Kingdom, while the final statistical analysis and supportive data listings were carried out by the clinical research and biostatistics sections of Merck Sharp & Dohme, in the United States.

A. Data Review

1. Worksheet Procedures

Data were recorded on study worksheets consisting of a top copy and two pressure-sensitive copies. Upon worksheet completion, the two pressure-sensitive copies were sent to the clinical research team at Hoddesdon. The top master copy was retained by the individual investigators for cross-reference purposes and was not collected until the end of the study. Each worksheet was logged into a computerized study monitoring system at the company on the day that the copies were received. This facilitated a continually updated report of worksheets in-house. Part of the logging process involved a complete review of the worksheet by the study monitor for completeness of data and assessment of the need for follow-up in the case of adverse experiences.

Missing or inconsistent data were referred back to the individual investigators for clarification, either by telephone or by letter, and any corrections were made to the worksheet and initialled. Edit lists were maintained for eventual inclusion with the case report forms (CRFs) returned to the investigator for signature. Worksheets for patients with serious or unexpected adverse experiences (including death) were passed to the adverse event coordinator on the day of receipt. Initial reports of adverse experiences were also sent to the company in the United States, and then any additional information required was obtained from the investigator. If the adverse experience was a rebleed requiring surgery, postsurgical follow-up forms were sent to the investigator to ensure completeness of information for such patients. At this stage, one of the copies of the worksheet was sent to the department of the coordinating investigator for duplicate data coding and entry, independent of the biostatistics section coding and data entry.

2. Data Procedures

Data were coded at both the company and the coordinating center in accordance with preestablished data coding guidelines set up by the biostatistics section at Hoddesdon. Identical SIR software (SIR, 1986) was used for data entry into a database, both at the company and at the coordinating center. A Compaq microcomputer was used for data processing purposes. After initial data entry by the biostatistics section at Hoddesdon, data were reentered by the clinical study monitors at the company, using the screen verification facility available within the SIR software to check entries against the values already held in the company database. Any discrepancies in the database were checked against the source worksheet and corrected as necessary. At several points during the study, a computer-run batch comparison was made between the databases at the company and the coordinating center in order to check the equivalence of patient allocation numbers and the consistency of data interpretation. Errors/inconsistencies were corrected after referring to the source worksheet and after mutual agreement between the company and the coordinating center.

On completion of data entry, the biostatistics department at Hoddesdon carried out further data correction procedures. Screening tables of all fields were used to identify remaining inconsistencies and were sent to the study monitor for review. An edit log was maintained at all times to document the changes and corrections made. Case records were frozen on a center-by-center basis by the biostatistics section, at the request of the study monitor. This prevented any further update of the frozen cases via the data-entry screens. Printed case report forms were then generated via the SIR system, and checked against the edited worksheet by the study monitor. Necessary edits were marked on the case report forms and also indicated on a cover sheet. Any marked edits were then made in the database by a senior member of the biostatistics department using a restricted-access entry screen. The case report forms, together with relevant edit log, were taken to the investigator for signature. If further edits were required, the case report forms were sent back to the company for database corrections and subsequently returned to the investigator for signature. At the end of the study, all final case report forms were sent to the regulatory affairs department. Copies of the case report forms were kept at the company and at the investigator sites.

B. The Interim Stage

While these procedures were taking place, study recruitment was regularly reviewed as patient accrual approached 500 patients, at which time the interim analysis was to be performed. A date was established when all worksheets for completed patients would be collected. An up-to-date list of patient numbers allocated to each investigator was stored in a "monitoring" database. When worksheets were received in-house, the records in the monitoring database were updated. The information was printed out and sent to each investigator in advance of the agreed cutoff date in order to obtain all outstanding available information which was then utilized to update the database. The mortality status of each patient was agreed upon quickly between the company and the coordinating investigators and the data file forwarded with a copy of the random treatment allocation schedule to an independent academic statistician for analysis. The results were produced with minimum delay and returned to both the company and the coordinating investigator in the form of "trial to continue."

C. The Final Analysis Stage

An audit was performed on the final database, after which the database was frozen. The data were downloaded at the company in the United Kingdom onto diskettes in the form of flat data files which were then sent to the United States for the final statistical analyses and production of the clinical study report (CSR). After validation procedures were carried out on the diskettes, the data were uploaded onto an IBM mainframe computer for analysis using the SAS system (SAS, 1985). Any further data inconsistencies identified during the analysis stage were fully documented and edited. A log was maintained of all changes made to the database.

IV. STATISTICAL ANALYSES

A. Interim Analysis After 500 Patients

1. Methodology

At the interim analysis stage, the study would be stopped and Famotidine declared superior to placebo if the difference in the event rates was significant at a nominal two-sided level of 0.1%. If this was not the case, a two-sided test at a nominal 5% level would be applied and the study terminated if the Famotidine event rate was significantly worse than the placebo rate. If neither criterion was met, recruitment would proceed to the intended 1000 patients and a nominal two-sided test at the 5% level would then be carried out.

If the final test performed favored Famotidine, the result would be delcared significant at the 5% level and the nominal two-sided p-value quoted. Should the test favor placebo, the overall significance level would be stated to be approximately 8% (McPherson, 1974), but other properties of the procedure (see below) would be discussed. In either event, a nominal 95% confidence interval for the difference between the two mortality rates, or appropriate statistics such as the corresponding odds ratio, would be reported.

2. Properties of the Procedure

a. Probability of Outcome in Favor of Famotidine. The mortality in the control group was assumed to be 10% and a reduction to 5% on Famotidine was postulated. The overall probability that Famotidine would be found superior to placebo was approximately 0.85. This would occur after exactly 500 patients if the rates observed at this point were approximately 11% and 3%, respectively.

b. Probability of Outcome in Favor of Placebo. If, in reality, the benefit of Famotidine was only marginal, resulting in, say, a mortality of 6% compared with a control rate of 8%, the chances that a midpoint analysis would favor placebo were approximately 1 in 500. The overall probability of this outcome at either of the two analyses was of the same order of magnitude.

B. Final Analysis After 1000 Patients

1. Methodology

All patients who received study medication were included in the efficacy analyses. The primary outcome measure analyzed was death from any cause prior to discharge. Secondary endpoints analyzed included surgery (GI) and rebleeds prior to discharge. All statistical tests were two-tailed with $\alpha = 0.05$ level of significance. All p-values were rounded to three decimal places and statistical significance was declared if the rounded p-value was less than or equal to 0.050.

a. Deaths. The proportions of deaths occurring before discharge were compared between the treatment groups using a Pearson chi-square test (Everitt, 1980). It was expected to demonstrate a halving of mortality from the level of around 20% seen in this high-risk group to 10% (Jones et al., 1973). This was amended for 10% to 5% differences. Results were also given by individual centers. The effect of various concomitant factors: for example, initial source of bleeding [gastric (pyloric patients were included in the gastric category), duodenal, other], age (<65, $\geqslant 65$), sex, prior nonsteroidal anti-inflammatory drug (NSAID) use (none, 1 to 7 days, >7 days), admission symptoms [hematemesis ($\pm$melena), melena only], shock (systolic blood pressure <100 mm, $\geqslant 100$ mm), stigmata (oozing, visible vessels, clot, slough), and initial hemoglobin (<10 g/dL, $\geqslant 10$ g/dL) on proportions of deaths before discharge was assessed using the Cochran–Mantel–Haenszel statistic (Fleiss, 1973). Times of deaths were displayed (death while on study treatment or death after treatment withdrawal but prior to discharge).

b. Surgery. Proportions of patients requiring surgery (GI) and outcome of surgery (GI) were analyzed in a similar manner to deaths (see above).

c. Rebleeds. The proportions of patients experiencing a rebleed prior to discharge, the distribution of the number of rebleed episodes, and the time to rebleed were compared between the treatment groups using methods similar to those described above. (Time to rebleed was taken as the time to the first rebleed from the start of IV therapy.) The rate of rebleeding in a population such as this would be estimated at 40% as described by Jones et al. (1973) and Macleod and Mills (1982). A summary of clinical signs of rebleed (hematemesis, hypovolemia, and fall in hemoglobin) was displayed for both treatment groups. Summary statistics were provided for time until discharge for each treatment group over all centers and for each center within each treatment group. (Time until discharge = discharge rate − start of IV date.)

d. Additional Analyses. In addition, a supplemental analysis was performed to assess how the concomitant factors previously outlined jointly affect the treatment differences. To do this, a logistic regression backward elimination procedure (Harrell, 1986) was adopted to determine a predictive model from the concomitant factors previously outlined for each of the three response variables (i.e., death prior to discharge, GI surgery, and rebleed prior to discharge). The significance level for keeping parameters in the model was 0.05. The corresponding parameter estimates obtained were then resubstituted as a linear model to determine predictive probabilities. The logistic transform, $e^{-x}/1 + e^{-x}$, was used for this purpose. Applying this transform to obtain predictive probabilities of $\leqslant 50\%$ or $>50\%$ is equivalent to the sum of the betas in the linear model being $\leqslant 0$ or >0, as described in Cox (1970) and McCullagh (1980). The resubstitution bias that can occur was not considered to be a problem for a trial of this size. Contingency tables were then formed for the actual numbers of deaths (surgery/rebleed) versus the predicted numbers and the ability of the model to predict the response variable assessed (Cox, 1970; McCullagh, 1980). The logistic regression approach has fewer assumptions than the linear discriminant model and for this reason was the model of choice.

e. Safety. Adverse experience data were analyzed using the Pearson chi-square statistic (Everitt, 1980). Differences between treatment groups for demographic variables were assessed using the Pearson chi-square test (for dichotomous variables) or the Cochran–Mantel–Haenszel statistic as appropriate (Everitt, 1980; Fleiss, 1973).

2. Results of the Final Analysis

At the time of completion of this section, the study was unfinished. The methodology outlined in the preceding section was performed as a prototype analysis on half of the patients without knowledge of treatment allocations, in preparation for the full analysis. The first half of the patients were assigned treatment

A and the second half were assigned treatment B. These "artificial" results will not be displayed here.

V. CONCLUSION

After analysis of data from 500 patients, there was no early evidence of an overwhelming benefit with active treatment in reducing the frequency of mortality. Similarly, there was no early evidence to indicate that the active treatment rate was significantly worse than that of the control group. This conclusion led to a decision to continue the trial to full course.

VI. DISCUSSION

Minimization of bias and maintenance of data integrity are always important concerns in the conduct of any clinical trial. The trial described here was carefully controlled to eliminate bias and to collect good-quality data. The study was randomized so that each patient had the same chance as any other patient of being assigned to either of the two treatments, and both the patients and the investigators were blinded as to the actual treatment received. The criteria for inclusion/exclusion in the study were carefully defined and the endpoints of interest—death, rebleed, and surgery (GI) prior to discharge—were objective binary responses. Data processing throughout the trial was conducted in a blinded fashion.

To minimize bias at the interim analysis stage, the data from the 500 patients along with the corresponding allocation schedule of treatments were sent to an independent outside academic statistician for analysis of mortality and the decision rule to either continue or stop the trial was evaluated in a timely fashion. In this case a decision of "trial to continue" was conveyed to the clinical research team without releasing any details of the actual analysis results. These results were kept on file by the independent statistician until the trial was completed.

The data were thoroughly checked for errors and inconsistencies as case record forms came in-house. Entry into the database was checked by means of a double-entry system. Data interpretation was also checked by independent coding and entry at both the company in the United Kingdom and the coordinating center. These procedures helped to ensure data integrity. The study was conducted on a carefully defined patient population of sufficient size and power to detect clinically meaningful differences between treatment groups with respect to mortality rates. This is the first such trial of H_2-receptor antagonists to fulfill these characteristics.

ACKNOWLEDGMENTS

The author would like to acknowledge the clinical research group at Merck Sharp & Dohme, Hoddesdon, United Kingdom, in particular, Nigel Freemantle, and the participating investigators, for providing information necessary to complete this summary.

REFERENCES

Collins, R., and Langman, M. J. S. (1985). Treatment with histamine H_2 antagonists in acute upper gastrointestinal hemorrhage: implications of randomized trials. *N. Engl. J. Med. 313:* 660–666.

Cox, D. R. (1970). *The Analysis of Binary Data,* Chapman & Hall, London.

Everitt, B. (1980). *The Analysis of Contingency Tables.* Chapman & Hall, London.

Fleiss, J. L. (1973). *Statistical Methods for Rates and Proportions,* 2nd ed., Wiley, New York.

Green, F. W., Kaplan, M. M., Curtis, L. E., and Levine, R. H. (1978). Effect of acid and pepsin on blood coagulation and platelet aggregation (a possible contributor to prolonged gastroduodenal mucosal hemorrhage). *Gastroenterology 74*(1): 38–43.

Harrell, F. E., Jr. (1986). The Logist Procedure, *SAS Supplementary Manual,* SAS Institute, Cary, N.C., Chap. 23.

Jones, P. F., Johnston, S. J., McEwan, A. B., Kyle, J., and Needham, C. D. (1973). Further hemorrhage after admission to hospital for gastrointestinal hemorrhage. *Brit. Med. J. 3:* 660–664.

Macleod, I. A., and Mills, P. R. (1982). Factors identifying the probability of further hemorrhage after acute upper gastrointestinal hemorrhage. *Brit. J. Surg. 69:* 256–258.

McCullagh, P. (1980). Regression models for ordinal data (with discussion). *J. R. Stat. Soc. B 42:* 109–142.

McPherson, K. (1974). Statistics: the problem of examining accumulating data more than once. *N. Engl. J. Med. 290:* 501–502.

Ostro, M. J., Russell, J. A., Soldin, S. J., Mahon, W. A., and Jeejeebhoy, K. N. (1985). Control of gastric pH with cimetidine: Boluses versus primed infusions. *Gastroenterology 89:* 532–537.

Pocock, S. J. (1977). Group sequential methods in the design and analysis of clinical trials. *Biometrika 64:* 191–199.

Pocock, S. J. (1982). Interim analysis for randomized clinical trials: the group sequential approach. *Biometrics 38:* 158–162.

SAS (1985). *SAS Users Guide: Basics, Statistics,* Version 5, SAS Institute, Cary, N.C.

SIR (1986). *SIR Reference Manual,* Version 2.1.3, Division of ISI, SIR Inc., USA.

Storey, D. W., Brown, S. G., Swain, C. P., Salmon, P. R., Kirkham, J. S., and Northfield, T. C. (1981). Endoscopic prediction of recurrent bleeding in peptic ulcers. *N. Engl. J. Med. 305:* 915–916.

Vellacott, K. D., Dronfield, M. W., Atkinson, M., and Langman, M. J. S. (1982). Comparison of surgical and medical management of bleeding peptic ulcers. *Brit. Med. J. 284:* 548–550.

VII

APPLICATIONS IN OTHER AREAS OF CLINICAL RESEARCH

18

Sample Size Reestimation in Clinical Trials

Weichung Joseph Shih

Merck Sharp & Dohme Research Laboratories, Rahway, New Jersey

I. INTRODUCTION

Estimation of the required sample size is a key issue for almost all clinical trials. Traditionally, there have been two distinct designs, fixed and sequential sample size designs (Meinert, 1986). Strictly speaking, a fixed sample size design is one in which the investigator specifies the required sample size before starting the trial. A classical sequential design is one in which patient enrollment continues until the observed test-control treatment difference exceeds a predefined boundary value (Wald, 1947) or the number of patients exceeds a prespecified limit (Bross, 1952; Armitage, 1957). The drawback of a fixed sample design is that the sample size estimation depends on previous data or some guesswork of the parameters, which can be very unreliable. The use of classical sequential designs, on the other hand, is limited to situations where outcome assessment can be made shortly after patients are enrolled in the trial. For most trials in which long periods of follow-up are required, the so-called group sequential design has become popular [see, e.g., Lan and DeMets, (1983), O'Brien and Fleming (1979), Pocock (1977, 1982), Geller and Pocock (1987), and Gould and Pecore, (1982)]. However, the focus of group sequential methods has been on the early stopping rules of a clinical trial to fulfill ethical concerns. These designs appear frequently in clinical trials involving cancer, myocardial infarction, and other type of life-threatening diseases, where mortality is the endpoint. For comparative trials, group sequential methods require that the treatment codes be broken at the interim stage and significance tests be repeatedly conducted on the accumulating data. Consequently, the type I error rate at each analysis stage has to be adjusted so that the overall type I error rate can be maintained at a predetermined level (Armitage et al., 1969).

The purpose of this chapter is to discuss sequential methods for sample size reestimation, as opposed to early stopping, in clinical trials. In many clinical trials, especially those with nonfatal diseases, investigators would like to devise a procedure at an interim stage to gather updated information on the adequacy of the planned sample size. This situation frequently occurs when the natural history of the disease is not well known or the therapy under study is a new class. In these circumstances, investigators are often uncertain about the assumed values of parameters that were used initially for the calculation of the (provisional) sample size at the planning stage, since these parameter values usually are obtained from some other studies with perhaps different patient populations, diagnosis criteria, or other study conditions. As a result, the sample size that was estimated initially does not necessarily assure the width of the confidence interval (for estimation) or the required power (for hypothesis testing). It is therefore desirable to monitor the trial to assure that the basic design assumptions are reasonably close to being met, and to construct procedures to reestimate the sample size with use of the observations available at an interim stage.

Since our goal is sample size reestimation, the only decision that will be taken is the determination of how many, if any, observations are needed beyond those originally planned. If no further observations are needed, the sample size planned is adequate and the trial will be carried to completion. In Section II we start with a review of the simple one-sample normal case, which was proposed by Stein (1945). We also extend Stein's procedure to the two-sample case. This extension is based on unmasking the treatment codes. For double-blind clinical trials, however, it is also strongly desirable to maintain the integrity of the trial by keeping the treatment codes blinded at the interim stage so that conscious or unconscious bias is best prevented. [In fact, many clinical trials sponsored by pharmaceutical industries have already implemented in-house blinding procedures in addition to the double-blindness (i.e., the so-called triple-blind trials) to further enhance unbiasness.] Section III is the main result of this chapter, in which we introduce a procedure for the normal case that meets the need of maintaining the blindness. In Section IV we review a similar procedure developed by Gould (1991) for the binary case and discuss some of the difficulties in the use of it. In the latter the procedures (Sections III and IV), since the sample size reestimation is made without the knowledge of patient treatment identifications, no treatment comparison will be made. The type I error rate will not be materially affected. More discussion on the implementation of the new procedures is included in Section V.

II. STEIN'S PROCEDURE

A. One-Sample Case

Stein (1945) proposed a method of two-stage sampling which assures that the final confidence interval will be no larger than a specified amount. The procedure is rather cumbersome in its original form, but a simplified version of it, with the same spirit, can be given as follows. Specifically, let the measurement be denoted as Y and assume that Y has a normal distribution with mean μ and standard deviation σ. We would like to take a random sample of size n from Y such that if $\bar{y}$ is the mean of the whole sample, $P\{|\bar{y} - \mu| \geqslant d\} \leqslant \alpha$, where d and α are chosen quantities.

Stein's method is as follows. First take n_1 observations, $y_1, y_2, \ldots, y_{n_1}$, which supplies its sample mean $\bar{y}_1$ and standard deviation s_1 as estimates of μ and σ, respectively. The half-width of the $(1 - \alpha)$ confidence interval based on $\bar{y}_1$ is

$$t_{(n_1-1)} \left(\frac{s_1^2}{n_1} \right)^{1/2} \tag{1}$$

where t_r is the $(1 - \alpha/2)$th percentile of the t distribution with r degrees of freedom. If (1) is less than or equal to the desired half-width d, the sample is already sufficiently large. If not, additional observations are taken so that the total sample size n is at least as great as

$$t_{(n_1-1)}^2 \frac{s_1^2}{d^2} \tag{2}$$

Stein (1945) provided details of the properties of this procedure. In the following, we extend this procedure to the two-sample case and follow a similar proof.

B. Two-Sample Case

Let the measurements be denoted as X and Y, which are independent and have normal distributions with means μ_x and μ_y, respectively, and the same standard deviation σ. We would like to take random samples of size n from each of the populations such that if $(\bar{x} - \bar{y})$ is the difference of the means of the whole samples, $P\{|(\bar{x} - \bar{y}) - (\mu_x - \mu_y)| \geqslant d\} \leqslant \alpha$, where d and α are chosen quantities.

The sequential sampling procedure is as follows. First take n_1 observations and obtain the sample means and standard deviations, $(\bar{x}_1, s_x)$ and $(\bar{y}_1, s_y)$, from each of the populations. Since X and Y have the same standard deviation σ, a combined estimate of σ^2 is $s_p^2 = n_1(s_x^2 + s_y^2)/2(n_1 - 1)$. The half-width of the $(1 - \alpha)$ confidence interval based on $(\bar{x}_1 - \bar{y}_1)$ is

$$t_{(2n_1-2)} \left(\frac{2s_p^2}{n_1} \right)^{1/2} \tag{3}$$

As in the previous case, if equation (3) is less than or equal to the desired half-width d, the sample is already sufficiently large. If not, additional observations are taken so that the final sample size n per group is at least as great as

$$t_{(2n_1-2)}^2 \frac{2s_p^2}{d^2} \tag{4}$$

The proof of this procedure follows similarly from that of Stein (1945) for the one-sample case. Throughout the proof, the quantities d, α, and n_1 are fixed. The total sample size per group, n, is not fixed, but is a random variable, since its value depends on the value of s_x and s_y (hence s_p) that turn up in the first sample. Nevertheless, for fixed s_p, n is fixed, and the quantity

$$(\bar{x} - \bar{y}) - (\mu_x - \mu_y)$$

is normally distributed with mean zero and variance $2\sigma^2/n$. Hence this quantity follows the normal distribution whether s_p is fixed or not. Moreover, by a well-known property of the normal distribution, the distribution is independent of that of s_p. Consequently,

$$\frac{n^{1/2}[(\bar{x} - \bar{y}) - (\mu_x - \mu_y)]}{(2)^{1/2} s_p}$$

follows the t distribution with $2(n_1 - 1)$ degrees of freedom. By definition of $t_{2(n_1-1)}$ it follows that

$$P\left[\frac{n_{1/2}[|(\bar{x} - \bar{y}) - (\mu_x - \mu_y)|]}{(2)^{1/2} s_p} \geqslant t_{2(n_1-1)} \right] = \alpha \tag{5}$$

This is the key result in the proof. Further, by the way in which the value n was calculated, we always have

$$n \geqslant \frac{t_{(2n_1-2)}^2 2s_p^2}{d^2} \quad \text{or} \quad \frac{n^{1/2}}{(2)^{1/2} s_p} \geqslant \frac{t_{2(n_1-1)}}{d}$$

Hence, from (5),

$$P\left[\frac{t_{2(n_1-1)} |(\bar{x} - \bar{y}) - (\mu_x - \mu_y)|}{d} \geqslant t_{2(n_1-1)} \right] \leqslant \alpha$$

That is,

$$P[\,|(\bar{x}-\bar{y})-(\mu_x-\mu_y)|\geqslant d]\leqslant\alpha$$

Notice that in this procedure, the within-group variances s_x^2 and s_y^2 are calculated with the treatment identifications known. The final confidence interval estimation will be based on these stage-1 within-group variances. Furthermore, the procedure permits stopping of the trial at the interim stage if the sample size, n_1 per group, is already sufficient. These are important aspects when comparing this procedure with the new ones in Sections III and IV.

C. Example

In a hypertension trial comparing a test treatment versus a control with respect to blood pressure change from baseline, we require $d = 4$ mmHg and $\alpha = 0.05$. From previous information, σ is guessed as about 10 mmHg, although this guess may be in error. The first step in applying the foregoing method is to select a value of n_1, the size of the initial sample. For this, it is helpful to know how large the final sample per group, N, would have to be if the assumed value of σ happened to be correct. This value is

$$N = 2\left(\frac{\sigma}{d}t\right)^2 = 2\left(\frac{10}{4}\times 2\right)^2 = 50$$

where $t = 2$ is taken from the normal approximation to the t distribution. Suppose that n_1 is taken as 30. With 30 observations per group, we usually can estimate σ reasonably well.

When the first set of samples is taken, s_p is found to be 12 mmHg. Since $t_{28,0.975}$ is 2.05, we have

$$t_{(2n_1-2)}\left(\frac{2s_p^2}{n_1}\right)^{1/2} = 2.05\times\left(2\times\frac{114}{30}\right)^{1/2} = 5.65$$

so that the sample size of 30 per group size gives a confidence interval of half-width 5.65 instead of 4. Hence we need to increase the sample size. According to equation (4), the final sample size per group should be

$$n = t^2\times 2\times\frac{s_p^2}{d^2} = (2.05)^2\times 2\times\left(\frac{12}{4}\right)^2 = 75.65$$

That is, we need to take 46 additional observations per group after the interim stage.

III. TWO-SAMPLE NORMAL CASE WITHOUT UNBLINDING

The method in Section II allows us to take a smaller sample than what was planned if s_p turns out to be smaller than the initial guess of σ. This may have some advantage in saving resources from the efficacy point of view. But in almost all clinical trials, we need to cumulate safety information as well. Early stopping a trial, except for safety reasons, may not be so desirable. Moreover, the previous method requires identification of the treatment group membership of the individual patients. As discussed earlier, maintaining the blindness is very important in conducting clinical trials. In the following we introduce a method developed by Gould and Shih (1991) that does not require the identification of patients' treatment group memberships. The key technique is to treat the problem as an incomplete data problem of a mixture distribution and utilize the EM algorithm to estimate the parameters.

A. Procedure

Specifically, we have two normal populations with means μ_1 and μ_2 and common variance σ^2 (all unknonwn) and are interested in testing H_0: $\mu_1 = \mu_2$ versus H_A: $\mu_1 < \mu_2$. At the planning stage, one assumes a value for σ (denote it by $\sigma*$) and specifies the alternative hypothesis with a least, clinically meaningful difference between treatment groups, $\delta* = \mu_2 - \mu_1 > 0$, for which the trial intends to detect with a desired power $1 - \beta$ and a type I error rate α. From this setup, a sample size per treatment group, with equal allocation, can be obtained by the normal approximation formula

$$n = 2(Z_\alpha + Z_\beta)^2 \left(\frac{\sigma*}{\delta*} \right)^2 \tag{6}$$

where Z_p is the $(1 - p)$ percentile of the standard normal distribution.

Notice that in the setup above only $\sigma*$ is an assumed value and needs to be monitored and verified; other elements, α, β, and $\delta*$, are design specifications and do not change with the data. The value $\delta*$ specified in the alternative hypothesis reflects the research interest. Our goal is not to estimate the true δ, but rather, to estimate σ and to monitor the sample size curve as shown in Figure 1. (More explanation of Figure 1 will be given later.) Also notice that we use a one-sided test here. This is certainly not a requirement for the procedure. For a two-sided test we replace α by $\alpha/2$ in equation (6).

After the trial has progressed to a point where a reasonable estimate of σ (denoted by $\hat{\sigma}$) can be made, one may reconsider the sample size estimation solely to assure that the intended power will be met in testing the specific alternative hypothesis. As in the previous two-stage sampling methods, we also recommend doing this reestimation only once, perhaps after data from approximately $n_1 = n/2$ patients per group are available. (Simulation results shown later indicate that $n_1 = 50$ is adequate.) Based on the updated estimates the revised sample size per group is then

$$N = n \left(\frac{\hat{\sigma}}{\sigma*} \right)^2 \tag{7}$$

That is, we choose N such that

$$P(\text{Reject } H_0 \,|\, \delta, \sigma^*, n) = P(\text{Reject } H_0 \,|\, \delta, \hat{\sigma}, N) \qquad \text{for all } \delta \tag{8}$$

if $n > N$, the planned sample size is large enough, and the trial will proceed as planned. If $N > n$, the trial will increase its size by additional patients. (See examples and more discussion later for some extreme cases in implementation.) Equation (8) is also a simple illustration of the fact that both the type I error rate (i.e., for $\delta = 0$) and power (i.e., for $\delta = \delta^* > 0$) are not materially affected by the procedure. Gould and Shih (1991) provide more rigorous investigation on the minuteness of the change of the type I error rate. This also indicates that blinding at the interim stage is a sufficient but not a necessary condition for "unaffecting" the type I error rate. What the blinding does best is to prevent all possible conscious or unconscious bias. Hence we keep the trial blinded as a principle to maintain the integrity of the double-blindness. Of course, the power curve is an approximation since the sample size formula itself is.

The remaining question is the estimation of σ based on the n_1 patients per group available at the interim stage. Of course, without knowing treatment group memberships, we use randomization to establish approximately equal number of patients in the treatment groups. Let z denote the outcome measurement. We can form the data as (z_i, I_i), $i = 1, \ldots, 2n_1$, where $I_i = 1$ if the ith patient belongs to the group that has population mean μ_1 and $I = 0$ otherwise. Since we do not unblind the treatment group identification, the I_i's are randomly missing in Rubin's sense (Rubin, 1976). To estimate σ we use the well-known EM algorithm (Dempster et al., 1977).

The complete-data log-likelihood function is proportional to

$$n_1(\log \sigma^2) + \frac{\Sigma[(z_i - \mu_1)^2 I_i + (z_i - \mu_2)^2(1 - I_i)]}{2\sigma^2} \tag{9}$$

where the summation is from $i = 1, \ldots, 2n_1$. From equation (9) we can easily derive the following E (expectation) and M (maximization) steps:

E-step:

$$\begin{aligned} \hat{I}_{i,e} &= E(I_i \,|\, z_i, \hat{\mu}_{1,e}, \hat{\mu}_{2,e}, \hat{\sigma}_e^2) \\ &= P(i\text{th patient belongs the control group} \,|\, z_i) \\ &= \frac{\exp[-(z_i - \hat{\mu}_{1,e})^2/\hat{\sigma}_e^2]}{\exp[-(z_i - \hat{\mu}_{1,e})^2/\hat{\sigma}_e^2] + \exp[-(z_i - \hat{\mu}_{2,e})^2/\hat{\sigma}_e^2]} \\ &= \frac{1}{1 + \exp[(\hat{\mu}_{1,e} - \hat{\mu}_{2,e})(\hat{\mu}_{1,e} + \hat{\mu}_{2,e} - 2z_i)/\hat{\sigma}_e^2]} \end{aligned} \tag{10}$$

for $i = 1, \ldots, 2n_1$.

M-step:

$$\hat{\mu}_{1,m} = \frac{\Sigma z_i \hat{I}_{i,e}}{\Sigma \hat{I}_{i,e}}$$

$$\hat{\mu}_{2,m} = \frac{\Sigma z_i (1 - \hat{I}_{i,e})}{2n_1 - \Sigma \hat{I}_{i,e}}$$

$$\hat{\sigma}_m^2 = \frac{1}{2n_1} \sum [(z_i - \hat{\mu}_{1,m})^2 \hat{I}_{i,e} + (z_i - \hat{\mu}_{2,m})^2 (1 - \hat{I}_{i,e})] \tag{11}$$

The EM algorithm starts with some initial values for the parameters ($\hat{\mu}_{1,e}$, $\hat{\mu}_{2,e}$, $\hat{\sigma}_e^2$) in the E-step to obtain the estimates of the missing data I_i, $i = 1, \ldots, 2n_1$. With the use of these estimates of I_i from the E-step, we obtain estimates $\hat{\mu}_{1,m}$, $\hat{\mu}_{2,m}$ and $\hat{\sigma}_m^2$ in the M-step. These estimates of the means and the common variance will then be used in the next E-step, and so on. The iterative process continues until convergence occurs. At convergence, we obtain the maximum likelihood estimate (MLE) $\hat{\sigma}$ of σ. Notice that the process also involves the estimation of μ_1 and μ_2. However, it is known [e.g., Fowlkes (1979)] that the accuracy of the estimation of μ_1 and μ_2 cannot be assured because of their sensitivity to the starting values. This property actually works toward the benefit of the proposed procedure since, as asserted earlier, we intend to prevent comparison between treatment group means at the interim stage. We shall demonstrate that the estimation of σ, which is our goal, works quite well despite the poor estimation of μ_1 and μ_2.

For the choice of the initial values of the parameters for starting the EM algorithm, we have the following suggestion adopted from Fowlkes (1979). Let $z_{(1)} < z_{(2)} < \cdots < z_{(2n_1)}$ be the ordered data and $p_i = (1 - 0.5)/2n_1$ for $i = 1, \ldots, 2n_1$. Take the quantiles of the unit normal calculated by $q_i = \Phi^{-1}(p_i)$, where Φ^{-1} is the inverse of the standard normal distribution function. Then fit the simple linear regression by least squares to the points $[(q_i, z_{(i)}), i = 1, \ldots, 2n_1]$. Denote the intercept and slope of the fitted line as (a, b) calculated by

$$b = \frac{\Sigma q_i z_{(i)} - (2n_1)\overline{qz}}{\Sigma q_i^2 - (2n_1)\overline{q}^2} \qquad a = \overline{z} - b\overline{q}$$

The initial values of σ, μ_1, and μ_2 are then

$$\hat{\sigma}_e = b \qquad \hat{\mu}_{1,e} = a - \frac{b}{c} \qquad \hat{\mu}_{2,e} = a + \frac{b}{c} \tag{12}$$

where c is some chosen constant. The choice of c influences the estimation of the means but not the variance. In practice, a choice of c might be considered as $c = 2b/\delta*$ such that $\hat{\mu}_{2,e} - \hat{\mu}_{1,e}$ is close to $\delta*$. However, since the true δ is unknown, being close to $\delta*$ does not guarantee success. We therefore use another value for c as follows. In most clinical trials that involve normal approximation for the sample size estimation, the inverse of the coefficient of variation $\lambda = \delta/\sigma$ usually ranges approximately from 0.20 to 0.50 (which correspond to about 430 and 70 patients per group, respectively, for power = 0.90, one-sided $\alpha = 0.05$, or about 400 and 60 patients per group for power = 0.80, two-sided $\alpha = 0.05$). Hence we take the middle value 0.35 in this range and convert it to $c = 2 \times (1/0.35) = 5.71$. In the next section we use simulations to examine the performance of the proposed procedure with this choice of c in the estimation of σ.

B. Simulation Results

We have undertaken a simulation study to examine the MLE of σ, and the sample size reestimation. We studied the following combination of situations: $\sigma = 1, 3, 5, 10, 20$; $n_1 = 50$ and 100. In each of the situations, $\mu_1 = 0$ and μ_2 varies so that the inverse of the coefficient of variation, $\lambda = (\mu_2 - \mu_1)/\sigma = \delta/\sigma$, ranges from 0.20 to 0.50. In our experience, these wide ranges of σ and λ cover most of the conditions in clinical trials involving normal approximation for sample size estimation. In addition, we also add $\lambda = 0$ for the case when the null hypothesis is true. The choice of the constant c in (12) was 5.71, as discussed previously, representing situations of good estimation (for $\lambda = 0.35$), overestimation (for $\lambda = 0.20$ and $\lambda = 0$), and underestimation (for $\lambda = 0.50$) in the setting of initial values, respectively. The normal variates were generated by the NORMAL substitute of SAS (1990). One hundred replicates were run in each of the situations, which provided standard errors of the means (SEM) within the range of 0.010 (for $\sigma = 1$) to 0.221 (for $\sigma = 20$) in the estimation of σ; or SEM/σ = 0.01 for all the cases (see Table 1).

Table 1 MLE of σ Based on $n_1 = 50$[a]

	True σ				
λ	1	3	5	10	20
0	0.947 (0.010)	2.815 (0.030)	4.776 (0.055)	9.356 (0.092)	18.747 (0.209)
0.20	0.953 (0.010)	2.837 (0.031)	4.826 (0.047)	9.723 (0.092)	18.792 (0.221)
0.35	0.945 (0.010)	2.848 (0.036)	4.890 (0.043)	9.560 (0.107)	19.304 (0.219)
0.50	0.959 (0.013)	2.941 (0.028)	4.907 (0.055)	9.862 (0.097)	20.003 (0.157)

[a] Mean and standard error of the mean of 100 simulation runs. $\mu_1 = 0$, μ_2 varies so that $\lambda = (\mu_2 - \mu_1)/\sigma = 0, 0.20, 0.35$, and 0.50 for different σ.

In all the situations, convergence (i.e., maximum absolute differences between successive steps of the estimate of μ_1, μ_2, and σ is less than 0.001) was achieved in an average of 40 to 60 iterations (with standard error about 4.4). Table 1 summarizes the MLE of σ for the combinations of true λ and σ, using $n_1 = 50$ observations per group. We can see that, in general, the procedure tends to slightly underestimate σ, but the estimation is quite satisfactory in all the situations. Using $n_1 = 100$ improved the estimation of σ moderately (not shown here). These results suggest that, as in the usual maximum likelihood estimation case, we would correct the small-sample bias by replacing the denominator $2n_1$ in equation (11) with $2(n_1 - 1)$ when using $n_1 = 50$, but this correction is not necessary for $n_1 = 100$.

C. Example

By using formulas (6) and (7), we illustrate the effect in the following numerical example. Assume that we require power $= 0.90$ and $\alpha = 0.05$ (one-sided) and are interested in detecting $\delta^* = 0.30$. Then the planned sample size would be 430 patients per group if the assumed $\sigma^* = 1.5$, or would be 122 per group if $\sigma^* = 0.80$. However, the true sample size required in 192 patients per group for the (unknown) true $\sigma = 1$. The proposed procedure, using an interim analysis when 50 patients per group are available, will reestimate the required sample size to be 188 per group. Notice the closeness of the reestimation to the true sample size required. According to the procedure, we would then increase the sample size by about 66 ($= 188 - 122$) patients per group if the originally planned sample size was 122 per group (under the initial assumption of $\sigma^* = 0.80$), or would retain the planned size if it was 430 per group (under the initial assumption of $\sigma^* = 1.5$).

The example above is a special case of the illustration in Figure 1. In the figure, the reestimated sample size is compared with the true sample size and the planned sample sizes for different alternative hypothesis δ^*. The reestimated sample sizes are very close to the true sample sizes in all the conditions studied. Depending on the assumed σ^* at the planning stage and the specific alternative hypothesis fixed by the researcher, the effect of the sample size reestimation procedure can be substantial in securing the desired power of a clinical trial.

IV. TWO-SAMPLE BINARY CASE WITHOUT UNBLINDING

Gould (1991) has proposed a procedure of sample size reestimation for the binary case. Notice that in the normal case, the sample size is adjusted at the interim stage, according to the comparison between the variance assumed in the design and the variance obtained from the interim data, and the adjustment is made independently from the difference of means expressed in the alterna-

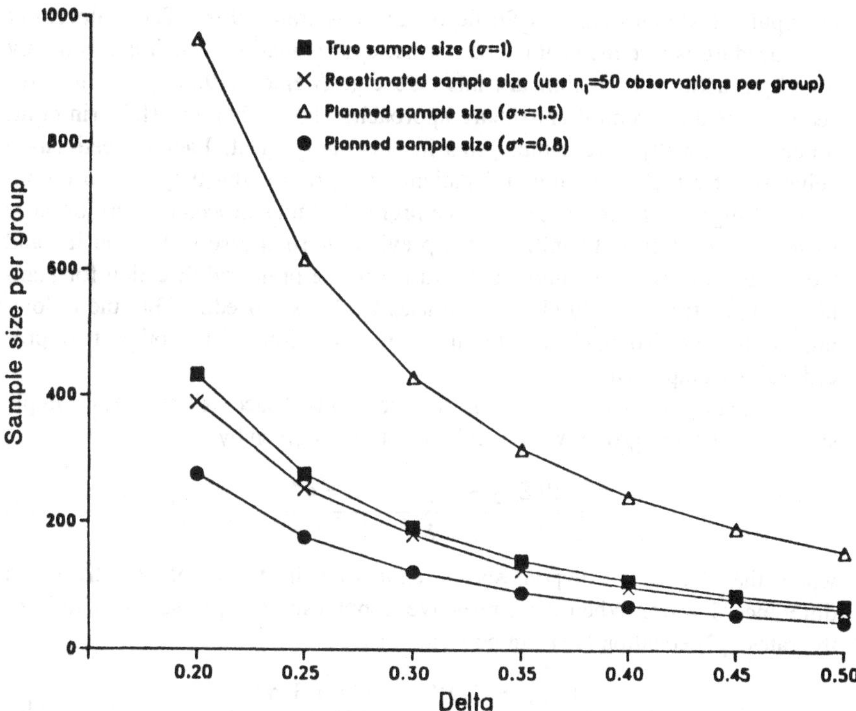

Figure 1 True, planned, and reestimated sample size versus delta power = 90%, $\alpha = 0.05$ (one-sided).

tive hypothesis. The procedure works well since mean and variance are distinct parameters in the normal case. In the binary case, however, the variance is a function of the mean. This is the basic technical difficulty for extending the procedure in Section III to the binary case. Another difficulty is that different expressions of the alternative hypothesis (in terms of difference or ratio) may lead to opposite decisions based on the same interim information. In this section we discuss these problems in details and give cautions for those who intend to apply Gould's procedure for their studies.

Denote p_1 and p_2 as the true "success" rates in the two treatment groups, respectively. At the planning stage, one specifies values for p_1 and p_2 (denote them by $p_1{}^*$ and $p_2{}^*$) for the alternative hypothesis, which is either expressed by the difference, $\delta^* = p_1^* - p_2^*$, or by the ratio $\gamma^* = p_1^*/p_2^*$, with power $1 - \beta$ and type I error rate α.

Lachin (1977) compared three estimation procedures of the sample size: Schork and Remington (1967), Halperin et al. (1968), and Lachin (1977). The Remington procedure uses a crude normal approximation, which is also used in popular textbooks such as Snedecor and Cochran (1967). The Halperin et al. procedure is a refinement of the normal approximation, which is commonly used by practitioners in clinical trials [see e.g., Meinert (1986)]. Lachin's procedure uses a noncentral chi-square approach. The Lachin and Halperin et al. procedures usually give sample size in close agreement, Lachin's estimation being slightly higher (within +2 patients per group). But they both are consistently higher than Remington's. We prefer Lachin's procedure here because its form is simpler and similar to the previous normal case in Section III, and the sample size result is more conservative in the preferred direction for planning clinical trials. Gould (1991) also uses Lachin's procedure. But the following discussion also applies with minor modifications if the other two procedures are employed.

Specifically, let $\sigma = (p_1 + p_2)/2$ be the pooled "success" rate. The sample size per treatment group, with equal allocation, is given by

$$n = \frac{2(Z_{\alpha/2} + Z_\beta)^2 \sigma^*(1 - \sigma^*)}{\delta^{*2}} \tag{13}$$

when the alternative hypothesis is expressed in terms of the treatment difference $\delta = \delta^*$. When the alternative hypothesis is expressed as a ratio of the rates, γ^*, equation (13) can be written as

$$n = \frac{\tfrac{1}{2}(Z_{\alpha/2} + Z_\beta)^2 (1 - \sigma^*)(1 + \gamma^*)^2}{\sigma^*(1 - \gamma^*)^2} \tag{14}$$

where Z_p is the $(1 - p)$ percentile of the standard normal distribution.

Equation (13) has been given in Lachin (1977, 1981), and equation (14) is obtained by the following one-to-one mappings among (σ, δ), (σ, γ), and (p_1, p_2):

$$p_1 = \frac{2\sigma\gamma}{1 + \gamma}, \qquad p_2 = \frac{2\sigma}{1 + \gamma} \tag{15}$$

$$p_1 = \sigma + \frac{\delta}{2}, \qquad p_2 = \sigma - \frac{\delta}{2} \tag{16}$$

$$\delta = \frac{2\sigma(\gamma - 1)}{\gamma + 1} \tag{17}$$

Gould (1991) noted that only the pooled rate, σ^*, is an assumed value in equation (13) or (14) which needs to be monitored and verified with the data and that other elements, α, β, and δ^* (or γ^*), are design specifications that should not change with the data. This is so since the value δ^* (or γ^*) specified in the alternative hypothesis reflects the research interest a priori, as in the normal case where the variance needs to be monitored and the clinically meaningful difference of the means for testing is prespecified and does not change.

There are, however, several potential difficulties with the binary case in practice, as we caution in the following.

First, the two expressions, difference and ratio of the rates, for the alternative hypothesis may give different indications of sample size adjustment from the same interim information. Specifically, the reestimated sample size per group, N, for testing the same alternative hypothesis under the same condition of power and type I errors, based on a pooled rate $\hat{\sigma}$ (from an interim sample of $n_1 = n/2$ patients per group, say), is a multiple of the originally planned sample size, n, as

$$N = f \times n$$

where the multiplier

$$f = f_d = \frac{\hat{\sigma}(1 - \hat{\sigma})}{\sigma^*(1 - \sigma^*)} \tag{18}$$

when the alternative hypothesis is expressed in terms of δ, and

$$f = f_r = \frac{\sigma^*(1 - \hat{\sigma})}{(1 - \sigma^*)\hat{\sigma}} \tag{19}$$

when the alternative hypothesis is expressed in terms of γ.

The procedure says that if the factor $f \geqslant 1$, the sample size will be increased to N per group; otherwise, the original sample size is large enough and the trial will continue as initially planned to the completion of n patients per group.

A potential problem is that (18) and (19) may indicate different directions as whether or not to increase sample size. For example, suppose that the assumed pooled rate is $\sigma^* = 0.3$ at the planning stage and the observed pooled rate is $\hat{\sigma} = 0.5$ at the interim stage. Then $f_d = (0.5 \times 0.5)/(0.3 \times 0.7) > 1$, but $f_r = (0.3 \times 0.5)/(0.7 \times 0.5) < 1$.

Second, the practitioners may find the specification of a clinically important difference (or ratio) of the rates not so easy, since the importance of the magnitude depends on the prevalence and the severity of the disease under study, and the disease prevalence varies in time and geographic regions. Investigators from different regions participating in a multicenter study would naturally have different opinions on the magnitude of importance for δ or γ. Small δ or γ can be very important for regions where the disease has high prevalence rate, but not as important for regions with low prevalence rate. As a consequence, medical researchers often request the detection of a true difference (or ratio) of the rates at the end of a study, whatever it may be, even though they agreed upon a δ^* or γ^* in the beginning of the study. For this we caution that in the sample size reestimation process, we are monitoring the power/sample size from the data, not monitoring the alternative hypothesis. We would never know whether the alternative hypothesis is reasonable or not until we break the treatment codes. We further illustrate this discussion numerically as follows.

Figure 2 shows several sample size curves as function of the alternative hypothesis γ^* and the pooled rate σ for power = 0.90 and type I error $\alpha = 0.05$ (two-sided). For example, suppose we assume that $\sigma^* = 0.7$ and specify $\gamma^* \geqslant 1.3$ at the planning stage (which is equivalent to specifying possible values for p_1 and p_2 in the range of $p_1 \geqslant 0.79$ and $p_2 \leqslant 0.61$). This requires the trial to start with 133 patients per group in the plan. At the interim stage, say, after half of the patients have the results, the pooled rate $\hat{\sigma}$ turns out to be 0.5. Then to detect the same ratio, 1.3, the sample size needs to be increased to 309 per group. Of course, when the pooled rate decreases from 0.7 (the assumed value) to 0.5 (the observed value at the interim stage), there could be several possibilities: it may be that the control group had a lower rate than what was expected; it may be that the active treatment group had a lower rate than expected; or it may be that both groups had lower rates. These scenarios would lead us to make different decisions regarding the sample size adjustment had we known which one is the fact. But since we do not know (due to the blinding of the trial), as long as we do not change the hypothesis, which we should not, the procedure calls for an increase of the sample size to 309 patients per group. This, in effect, implies that we are willing to take the third possibility as if it were the fact (i.e., both groups had lower than expected rates: $p_1 = 0.57$ and $p_2 = 0.43$).

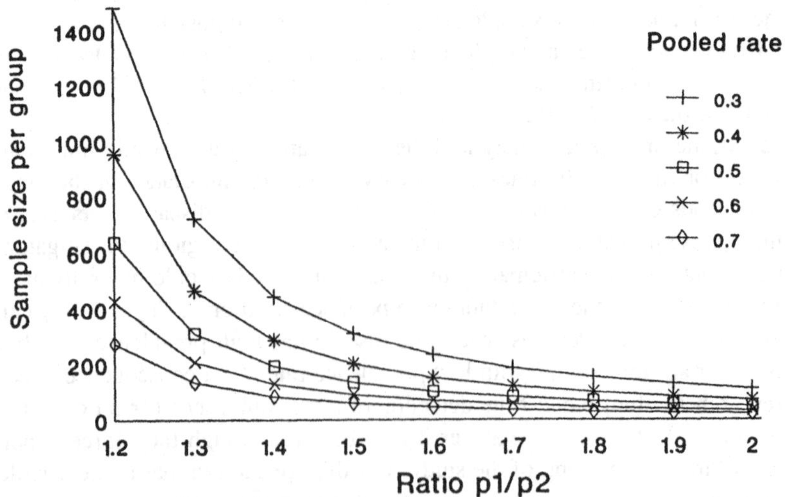

Figure 2 Sample size for binomial distribution.

We caution that it is possible that one of the other two scenarios was in fact true, in which case we would not increase the original sample size (113 per group) either because the original sample size is already large enough (when the control group has a lower rate) or because the alternative hypothesis does not hold (when the active treatment group has a lower rate). One should recognize that the sample size reestimation procedure of Gould (1991) is not intended for checking whether or not the alternative hypothesis is set up reasonably.

V. DISCUSSION

We have reviewed two types of sample size reestimation techniques in this chapter. The first is Stein's approach; the second is what we have proposed. The important difference between the two types is that Stein's procedure requires unblinding the treatment code but permits early stopping of the trial at the interim stage. Also, it does not utilize the full information in the final analysis. Our procedure maintains the blinding of the trial at the interim stage and, in principle, continues the trial to the completion of either the planned or the reestimated sample size. (Some flexibility of our method is discussed later.) Wittes and Brittain (1990) also considered an approach similar to ours, but in the context of pilot studies. Although Stein's method was demonstrated by confidence interval estimation, due to the cumbersomeness of its original form, it also works for the hypothesis-testing setting as well. We emphasize that the goal of our new procedure is to reestimate the sample size, not to end the trial early with acceptance or rejection of the null hypothesis. Hence the type I error rate is not affected materially by this procedure. [see Gould and Shih (1991) for detail]. The method is useful for clinical trials evaluating the efficacy of new drugs in treating nonfatal diseases, in which early stopping is not a concern.

The main idea used in Section III is formulating the problem in terms of a mixture of normal distributions and applying the EM algorithm to obtain the MLEs. Other estimation methods (e.g., moment estimator) or algorithms (e.g., Newton–Raphson) are also available in the literature [see e.g., Everitt and Hand (1980)], but the EM method has the advantage of its simplicity. The EM algorithm works well for the normal distribution, but not for the binomial case since the mean and the variance are distinct parameters in the former, but not the latter.

It was emphasized in Section III that this procedure does not estimate the true difference of treatment means, δ. The statistical power, which is required at the planning stage and then ensured at the interim stage, is under a fixed alternative hypothesis δ^*, specified by the researcher. Sample sizes are calculated based on δ^* since it is generally recognized that in clinical trials, the sample size should be made adequate to detect the least difference between treatment groups that is clinically meaningful, not solely to attain statistically significant results. Furthermore, the ultimate power would be greater if the (unknown) true difference is larger than δ^*, a case that we always would like to ensure in a trial. It is easy to find clinically meaningful changes in different continuous variables in the medical literature. For example, see Gometz and Cirillo (1985) for blood pressures; Dyck and O'Brien (1989) for nerve conduction velocity, and so on. It is, however, not so easy to define clinically meaningful changes in comparing probability of "success" such as cure rates of antibiotics, since it depends on the prevalence and severity of the disease.

Although the new procedure in Section III is applicable for multiple reestimations, we recommend it be performed only once, when enough patients (at least 50 per group, based on the simulation results) are available. This restriction of one reestimation is simply for administrative reasons, since adding new patients in multicenter clinical trials, if necessary, involves changes in many practical matters, such as contracts, budgets, perhaps number of centers, and so on. The earlier and fewer changes that have to be made, the better.

When the number of patients based on the reestimation is much larger than an affordable limit (say, N^* per group), one can calculate the power based on $\hat{\sigma}$, δ^*, and N^*, and decide the course of action for the trial. Depending on the conditions, such as the ultimate power, ease or difficulty of recruiting new patients or new investigators, and so on, a possible but rare decision in this case may be to bail out the trial without either rejection or acceptance of the null hypothesis.

On the other hand, in situations when the reestimated sample size is much smaller than the planned size (such as 188 versus 430 patients per group as illustrated in Section III.C), one may be encouraged to plan breaking the codes and comparing the treatment groups when the reestimated sample size is reached. In this case the proposed method can be used in conjunction with other group sequential methods, such as the α-spending function (Lan and DeMets, 1983; Hwang et al., 1990). In this case the type I error rate may need to be adjusted accordingly.

REFERENCES

Armitage, P. (1957). Restricted sequential procedures. *Biometrika 44*: 9–26.

Armitage, P., McPherson, C. K., and Rowe, B. C. (1969). Repeated significance tests on accumulating data. *J. R. Stat. Soc. A 132*: 234–244.

Bross, I. (1952). Sequential medical plans. *Biometrics 8*: 188–225.

Dempster, A. P., Laird, N. M., and Rubin, D. B. (1977). Maximum likelihood from incomplete data via the EM algorithm (with discussion). *J. R. Stat. Soc. B 39*: 1–38.

Dyck, P. J., and O'Brien, P. C. (1989). Meaningful degrees of prevention or improvement of nerve conduction in controlled clinical trials of diabetic neuropathy. *Diabetes Care 12*(9): 649–652.

Everitt, B. S., and Hand, D. J. (1980). *Finite Mixture Distributions,* Chapman & Hall, London.

Fowlkes, E. B. (1979). Some methods for studying the mixture of two normal (lognormal) distributions. *J. Am. Stat. Assoc. 74*: 561–575.

Geller, N. L., and Pocock, S. J. (1987). Interim analyses in randomized clinical trials: ramifications and guidelines for practitioners. *Biometrics 43*: 213–223.

Gometz, H. J., and Cirillo, V. J. (1985). Determination of the optimal dose of antihypertensive druves. *Progress in Pharmacology,* 6/1, Gustav Fisher, Stuttgart, pp. 125–133.

Gould, A. L. (1991). Interim analyses for monitoring clinical trials that do not affect the type I error rate. To appear in *Stat. Med.*

Gould, A. L., and Pecor, V. J. (1982). Group sequential methods for clinical trials allowing early acceptance of H_0 and incorporating costs. *Biometrika 69*: 75–80.

Gould, A. L., and Shih, W. J. (1991). Interim analyses for sample size reestimation without unblinding for normally distributed outcomes with unknown variance. Submitted for publication.

Halperin, M., Rogot, E., Gurian, J., and Ederer, F. (1968). Sample sizes for medical trials with special reference to long term therapy. *J. Chronic Dis. 21*: 13–23.

Hwang, I. K., Shih, W. J., and DeCani, J. S. (1990). Group sequential designs using a family of type I error probability spending rate functions. *Stat. Med. 9*: 1439–1445.

Lachin, J. M. (1977). Sample size determination for $r \times c$ comparative trials. *Biometrics 33*: 315–324.

Lachin, J. M. (1981). Introduction to sample size determination and power analysis for clinical trials. *Controlled Clin. Trials 2*: 93–113.

Lan, K. K. G., and DeMets, D. L. (1983). Design and analysis of group sequential tests based on the type I error spending rate function. *Biometrika 74*: 149–154.

Meinert, C. L. (1986). *Clinical Trials: Design, Conduct, and Analysis,* Oxford University Press, New York.

O'Brien, P. C., and Fleming, T. R. (1979). A multiple testing procedure for clinical trials. *Biometrics 35*: 549–556.

Pocock, S. J. (1977). Group sequential methods in the design and analysis of clinical trials. *Biometrika 64*: 191–199.

Pocock, S. J. (1982). Interim analyses for randomized clinical trials: the group sequential approach. *Biometrics 38*: 153–162.

Rubin, D. B. (1976). Inference and missing data. *Biometrika 63*: 581–592.

SAS (1990). *SAS User's Guide: Statistics,* Version 6 edition, SAS Institute, Cary, N.C.

Schork, M. A., and Remington, R. D. (1967). The determination of sample size in treatment control comparisons for chronic disease studies in which drop-out or non-adherence is a problem. *J. Chronic Dis. 20*: 223–239.

Snedecor, G. W., and Cochran, W. G. (1967). *Statistical Methods,* 6th ed., Iowa State University Press, Ames, Iowa.

Stein, C. (1945). A two-sample test for a linear hypothesis whose power is independent of the variance. *Ann. Math. Stat. 16*: 243–258.

Wald, A. (1947). *Sequential Analysis,* Wiley, New York.

Wittes, J. and Brittain, E. (1990). The role of internal pilot studies in increasing the efficiency of clinical trials. *Stat. Med. 9*: 65–72.

19

Interim Analysis in the Development of an Anti-Inflammatory Agent

Sample Size Reestimation and Conditional Power Analysis

Ronald Pedersen and Robert R. Starbuck

Wyeth-Ayerst Research, Radnor, Pennsylvania

I. BACKGROUND

Rheumatoid arthritis is characterized by a gradual accumulation of damage to joints. This damage includes erosion of bone and joint space narrowing resulting from loss of cartilage. The adjuvant-injected rat shares a number of symptomatic and pathological features with the human arthritis patient, including damage to bone and cartilage. A developmental nonsteroidal anti-inflammmatory drug (NSAID) was compared to other NSAIDs and to aspirin in experiments in rats with established Freund's adjuvant arthritis. This experimental compound was found to arrest or retard the progression of disease to a greater degree than the other compounds in these experiments. In humans, early studies indicated that the compound was effective in relieving the signs and symptoms of rheumatoid arthritis and degenerative joint disease. These findings suggest that this compound could effectively retard the progression of joint disease associated with rheumatoid arthritis in humans.

II. PROTOCOL

A. Original Plan

The objective of the protocol was to evaluate the long-term effects of the test drugs in patients with active rheumatoid arthritis, including the drugs' ability to retard, arrest, reverse, and/or cure the joint damage associated with rheumatoid arthritis. Two doses of the experimental NSAID were to be compared with the recommended dose of a standard NSAID. The study design called for a double-blind, randomized, parallel group multicenter trial. Eligible patients were to receive treatment for up to 3 years.

Two primary measures of efficacy were planned. One was the rate of radiologic changes of the hands and wrists; the other was the frequency of disease remission, as measured by the American Rheumatism Association (ARA) criteria for remission of rheumatoid arthritis. These include the duration of morning stiffness, fatigue, joint pain, joint tenderness, pain on motion, soft tissue swelling in joints or tendon sheaths, and the erythrocyte sedimentation rate.

The planned approach for analysis was for an outside independent consultant to test at five intervals using Pocock's (1982) decision boundaries. The required p-values and the number of completed patients expected at each interim analysis are shown in Table 1 for an overall significance level of 5% and power of 90%.

These interim analyses were to be performed on the radiologic data accumulated during the trial and on the proposed ARA remission criteria. If the radiographic results were favorable but the ARA criteria had not reached statistical significance, a consultation with the Food and Drug Administration (FDA) prior to terminating the trial was planned.

B. Modified Approach—Rationale

Three years after protocol enrollment began, when 1300 patients had been enrolled, a complete review of the developmental program for this product was undertaken. Much attention was given to the primary endpoint of radiologic change in the hands and wrists. It was decided that the sample size should be reassessed and that the interim analysis strategy included in the original protocol should be modified. (*Note:* At this point no interim analyses of x-ray

Table 1 Original Interim Analysis Schedule

Nominal significance level for five repeated tests	Number of completed patients
0.010	405
0.017	810
0.017	1215
0.017	1620
0.021	2025

data had been performed and only some of the x-ray films had been evaluated.)

It was concluded that five interim analyses would be logistically difficult, and spreading the error rate ($\alpha = 0.05$) nearly evenly over five interim looks would result in little sensitivity to detect real treatment differences at any one of the five looks. Therefore, formal analysis only at the end of the trial was considered preferable. Early termination for efficacy based on the data available was excluded from the plan. A portion of the existing data would be examined to refine sample size estimates as part of a reevaluation of the feasibility of the study.

A. Final Interim Analysis Plan

The following proposed amendment to the statistical analysis strategy was discussed with the FDA and, ultimately, implemented. This process is outlined in Figure 1. Two hundred ninety-six pairs of x-ray films, taken at baseline and 1 year (or at termination between 6 months and 1 year) and 150 pairs taken at baseline and 2 years (or at termination between 1.25 and 2 years) were to be summarized as follows: The slope of the control group would be used to obtain a refined estimate of the sample sizes required to detect a 25% or 12.5% difference in slopes between the high-dose experimental drug group and the control drug group using a two-tailed test with 90% power. These choices reflected the belief that the patients receiving the experimental NSAID might have up to 25% less erosion and joint space narrowing per year, compared to the patients receiving the standard NSAID.

The feasibility of enrolling the required numbers of patients was to be determined on the basis of these refined sample sizes. If the study was not considered feasible, study enrollment would be closed and the trial would be concluded. If the additional enrollment was considered feasible and the required number of patients had already been enrolled, enrollment would be closed and the study would be concluded; otherwise, the likelihood of obtaining a statistically significant finding, were the projected sample size obtained, would be evaluated as discussed by Ware et al. (1985). If this likelihood were acceptably high, the enrollment would continue to the refined sample size; otherwise, the trial would be concluded. The trial would not be stopped for success, so the type I error rate would not be altered. The conditional power analyses to determine the likelihood of a significant result would focus on the comparison of the high-dose experimental group with the control group.

III. MONITORING AND DATA COLLECTION

When the modified plan for interim analyses was approved, 1421 patients had been enrolled; the enrollment status and the status of the x-ray readings are

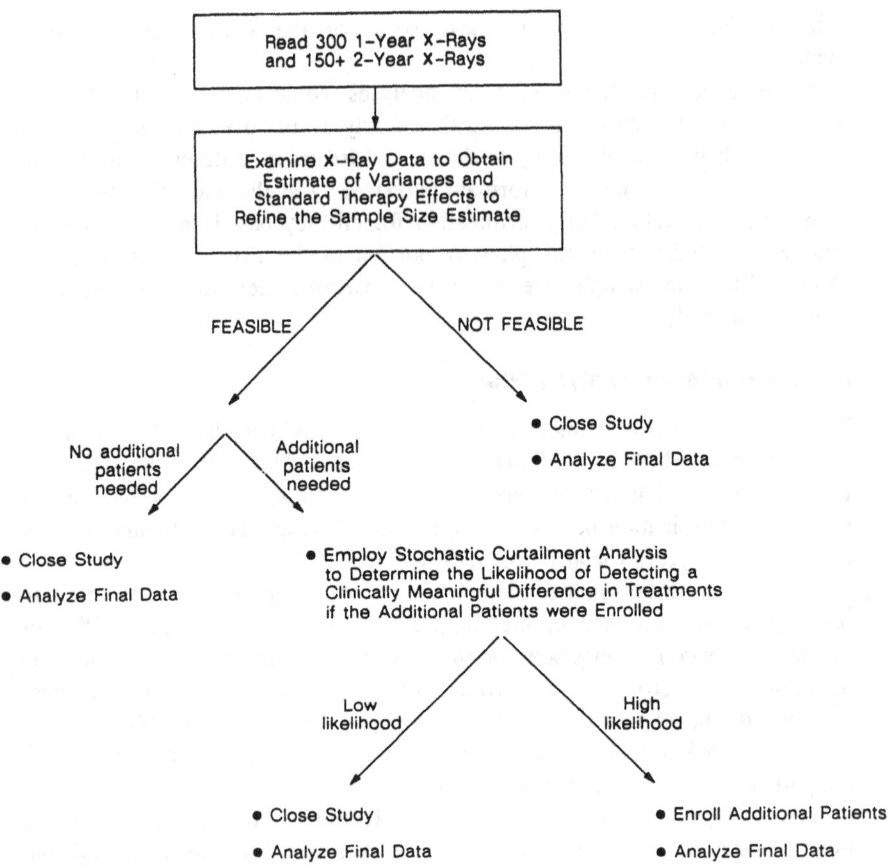

Figure 1 Interim analysis plan.

shown in Table 2. Because the x-rays films were read in pairs (baseline and those taken during therapy), and because each pair had to be read by three radiologists, considerable time would have passed before additional x-ray data could become available. The decision was made to proceed with reestimation of sample size and stochastic curtailment analysis with the 445 pairs available at that time.

The intended key analysis variable was the sum of erosions and joint space narrowings, averaged over all three readers. The agreement among readers was tested by computing Cronbach's coefficient α (Lord and Novick, 1968). For the combined total of erosion and joint space narrowings, Cronbach's α was found to be 0.92, which is considered to indicate very good agreement among readers.

Table 2 Enrollment at Time of Protocol Review

Number of patients		Time (yr) period	Number of x-rays Taken	Number of x-rays Read
Number enrolled	1421	½–1	815	295 (36%)
Completed 1 year	655	1¼–2	477	150 (31%)
Completed 2 years	401	2¼–3	247	0
			1539	445 (29%)

Those patients with follow-up x-ray films at both the 1-year and 2-year visits had their baseline read twice. The recommended method of reading the x-rays in pairs (Fries et al., 1986) is intended to produce reliable estimates of the change within the pair only; therefore, the following adjustment was made for these patients. The baseline score was taken to be the average of the two readings, and the 1- and 2-year scores were adjusted to maintain the difference from the matched baseline reading. The adjusted pooled data were used in all subsequent analyses.

IV. STATISTICAL METHODS AND RESULTS

A. Sample Size Reestimation

Both the raw data and the logarithmically transformed values (plus ½) were considered in the sample size reestimation. The logarithmically transformed data seemed more appropriate for this analysis, however, because these data were more nearly normal in their distribution and the variance was less correlated with the mean. The results of the estimates based on the logarithmically transformed data were therefore given greater consideration in the decision process.

To estimate the sample size, regressions were fitted to each person in the control group and the mean $\hat{b}_2$, and variance s_2^2, of these slopes were obtained for the observed portion of the sampled data, as described below. The number of patients required in each treatment group was then

$$n = \frac{2s_2^2(Z_{0.025} + Z_{0.1})^2}{(\hat{b}_2 - \hat{b}_1)^2}$$

Consideration was given to $b_1 = 0.75b_2$ and $b_1 = 0.875b_2$ in these calculations.

B. Conditional Power Calculation [Following Ware (1988)]

Each patient was to have an x-ray evaluation at baseline and at the end of 1, 2, and 3 years on double-blind therapy. Upon completion of the study the rate of joint score degeneration will be estimated by the slope estimate

$$\hat{b}_{ij} = \Sigma w_{ijk} y_{ijk}$$

where

$$w_{ijk} = \frac{x_{ijk} - \bar{x}_{ij}}{\Sigma(x_{ijk} - \bar{x}_{ij})^2}$$

for the $i = , \ldots , n_j$ patients in the $j = 1, 2$ treatment groups for the $x_{ijk}(k = 1, 2, 3, 4)$ times. The mean slope will be estimated for the jth group as

$$\bar{b}_j = \frac{\sum_{i=1}^{n} \hat{b}_{ij}}{n_j} \qquad j = 1, 2$$

with sample variance estimated as

$$s_j^2 = \frac{\sum_{i=1}^{n} (\hat{b}_{ij} - \bar{b}_j)}{n_j - 1}$$

The hypothesis of equal treatment effect will be tested by computing

$$t = \frac{\bar{b}_1 - \bar{b}_2}{\sqrt{s_1^2/n_1 + s_2^2/n_2}} \quad \text{or approximately} \quad z = \frac{\bar{b}_1 - \bar{b}_2}{\sqrt{\sigma_1^2/n_1 + \sigma_2^2/n_2}}$$

Partway through the study partial information is available on those patients who have had at least one double-blind x-ray. At that time, the estimated slopes will have a conditional distribution given the observed data, y_{ijo}, of the form

$$f(\hat{b}_{ij} \mid \mathbf{y}_{ijo}) \sim N(\mu_{ij}, \sigma_{ij}^2)$$

To calculate the conditional power we need $E(b_{ij} \mid \mathbf{y}_{ijo})$, and $\text{var}(b_{ij} \mid \mathbf{y}_{ijo})$. In treatment group j, letting $\mathbf{x}' = [0, x_{ij1}, x_{ij2}, x_{ij3}]$,

$$E(\mathbf{y}_{ij}) = \beta_0 + \mathbf{x}\beta_j = \mu_j \qquad \text{and} \qquad \text{var}(y_i) = \Sigma_{4\times4}$$

The conditional means, ν_{ij}, variances, σ_{ij}^2, and conditional variances, δ_{ij}^2, of the slopes can be calculated as

$$E(b_{ij} \mid \mathbf{y}_{ijo}) = \underset{\text{observed}}{\Sigma w_{ijk} y_{ijk}} + \underset{\text{unobserved}}{\Sigma w_{ijk}^* y_{ijk}^*} = \nu_{ij}$$

$$\text{var}(b_{ij}) = (\mathbf{x}'\Sigma\mathbf{x})^{-1} = \sigma_{ij}^2$$

$$\text{var}(b_{ij} \mid \mathbf{y}_{ijo}) = \mathbf{w}_{ij}^* \text{cov}(\mathbf{y}_{ij}^* \mid \mathbf{y}_{ijo}) \mathbf{w}_{ij}^* = \delta_{ij}^2$$

where $\mathbf{y}^*$ and $\text{cov}(\mathbf{y}_{ij}^* \mid \mathbf{y}_{ijo})$ are determined for group j as follows: Partition $\Sigma_{4\times 4}$ and μ into

$$\begin{bmatrix} \Sigma_{11} & \Sigma_{12} \\ \Sigma_{21} & \Sigma_{22} \end{bmatrix} \quad \text{and} \quad \begin{bmatrix} \mu \\ \mu^* \end{bmatrix}$$

Letting t equal the number of completed observations and t^* equal the number of expected additional observations, Σ_{11} is $t \times t$, Σ_{22} is $t^* \times t^*$, μ is $1 \times t$, and μ^* is $1 \times t^*$. Then

$$\text{cov}(\mathbf{y}_{ij}^* \mid \mathbf{y}_{ij}) = \Sigma_{22} - \Sigma_{21}\Sigma_{11}^{-1}\Sigma_{12},$$

and

$$\mathbf{y}_{ij}^* = E(Y_{\text{unobs}} \mid Y_{\text{obs}}) = \mu^* + \Sigma_{21}\Sigma_{11}^{-1}(\mathbf{y} - \mu)$$

The conditional probability of rejecting H_0 (using the large-sample normal approximation),

$$P\left[\frac{\bar{b}_1 - \bar{b}_2}{\sqrt{\sigma_1^2/n_1 + \sigma_2^2/n_2}}\right] > 1.96$$

can be shown to be

$$1 - \Phi\left[\frac{1.96(\Sigma\sigma_{i1}^2/n_1^2 + \Sigma\sigma_{i2}^2/n_2^2)^{1/2} - (\Sigma\nu_{i1}/n_1 - \Sigma\nu_{i2}/n_2)}{(\Sigma\delta_{i1}^2/n_1^2 + \Sigma\delta_{i2}^2/n_2^2)^{1/2}}\right]$$

where $\Phi(z)$ is the cumulative normal density function for a $N(0,1)$ distribution.

C. Estimating the Covariance Matrix

Various approaches to estimating the covariance matrix for longitudinal models are discussed by Ware (1985). We felt that the random coefficient growth model was appropriate for these data. Based on this model we are able to estimate the covariance matrix as

$$\mathrm{var}(\mathbf{y}_{ij}) = \mathbf{x}\Gamma\mathbf{x}' + \sigma_e^2\mathbf{I}$$

where

$$\mathbf{x} = \begin{bmatrix} 1 & 0 \\ 1 & x_1 \\ 1 & x_2 \\ 1 & x_3 \end{bmatrix} \qquad (x_t\text{: observed or expected time of observation})$$

and

$$\Gamma = \begin{bmatrix} \sigma_{\beta 0}^2 & \sigma_{\beta\beta 0} \\ \sigma_{\beta\beta 0} & \sigma_\beta^2 \end{bmatrix}$$

Estimates of $\sigma_{\beta 0}^2$, $\sigma_{\beta\beta 0}$, σ_β^2, and σ_e^2 were obtained following Halperin et al. (1987), as described below.

The error variance was estimated as the average mean-squared error from the individually fit regressions. The variances and covariance of the true intercept and slope, $\sigma_{\beta 0}^2$, σ_β^2, and $\sigma_{\beta\beta 0}$ were estimated through the following relationships:

$$\hat{s}_{b0}^2 = \sigma_{\beta 0}^2 + n_j^{-1} \sum_{j=1}^{n} \left(\frac{1}{m_{ij}} + \frac{\bar{x}_{ij}^2}{s_{ij}^2} \right) \sigma_e^2$$

$$\hat{s}_b^2 = \sigma_\beta^2 + n_j^{-1} \frac{\sum_{j=1}^{n} \sigma_e^2}{s_{ij}^2}$$

$$\mathrm{cov}(\hat{b}_0, \hat{b}) = \sigma_{\beta 0} - n_j^{-1} \frac{\sum_{j=1}^{n} \bar{x}_{ij}\sigma_e^2}{s_{ij}^2}$$

where $\bar{x}_{ij}$ is the average of the m_{ij} times of measurement for the ith individual in the jth group, and s_{ij}^2 is the sum of squares of deviations of the m_{ij} times from their mean.

D. Treatment of Completed, Ongoing, and Unobserved Patients

Patients who dropped out of the trial had zero conditional variance; their slope and variance estimates were unconditional. Ongoing patients were treated by assuming that they would complete the study with future visits at the scheduled timepoints. Unobserved patients (those with no follow up x-ray films read) were assigned the average conditional and unconditional variance estimates for their treatment group. The average conditional slope estimate was used to estimate the slope for unobserved patients in the standard therapy group. Three possible outcomes were considered for the slope estimate for the unobserved data in the experimental therapy group. These estimates were (1) the average estimate for the observed patients, (2) 25% less than the standard therapy group average, and (3) 12.5% less than the standard therapy group average.

E. Results

Patients fell into one of three subgroups, based on the availability of pairs of x-ray films. These groups are (1) baseline/1-year pair only, (2) baseline/2-year pair only, and (3) both pairs available. The mean scores of the total of erosions and joint space narrowings for the standard NSAID group and the high-dose experimental NSAID group are shown in Table 3.

The mean and variance estimates of the rate of disease progression in the control group, based on the unweighted average of the individually fitted regressions, are shown in Table 4. The results for both the raw data and the

Table 3 Total of Erosions and Joint Space Narrowings

		Baseline	Year 1	Year 2
	Group[a]	Mean (std)	Mean (std)	Mean (std)
		Raw data		
Standard NSAID	1 ($n = 63$)	15.4 (19.1)	18.0 (19.9)	
	2 ($n = 11$)	21.3 (27.6)		25.3 (28.5)
	3 ($n = 25$)	14.0 (20.8)	16.5 (23.3)	16.8 (22.9)
Experimental NSAID	1 ($n = 44$)	12.6 (13.7)	15.1 (15.4)	
	2 ($n = 14$)	8.0 (11.4)		11.4 (17.4)
	3 ($n = 36$)	11.0 (11.9)	14.2 (13.8)	17.5 (17.0)
		Log-transformed data		
Standard NSAID	1 ($n = 63$)	2.03 (1.38)	2.24 (1.37)	
	2 ($n = 11$)	1.98 (1.80)		2.32 (1.77)
	3 ($n = 25$)	2.17 (2.17)	2.22 (1.19)	2.03 (1.38)
Experimental NSAID	1 ($n = 44$)	1.93 (1.26)	2.13 (1.28)	
	2 ($n = 14$)	1.35 (1.34)		1.61 (1.45)
	3 ($n = 36$)	1.96 (1.07)	2.23 (1.08)	2.39 (1.13)

[a] See text for group definitions.

Table 4 Reestimated Sample Size Requirements

Transformation	$\hat{b}_2^2$	s_2^2	n ($b_1 = 0.75b_2$) (per group)	n ($b_1 = 0.875b_2$) (per group)
None	2.52	17.39	920	3680
Log	0.197	0.091	790	3159

logarithmically transformed data are shown. The table also shows the refined sample size estimates for detection of differences of 12.5% and 25% differences in slope between the standard drug and the experimental drug.

Note that the sample size of 790 is the number of patients required in the high-dose experimental group and in the standard therapy group. The original plan called for a low-dose experimental group to have 50% higher enrollment than for the high-dose experimental group or standard therapy group due to a prior expectation of a higher dropout rate in the low-dose experimental group. Examination of patient termination records, however, indicated similar dropout rates for all three groups. If equal-sample-size goals were set, a total of 2370 evaluable patients would be needed. To attain this number, approximately 3555 patients would have to be enrolled, since a third of enrolled patients drop out before the first scheduled follow-up x-ray film.

F. Disease Progression Rate Estimates

The slope and intercepts for the 94 patients receiving a high dose of the experimental drug and the 99 patients receiving the standard drug were obtained through linear regression on each patient's values. The unweighted averages, variances, and covariances of the intercept ($\hat{b}_0$) and slope ($\hat{b}$) for each group are shown in Table 5. The results indicate that the rate of disease progression,

Table 5 Unweighted Intercept ($\hat{b}_0$) and Slope ($\hat{b}$) Estimates

	n	$\hat{b}_0$	$\hat{s}_{b0}^2$	$\hat{b}$	$\hat{s}_b^2$	$\hat{s}_{bb0}$
			Raw data			
Standard	99	15.75	421.4	2.52	17.38	12.16
Experimental	94	11.28	161.5	2.88	21.55	19.08
			Log data			
Standard	99	2.02	1.862	0.196	0.091	−0.044
Experimental	94	1.86	1.472	0.213	0.146	−0.041

Table 6 Conditional Mean and Variance Estimates

	$\hat{\sigma}_b^2$	$\hat{\delta}_b^2$	$\hat{\nu}$
	Raw data		
Standard	14.81	13.16	2.49
Experimental	18.57	16.58	2.61
	Log data		
Standard	0.070	0.063	0.1917
Experimental	0.122	0.109	0.2093

expressed as the total of erosions and joint space narrowings per year, was slightly lower in the standard therapy group (2.52) than in the experimental therapy group (2.88).

G. Conditional Power Calculation

Conditional power calculations were based on a final sample size of 790 in each group. The estimates of the variances of the slopes and the conditional means and variances of the slopes for each group are shown in Table 6; the resultant conditional power estimates for the three alternative hypotheses considered are shown in Table 7. The probability of rejecting H_0 if the current trend continues is very small. However, if the original alternative hypothesis is considered (i.e., that the rate of disease progression on the experimental NSAID is 25% less than the rate on the standard NSAID), the conditional power is reduced only to 75%, compared to the designed power of 90%.

V. CONCLUSION

It had taken more than 4 years to enroll 1421 patients. Unless the rate of enrollment could be accelerated substantially, it could have taken an additional 6 to 7 years to enroll a total of 3555 patients. Because (1) the observed data did not support the hypothesis that the experimental therapy is better than the

Table 7 Conditional Power Estimates

	Observed	$b_2 = 0.75b_1$	$b_2 = 0.875b_1$
Raw data	0.0005	0.743	0.217
Log data	0.003	0.748	0.229

standard therapy and (2) only very optimistic assumptions (not supported by the data) would have to be realized to have an acceptable level of power, the decision was made not to continue enrollment in the study.

VI. DISCUSSION

The clinical trial under consideration involved a substantial number of patients who would be studied for a long period of time at a substantial cost to the company in terms of human and financial resources. The science of how to evaluate radiological progression in clinical studies is relatively new and still evolving. The study was therefore initiated without the benefit of a substantial literature on which to base decisions on efficacy endpoints and sample size.

The interim examination of the data provided for a more credible estimation of sample size and an evaluation of the likelihood of achieving a significant finding had the trial continued to completion. The result of this examination was a well-informed decision to terminate the study. This decision (1) avoided unnecessarily exposing patients to treatments in an attempt to achieve an unlikely desired result and (2) resulted in a substantial savings of resources that could be redirected toward other clinical research.

REFERENCES

Fries, J. F., Bloch, D. A., Sharp, J. T., McShane, D. J., Spitz, P., Bluhm, G. B., Forrester, D., Genant, H., Gofton, P., Richman, S., Weissman, B., and Wolfe, F. (1986). *Arthritis Rheum. 29:* 1–9.

Halperin, M., Lan, K. K. G., Wright, E. C., and Foulkes, M. A. (1987). *Controlled Clin. Trials 8:* 315–326.

Lord, F. M., and Novick, M. R. (1968). *Statistical Theories of Mental Test Scores,* Addison-Wesley, Reading, Mass., pp. 87–95.

Pocock, S. J. (1982). *Biometrics 38:* 153–162.

Ware, J. H. (1985). *Am. Stat. 39:* 95–101.

Ware, J. H. (1988). A conditional power calculation for studies comparing rates of decline, *Invited Lecture,* Wyeth-Ayerst Research.

Ware, J. H., Muller, J. C., and Braunwald, E. (1985). *Am. J. Med. 78:* 635–643.

20

Use of Interim Analyses to Design Further Studies in Analgesic Drug Preference

Albert J. Getson, Katherine H. Lipschutz, Robert L. Davis, and Balasamy Thiyagarajan

Merck Sharp & Dohme Research Laboratories, West Point, Pennsylvania

I. INTRODUCTION

Much of the statistical literature on interim analyses provides methodology by which studies, such as mortality trials, can be terminated early with adequate evidence of overwhelming efficacy. However, most of the drugs developed do not involve mortality studies. For such compounds, governmental regulations require the sponsoring company to document efficacy in well-controlled clinical studies and to demonstrate safety in a large number of patients followed for an extended period of time. As a result, sponsoring companies usually have little interest in terminating a trial early and filing a new drug application (NDA) based on the interim results.

When beginning a drug development program, success is not a certainty. In new therapeutic areas, the appropriate measures of efficacy, the relevance of potential changes, and the estimates of variability may not be well-known. Even if fundamental issues concerning the design of the clinical program are not questioned, the decision to fully develop a compound may depend on other scientific, regulatory, and business concerns. Such issues as whether to stop the program as a failure, study a different patient population or build a new production facility are too costly to wait until study completion.

With unlimited resources and time, it would be appropriate for the sponsor to conduct a pilot trial, review the results, and then decide on the scope and direction of the final program. However, with such an approach there is a hiatus while waiting for the results of a pilot study. With the exception of sample size, pilot trials can be essentially identical in design to the definitive studies conducted for registration. Therefore, it seems unreasonable to stop patient accrual while waiting to start another trial. From this point of view, the most practical strategy is to start a single full-scale trial, take an early look at the data while the study continues, and based on the results, decide on the balance of the remaining trials in the program.

While a formal test of hypothesis is not necessary at the interim look, some measure of the eventual success of the trial is needed to provide a level of comfort to the decision making. When long-term safety data are needed, the traditional group sequential approach allowing for early termination of the study may not be an advantage. Furthermore, both the sponsor and the investigators may be willing to commit to completing the trial regardless of the results of the interim analysis. Under such conditions is it necessary to adjust the α-level for any interim look?

In this chapter the discussion focuses on the development of a new analgesic compound. The principal objective of the program was to register the compound with the claim that in acute circumstances, the relief of pain occurs faster with the new drug than with the standard treatment. As an alternative to starting the entire program, it was proposed internally to start one single-dose, double-blind dental pain study. The design of the study was standard and has been used by several sponsoring companies to document clinically the analgesic efficacy of new chemical entities. This study was designed to have sufficient power potentially to be a pivotal trial in demonstrating the faster onset of analgesic activity. It was agreed to look at the data after about one-third to one-half of the patients completed the trial. The trial would run to completion regardless of the outcome of this evaluation unless there were serious concerns regarding patient safety. The interim look would consist of summary statistics and an assessment of the probability that the trial at its conclusion would yield the appropriate significant results. The calculation of the latter was based on computations given by Gould (1987) and is similar to stochastic curtailing introduced by Lan et al. (1982). The details of the protocol and a description of the methodology are contained in the following sections.

II. PROTOCOL

The study described in this chapter was a single-dose, double-blind study comparing new drug (ND) 500 mg, long-acting standard therapy 1 (ST1) 500 mg, standard therapy 2 (ST2) 650 mg, and placebo in the treatment of outpatients experiencing moderate or severe postoperative dental pain. Three hundred patients were to participate in the study: 80 on each active treatment group and 60 on placebo. The primary objective of the study was to determine whether there was a faster onset of analgesic activity with the ND than with the two standard treatments, ST1 and ST2.

Patients who were scheduled for surgical extraction of one or more impacted third molars were selected for the study. Patients were instructed to rate their pain intensity and take study medication when they first began feeling moderate to severe pain following the surgery. Patients evaluated their pain response every 30 minutes for the first 2 hours and then hourly up to a total evaluation time of 12 hours. Patients rated their pain and pain relief using the following three scales:

1. *Pain intensity* (0 = none, 1 = slight, 2 = moderate, 3 = severe) rated immediately before and after treatment until the evaluation period was over or a backup analgesic was required
2. *Degree of pain relief* (0 = none, 1 = slight, 2 = marked, 3 = complete) at the specified time intervals after treatment
3. *50% pain relief* (1 = yes, 2 = no) at the same intervals

Pain intensity was expressed and analyzed as *pain intensity difference*, defined as the change in pain intensity from baseline. Pain intensity difference values ranged from −1 to 3.

The sample sizes in this study were chosen to provide 95% power to detect a true difference of 30 percentage points in the proportion of patients (60% versus 30%) responding to treatment, with response defined as at least 50% pain relief. Faster onset of analgesic activity could be inferred if significant differences between treatments were observed early (e.g., at 0.5 and 1.0 hour postdose).

The protocol called for an interim assessment of the data when about one-third to one-half of the patients completed the study. In this situation the purpose of the interim analysis was to provide information to help make a decision about continuing the development of ND by obtaining the probabilities that ND would have a significantly faster onset, and comparable extent and duration of analgesic effect compared to ST1 and ST2 when the trial was completed. Regardless of the outcome of the interim evaluation, the trial was to continue until completion except if there were serious concerns regarding patient safety. The interim analysis was conducted under the following guidelines:

1. The results would not be shared with the investigators.
2. The identity of test therapy received by individual patients would not be disclosed to either the clinical monitor or those supervising the trial.

3. The interim assessment would consist of a presentation of summary statistics overall by treatment group and a calculation of the probability that the observed differences between the groups would achieve statistical significance when the trial was completed.

Since this interim look was for the planning of future studies and would not affect the conduct of this trial, the size and power of the statistical tests described above remained unaffected.

III. MONITORING AND DATA COLLECTION

At Merck the in-house blinding procedures for all phase III trials and most phase II trials require that clinical monitors, statisticians, programmers, and data coordinators as well as the patients and off-site study investigators be kept blind to any individual treatment allocations and overall treatment results until all data from the study have been received, verified, and a clean file generated. When a planned or unplanned interim analysis is required, this blinding system must be circumvented and someone must be able to access information regarding which treatments were received by individual patients. Knowledge of treatment results, expected or unexpected, could lead to the introduction of bias into the trial either at the study site or from within the company. For this reason, the minimum amount of information required to meet the objectives of the interim analysis should be presented only to the few people responsible for making decisions about the drug's development.

For this study it was possible to devise a system where none of the people directly involved in monitoring the study knew which treatments were received by individual patients; however, identification of the treatment groups for overall summaries of the results was necessary for meaningful discussion and interpretation of the results. The allocation schedule was retrieved electronically by an assistant statistician who was not directly involved in the study and then merged with patient identification numbers in programs used in the analysis.

IV. STATISTICAL METHODOLOGY

Consider a study of two treatments with an objective to test $H_0: \mu_x = \mu_y$. Suppose that m_1 observations on x and n_1 observations on y are available at an interim stage and m_2 more observations on x and n_2 more observations on y could be obtained if the trial is completed as planned. At the interim look of the study with $m_1 + n_1$ observations accumulated, we are interested in the probability that H_0 will be rejected with the additional data $m_2 + n_2$ observations. It is assumed that the data from both stages follow the same distribution. Following Gould (1987), we have at the interim look

$$t = \frac{(a_1\bar{x}_1 - b_1\bar{y}_1) + (a_2\bar{x}_2 - b_2\bar{y}_2)}{\sqrt{(f_1 s_1^2 + f_2 s_2^2)/(f_1 + f_2)}}$$

where $a_k = m_k/(m_1 + m_2)$, $b_k = n_k/(n_1 + n_2)$, and $f_k = m_k + n_k - 2$, $k = 1, 2$. This is a simplified pooled t-statistic based on all the data and has $f_1 + f_2$ degrees of freedom. The quantities m_1, n_1, $\bar{x}_1$, $\bar{y}_1$, and s_1^2 are based on the data collected before the interim look and the quantities m_2, n_2, $\bar{x}_2$, $\bar{y}_2$, and s_2^2 all refer to data obtained after the interim look. A predictive density for $w = (a_2\bar{x}_2 - b_2\bar{y}_2)$ and s_2^2 given the data available at this interim look could be used to compute the probability that H_0 will be rejected with the additional data.

The predictive density of w and s_2^2 given $\bar{x}_1$, $\bar{y}_1$, and s_1^2 is proportional to

$$(f_2 s_2^2)^{(f_2/2)-1}\left[f_1 s_1^2 + f_2 s_2^2 + \frac{m_1 n_1 (w - \bar{w})^2}{a_2 n_1 + b_2 m_1}\right]^{-(f_1+f_2+1)}$$

where $\bar{w} = a_2\bar{x}_1 - b_2\bar{y}_1$. If

$$v = \frac{f_2 s_2^2}{f_1 s_1^2 + f_2 s_2^2}$$

and

$$u = (w - \bar{w})\sqrt{\frac{m_1 n_1 (f_1 + f_2)(1 - v)}{(a_2 n_1 + b_2 m_1) f_1 s_1^2}}$$

then u and v are independently distributed. Furthermore, u has a central t-distribution with $f_1 + f_2$ degrees of freedom and v has a beta distribution with parameters $f_2/2$, $f_1/2$. This forms the basis for the computation of the probability of rejecting H_0.

V. STATISTICAL ANALYSIS

One-hundred one patients received study medication. Three patients were excluded from the analysis because they remedicated within the first hour after receiving the study drug. Patients whose pain evaluations were not recorded at the correct time used the observation closest (within 30 minutes) to the prescribed evaluation time. For patients who withdrew from the study early or had incomplete data for any reason, missing values were estimated by using the last available value. The interim analysis for this study consisted of tables and graphs presenting summary statistics, as well as tables of conditional probability values that estimated the likelihood that significant differences between treatments would be observed at the end of the trial, given the difference that was observed at the interim analysis.

The hourly mean pain intensity differences, mean pain relief scores, and proportions of patients with at least 50% pain relief are summarized for each treatment group in Figures 1, 2, and 3, respectively. ND appears to be superior to ST1 from hour 1 through hour 9, particularly as measured by pain relief and 50% pain relief. ND also appears superior to ST2 from hour 1 through the end of the study. ST1 appears better than ST2 from 90 minutes through the end of the study. ND and ST1 provide consistently better relief than placebo, and although ST2 is superior to placebo through hour 4, it is similar to placebo thereafter.

Table 1 displays the conditional probability that at a particular hour ND will be significantly superior to each of ST1, ST2, and placebo at the conclusion of the trial. A larger probability corresponds to a greater confidence that the observed difference between ND and each of the other treatments will achieve significance at the conclusion of the trial.

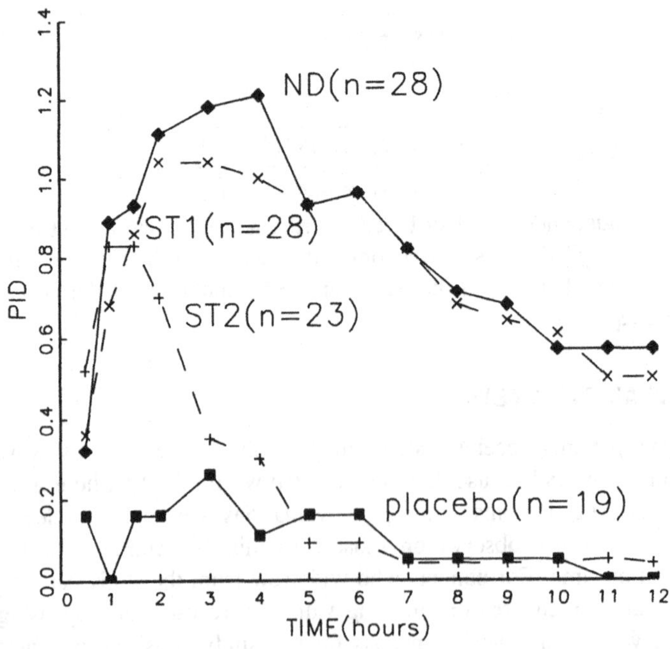

Figure 1 Mean pain intensity difference.

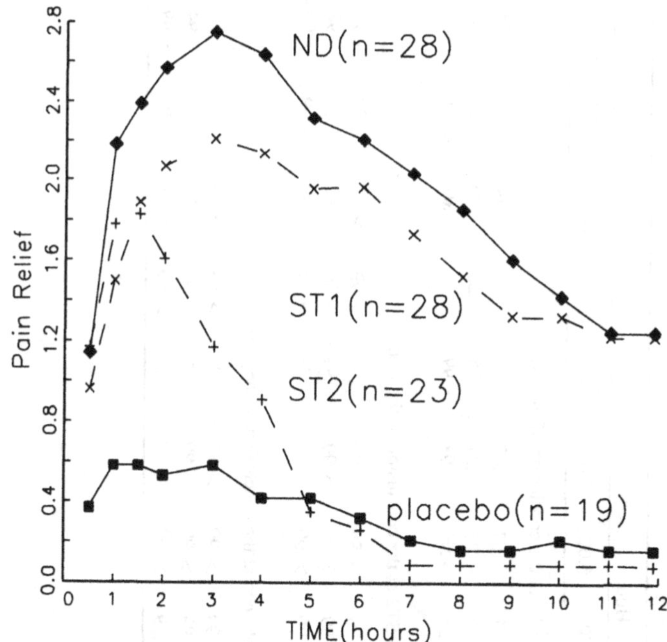

Figure 2 Mean pain relief.

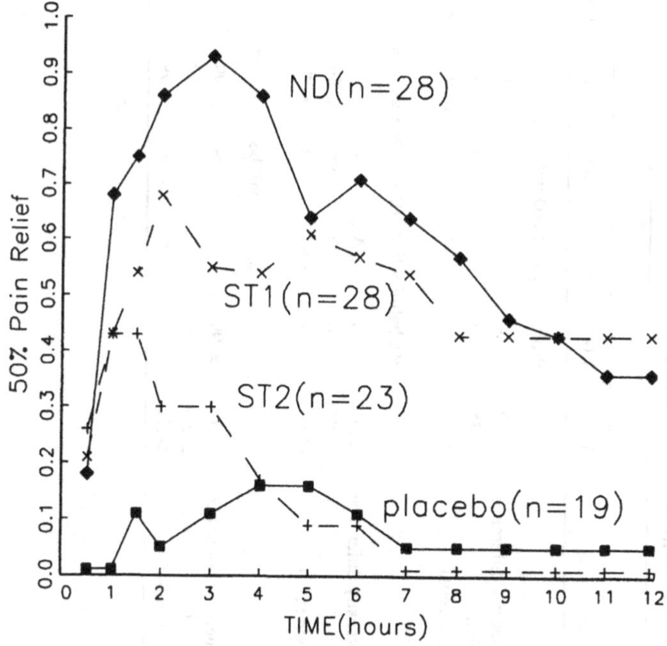

Figure 3 Percentage patients with 50% pain relief.

Table 1 Conditional Probabilities

Parameter	Hour													
	0.50	1.00	1.50	2.00	3.00	4.00	5.00	6.00	7.00	8.00	9.00	10.00	11.00	12.00
Probability that ND will be significantly superior to ST1 at the conclusion of the trial														
Pain intensity difference	.02	.66	.17	.18	.37	.80	.07	.07	.07	.14	.14	.14	.32	.32
Pain relief	.35	.90	.64	.60	.64	.50	.33	.25	.27	.35	.23	.10	.07	.06
50% Pain relief	<.02	>.99	>.99	>.99	>.99	>.99	.25	>.99	.98	>.99	.40	.07	<.01	<.01
Probability that ND will be significantly superior to ST2 at the conclusion of the trial														
Pain intensity difference	<.01	.20	.24	.94	>.99	>.99	>.99	>.99	>.99	>.99	>.99	>.99	>.99	>.99
Pain relief	.07	.56	.70	.95	>.99	>.99	>.99	>.99	>.99	>.99	>.99	.98	.97	.98
50% Pain relief	<.01	>.99	>.99	>.99	>.99	>.99	>.99	>.99	>.99	>.99	>.99	>.99	>.99	>.99
Probability that ND will be significantly superior to placebo at the conclusion of the trial														
Pain intensity difference	.73	>.99	>.99	>.99	>.99	>.99	>.99	>.99	>.99	>.99	>.99	>.99	>.99	>.99
Pain relief	>.99	>.99	>.99	>.99	>.99	>.99	>.99	>.99	>.99	>.99	.98	.95	.93	.94
50% Pain relief	>.99	>.99	>.99	>.99	>.99	>.99	>.99	>.99	>.99	>.99	>.99	>.99	>.99	>.99

VI. CONCLUSIONS

On the basis of this interim assessment the following conclusions were considered to be likely at the completion of this trial.

1. ND will have significantly better analgesia than the long-acting ST1 by the first hour after dosing, suggesting faster onset of relief. ND pain relief will remain superior to ST1 for nearly 4 hours, suggesting greater extent of relief. The duration of effect will be similar for ND and ST1.
2. The analgesic efficacy of ND will be equivalent to ST2 at 0.5, 1.0, and 1.5 hours post dose; thereafter, ND will be superior to ST2. These results suggest similar onset and greater extent and duration of effect for ND versus ST2.

VII. DISCUSSION

The results of this interim look were encouraging in that not only did the new compound provide faster pain relief, but the duration of effect was similar to that of long-acting standard therapy. These results provided information allowing management to start a full development program for the new compound, with the added benefit of having one of the two or three large clinical trials required for an NDA nearly complete. However, for this compound, the development was terminated for reasons unrelated to efficacy.

There are some risks to interim analyses. For one thing, the early data may not be representative of the study as a whole. At Merck we remind clinical monitors about the Schor–Davis rule (Davis, 1988), which states that "the best data from the best investigators always come in-house first!" Thus the early returns may be misleading, since they may reflect the best clinics. Conversely, an equally worrisome result is that the interim results may be *worse* than the final results. Another risk is that since the sample sizes are smaller in interim analyses, there may be limitations to the statistician's ability to investigate the impact of confounding factors on the results. This could be especially important if at the interim look there are unexpected results.

Pharmaceutical company statisticians should also worry about whether regulatory agencies will approve of the interim analysis in the first place. Reviewers may tend to regard any interim analysis as an opportunity for the sponsor to bias the trial. Regulatory agencies may also be concerned that the study population has been changed in midstream to achieve a more favorable result. Companies might also be required to supply reviewers a p-value adjustment on the grounds that any interim analysis provides an opportunity to stop the study early if the interim data look favorable. The statistician could head off that controversy by including a statement in the protocol to provide for an interim analysis at some small α and then make the appropriate adjustment in the final p-value when the study is completed. However, by choosing α to be infinitesimally small, the likelihood of rejecting H_0 is practically zero and in reality we would be conducting a no-penalty analysis. In general, these concerns are only cautions. This no-penalty approach is a realistic way to provide management with good information as soon as possible and should be a useful strategy in drug development.

REFERENCES

Davis, R. L. (1988). Some practical problems with interim analyses, *Biometrics Society Meeting*, Boston.

Gould, A. L. (1987). Scheduling interim analyses in group sequential trials, *ASA Proceedings of the Biopharmaceutical Section*, pp. 23–29.

Lan, K. K. G., Simon, R., and Halperin, M. (1982). Stochastically curtailed tests in long-term clinical trials, *Commun. Stat. C1:* 207–219.

21

A Sequential Trial of Dantrolene in Human Malignant Hyperthermia

Paula K. Norwood

R. W. Johnson Pharmaceutical Research Institute, Raritan, New Jersey

I. BACKGROUND

Dantrolene sodium is a direct-acting muscle relaxant that was first indicated in controlling the manifestations of clinical spasticity resulting from upper motor neuron disorders, including spinal cord injury, stroke, cerebral palsy, and multiple sclerosis. The initial new drug application (NDA) for a capsule formulation was approved in 1974. Malignant hyperthermia (MH) is a term used to describe a specific life-threatening episode initiated by use of certain general anesthetics. MH is rare: it has been reported as ranging from 1:15,000 to 1:50,000 patients exposed to general anesthetics. It was first recognized and reported in the 1960s. A familial pattern of incidence has been noted, and it is believed to be inherited as an autosomally recessive trait. It is more common in the United States in the western states than in other parts of the country.

Initial research in the use of dantrolene sodium in the treatment of MH was done in pigs. Several researchers, including Harrison (1975), Gronert et al. (1976), and Hall et al. (1977) reported dantrolene's effectiveness in treating malignant hyperpyrexia in a strain of swine inbred for susceptibility to porcine malignant hyperthermia. These researchers demonstrated dantrolene's effectiveness in porcine models of MH similar to human MH.

Malignant hyperthermia usually presents as a crisis in the operating room. The onset is often within 3 hours of administration of general anesthesia, during major surgery. The clinical signs of MH vary in severity and degree but include rapidly increased body temperature, restlessness, muscle rigidity, cyanosis, and skin mottling. It progresses to cardiac dysrhythmia and tachycardia and often to death due to cardiac arrest. Estimates of the mortality rate with the best palliative treatment available prior to the availability of dantrolene ranged from 60 to 75% of episodes.

With this background, human clinical trials of the efficacy and safety of dantrolene sodium in treating human MH were proposed. It is unusual for efficacy to be the only endpoint in a clinical trial. Typically, no more is known about the safety of a clinical treatment than is known about the efficacy, so that the approach and sample size are determined by both considerations. In this case, however, the primary indication for the drug required long-term treatment, and the long-term safety profile was relatively well understood. The treatment of MH required intravenous (IV) therapy of relatively short duration. The efficacy of dantrolene in preventing death due to malignant hyperthermia was the only endpoint of interest, provided that the treatment did not decrease the survival rate for some unanticipated reason.

Initial discussions of the proposed study were of an open nonrandomized trial, of fixed sample size, to test the hypothesis that the survival rate with dantrolene IV therapy is greater than 0.50. The choice of the comparative value of 0.50 as the historical survival rate was conservative compared to the reported survival rate of 0.25 to 0.40. It was also mathematically convenient. The sample size under consideration was 26, for good power to detect a difference between 0.50 and a theoretical survival rate for dantrolene sodium of 0.85. It was estimated that at least 3 years would be required to accrue 26 patients, if the protocol was established in a multicenter trial of approximately 100 centers.

There was no financial incentive for the company to undertake the required development. With an indication as rare as MH, the sales of the drug would be nominal. It would be unlikely ever to be great enough to recover the costs of developing a new indication with a new IV formulation. This was prior to the enactment of the Orphan Drug Act, which provides companies with tax relief for the money spent in development efforts of this kind. Therefore, any efforts to reduce the costs of development, including a possible reduction in the size of the clinical trial required, increased the chances of obtaining approval to undertake the project.

Without the requirement of establishing the safety profile other than not increasing the mortality due to malignant hyperthermia, and with the desire to minimize the clinical testing requirements, a sequential trial was proposed. Since no one wanted to increase the potential size of the trial beyond 26, the size of the proposed fixed trial, attention was restricted to closed sequential trials with the maximum sample size at or close to 26. Also, there was no interest in a two-sided test of hypothesis. Therefore, the lower bound of the sequential stopping rule was set at the point at which it would no longer be possible to reach the upper bound. Armitage calls these rules skew-restricted. In addition, two early stopping points were added to prevent the trial from continuing if the survival rate was much lower than anticipated.

Based on these considerations, a sequential study design was chosen and included in the study protocol. The following section is exactly as it appeared in the study protocol.

II. STATISTICAL ANALYSIS: DANTROLENE SODIUM IV COOPERATIVE STUDY

A. Inclusion Criteria

To include a patient in the formal analysis, the diagnosis of malignant hyperthermia must be confirmed on the basis of signs, symptoms, and laboratory data reported in the anesthetic history report, postrecovery studies reported in the case history report, and if necessary, the results of a muscle biopsy.

B. Exclusion Criteria

Even though the diagnosis of malignant hyperthermia is confirmed, a patient will be excluded from the analysis who had, prior to receiving dantrolene sodium IV, developed bradycardia, hypotension, fixed or dilated pupils, or cardiac arrest. A patient will also be excluded if there was a medically significant deviation (such as the use of a contraindicated drug) from the treatment regimen described in the protocol.

C. Method of Analysis

We propose a sequential scheme for the analysis of the efficacy of dantrolene sodium IV in reduction of the lethal effects of the malignant hyperthermia crisis. The trial would continue until any of the following criteria for stopping is achieved:

1. Stop the trial when there are

7	survivors out of	7 confirmed cases	(no deaths)
or 10	survivors out of	11 confirmed cases	(1 death)
or 12	survivors out of	14 confirmed cases	(2 deaths)
or 14	survivors out of	17 confirmed cases	(3 deaths)
or 16	survivors out of	20 confirmed cases	(4 deaths)
or 19	survivors out of	24 confirmed cases	(5 deaths)
or 20	survivors out of	26 confirmed cases	(6 deaths)
or 20	survivors out of	27 confirmed cases	(7 deaths)

Conclusion: The recovery rate with dantrolene sodium IV is significantly greater than 0.50.

2. Stop the trial when there are
   0 survivors out of 4 confirmed cases (4 deaths)
   or 1 survivor out of 6 confirmed cases (5 deaths)
   or after 8 deaths have occurred
   or after 27 confirmed cases are completed

   Conclusion: No significant difference between the survival rate with dantrolene sodium IV and 0.50 has been demonstrated.

This design is a modification of a skew-restricted sequential design described by Armitage (1960). It has (one-sided) significance level $\alpha = 0.025$ and power $1 - \beta = 0.95$ of detecting a difference between a Dantrium survival rate of 0.85 and the hypothesized survival rate of 0.50. As in any sequential design, it has the advantage that the trial is terminated early if large benefits are observed. Also, it has the disadvantage that the trial could go beyond the size of a fixed-size study of the same power.

To judge how many patients might be required, we have computed the probabilities tabulated below. These probabilities are based on the assumption that the true survival rate in malignant hyperthermia crisis is 0.90 if dantrolene sodium IV is used as described in the study protocol.

n	P (sample size $< n$)
7	0.48
11	0.72
14	0.86
17	0.93
20	0.96

III. DERIVATION OF METHOD

This design is a modification of the design given in Table 3.7 of Armitage (1975) for theta = 0.85 and $N = 27$. In the notation Armitage uses, the variable y is the difference between the number of surviving patients and the number of deaths. This, of course, is the natural variable to use in the mathematical development of boundaries for the stopping rule. The restatement given in the study protocol into the ratio of the number of survivors to the number of patients treated is a more natural statement of the stopping rule for the medical community.

The modifications to the design given by Armitage were derived as follows. The portion of the rule that says to stop after 8 deaths have occurred is the portion of the rule that results from the decision to do a one-sided test of hypothesis. This represents the line from which the upper boundary of the stopping rule cannot be reached. With no other modification, the addition of this rule makes the design a skew-restricted design of the type discussed by Armitage.

The additional two stopping points were added to provide for early stopping of the trial in the event that the survival with the use of dantrolene IV was much lower than anticipated. Both are above the point at which one would conclude that the survival rate is significantly lower than 0.50, and preclude reaching that conclusion. The choice of points was somewhat arbitrary. For the survival rate of 0.85 assumed for the purposes of planning the trial, the addition of these two points affects the power less than 0.001; the power remains greater than 0.95.

IV. RESULTS OF THE TRIAL

The results of the trial were reported by Kolb et al. (1982). It was an open multicenter study from September 1977 to May 1979 with anesthesiologists from 65 institutions in the United States and Canada acting as investigators. All of the investigators committed themselves to a standardized protocol and case report form that were approved by the appropriate institutional review boards.

Correct diagnosis of MH and adherence to protocol methodology were essential to evaluation of drug therapy. However, the clinical signs of MH vary in kind and degree, and the facilities and procedures for monitoring and laboratory tests differ among institutions. Furthermore, a crisis situation makes data collection and timing of laboratory tests difficult. Therefore, all cases reported from the study were reviewed by anesthesiologists considered expert in MH.

Clinical evidence (e.g., tachycardia, dysrhythmia, muscle rigidity, increased temperature, cyanosis, and/or mottling) prompted a suspicion of MH. The diagnosis was usually established by acid-base analysis and occasionally, when blood gases were not drawn, by correlation of the clinical picture with results of muscle biopsy (caffeine–halothane contractures). Presence of myoglobin in the urine and rise in creatine phosphokinase (CPK) furnished additional evidence of skeletal muscle damage. Patients who had a cardiac arrest or delay of more than 6 hours prior to treatment with intravenous dantrolene were excluded from statistical analysis.

During a period of 18 months, 21 patients with apparent MH were treated with IV dantrolene by 16 anesthesiologists in the study. Eight patients had good evidence supporting the diagnosis of unequivocal MH and were treated promptly. Three patients were diagnosed as probable MH and were treated promptly. Four patients were diagnosed as unequivocal MH but were treated late. These four patients therefore were excluded from the study. Three of these four died. All 11 patients with unequivocal or probable MH who were treated promptly survived. Six of the 21 patients were uncategorized as they had equivocal episodes unlikely to be MH. All six survived.

In monitoring the results of the trial for the purpose of the sequential analysis, only cases classified as unequivocal MH treated promptly were included. In some cases, confirmatory tests (e.g., muscle biopsy) were required with evaluation and confirmation of diagnosis made several days after treatment was completed. Hence eight unequivocal cases of MH, with all eight surviving, were accrued before the trial was stopped.

In summary, 15 patients with probable or unequivocal MH were identified, and 11 of these were treated promptly with IV dantrolene. Of these, eight had an unequivocal diagnosis of MH and three presented a less certain clinical picture and therefore were deemed "probable" for MH. Regardless of whether one accepts eight or 11 MH patients, there were no deaths. This satisfies the requirement to conclude that dantrolene therapy resulted in a statistically significant lower mortality than would be expected in this group of MH patients without the use of dantrolene.

This single multicenter sequential trial was the basis of the NDA filed for use of dantrolene sodium IV in the treatment of human malignant hyperthermia. Supporting data submitted included case reports of the compassionate use of Dantrium IV in less controlled clinical settings. The NDA was approved 4 months after termination of the trial, in September 1979.

V. SUMMARY

An open trial of dantrolene sodium IV was conducted to determine whether it increased the survival of malignant hyperthermia crisis above the hypothesized rate of 0.50. This was a very conservative hypothesis against a historical mortality rate reported at 0.60 to 0.75. A closed sequential design was chosen for the one-sided test of hypothesis.

Anesthesiologists from 65 institutions throughout the United States and Canada participated in the trial. During a period of 18 months, 21 patients with apparent MH were treated with IV dantrolene by 16 investigators. Of these 21 patients, eight patients with unequivocal MH were treated promptly. All eight survived. Seven survivors out of seven treated patients satisfied the stopping rule that had been established prior to the study. Delays in confirming diagnosis due to the follow-up testing required resulted in continuing the trial beyond the required 7. Upon successful treatment and confirmation of the eighth case the trial was stopped, with the conclusion that dantrolene sodium IV is effective in significantly reducing the mortality due to malignant hyperthermia.

ACKNOWLEDGMENTS

The author gratefully expresses her appreciation to Norwich Eaton Pharmaceutical for permission to publish the results of this trial.

REFERENCES

Armitage, P. (1975). *Sequential Medical Trials,* 2nd ed., Wiley, New York, p. 70.
Gronert, G. A., Milde, J. H., and Theye, R. A. (1976). *Anesthesiology 44*: 488.
Hall, G. M., Lucke, J. N., and Lister, D. (1977). *Anaesthesia 32*: 472.
Harrison, G. G. (1975). *Br. J. Anaesth. 47*: 62.
Kolb, M. E., Horne, M. L., and Martz, R. (1982). *Anesthesiology 56*: 254.

22

Randomized Play-the-Winner Designs and ECMO

Richard G. Cornell and David D. Cuthbertson

University of Michigan, Ann Arbor, Michigan

I. BACKGROUND

The mortality rate among infants with severe newborn respiratory failure was 80% or higher for many years. An alternative treatment, extracorporeal membrane oxygenation (ECMO), was introduced in 1977. Enough experience with individual cases had been gained by 1982 to undertake a randomized clinical trial. The potential existed for ECMO to lead to a survival rate of 80% or more, but it was not known if this high a success rate could be achieved in a clinical trial on infants with well-defined entry criteria. The possibility of bleeding and other adverse effects existed since ECMO is essentially a heart-lung machine, and its use involves the surgical bypass of both the heart and lungs.

With the potential for a high success rate for ECMO, an adaptive, randomized play-the-winner (RPW) design was selected for use during the first phase of experimentation. This allowed for convergence of allocations to the better treatment with high probability. Convergence to ECMO would be likely if its potential were realized, in which case the evaluation was to be continued with all patients assigned to ECMO.

An adaptive design was selected for the first phase to balance ethical and scientific concerns. This design allowed the expected number of patients assigned to the inferior treatment during the first phase to be minimized while maintaining the random allocation of treatments and other design features of a clinical trial.

The RPW design for the first phase did not ensure protection against a type I error in a hypothesis-testing context. The RPW is a treatment selection procedure as opposed to a hypothesis-testing procedure. A treatment selection procedure with an adaptive design was chosen despite the possibility of few patients on the inferior treatment, and consequently, of meager comparative data, because of the substantial past experience which indicated that the survival rate on standard intensive therapy was 20% or less.

Only one patient could be treated at a time with ECMO, and a patient was admitted to the study for randomization only if ECMO were available. The course of treatment, with either ECMO or conventional therapy, was only a few days. An adaptive design was feasible since the outcome of each case was known before the next treatment allocation was made.

Since the initial ECMO trial, the need has arisen to design another clinical trial for the comparison of ECMO with another treatment, but with ECMO as the treatment of last resort if patients deteriorate under the alternative treatment. Since ECMO has now been found to be effective in preventing death, whether used initially or as a treatment of last resort, the emphasis in this trial is not on the reduction of the expected number of deaths on the inferior treatment. However, an adaptation of the RPW approach, which allows for both the probability of a type I error and power to be controlled, is of interest to minimize the expected sample size. The design of this study is discussed after the initial RPW plan and ECMO trial are described.

II. THE DESIGN AND RESULTS OF THE ECMO STUDY

A. Objective

Wei and Durham (1978) studied RPW trials as a modification of the play-the-winner (PW) plan presented by Zelen (1969). This type of trial requires sequential recruitment of patients and a dichotomous response. The purpose of the first-phase RPW design in the ECMO trial was the selection of the best of two treatments with high probability while minimizing the expected number of patients allocated to the inferior treatment. The response was survival or death of the neonate. If the RPW phase led to selection of ECMO as the better treatment, a second phase in which all infants were assigned to ECMO was planned. The purpose of this continuation phase was to estimate the survival rate with ECMO precisely.

B. Eligibility Criteria

The eligibility criteria were established to select infants with newborn respiratory failure who had an 80% or greater chance of mortality despite optimal conventional therapy. In particular, to be eligible an infant had to fall in one of the following five categories: acute deterioration, unresponsive over a 3-hour period, barotrauma, diaphragmatic hernia, and high pulmonary insufficiency index. Additional details of the specification of these categories are given by Bartlett et al. (1985). Birthweight was required to be greater than 2 kg to ensure a high probability of surviving the ECMO surgical procedure.

C. Informed Consent

The randomized consent procedure introduced by Zelen (1979) was used in the RPW phase of this trial. Consent was not requested after randomization to conventional intensive therapy, since this was widely recognized as the best care available at that time. Consent was required after randomization to ECMO because of its experimental and invasive nature. Consent before randomization would not have been feasible. Even if consent had not been obtained after randomization to ECMO, an infant would have been regarded as assigned to ECMO in the analysis, following the intent to treat approach. However, consent was obtained for all assignments to ECMO.

D. Randomization Procedure

Allocation probabilities during the RPW phase of the trial changed based on the results with completed courses of treatment. The allocation procedure can be conceptualized with an urn model where a patient is assigned to either treatment (A or B) by random selection with replacement of either an A or a B ball from an urn containing u balls of each type initially. Each time a treatment response is observed a ball is added to the urn. An A ball is added following a success on treatment A or a failure on treatment B. Otherwise, a B ball is added. Each time a patient enters the trial a treatment is assigned by again selecting a ball at random from the urn with replacement.

The randomization was carried out by personnel in the department of biostatistics. Sealed envelopes were opened after a patient was found to be eligible for the trial. The separation of eligibility determination and randomization was made to avoid selection bias in the admission of patients to the trial. The potential for bias was also reduced by designating the treatments as A and B, without the biostatistician knowing the identity of the treatments. After each outcome was known, the biostatistician was notified that treatment A or B had been successful or unsuccessful, and new random assignments were prepared. The random selection was done in accord with the urn model, using a random number generated by a computer program.

E. Stopping Rule

Wei and Durham suggested a stopping rule for an RPW trial which calls for termination of the trial when the total number of balls added to the urn for either one of the treatments first reaches a prescribed integer r. This is the stopping rule used in the randomization phase of the ECMO trial. It has already been mentioned in the description of the urn sampling model that the design calls for u balls of each type in the urn initially. To design the ECMO trial it was necessary to select values of u and r that met design specifications in order to carry out the sequential adaptive randomization plan.

F. Design Specification

In their evaluation of RPW trials, Wei and Durham only consider the case where $u = 0$ in detail because their primary purpose was to compare the RPW plan with the PW plan, for which u is always zero. However, we wished to take $u > 0$ in the ECMO trial to reduce selection bias and to retain more nearly equal allocation probabilities longer.

We compared RPW plans for several pairs of r and u integers. In particular, we tabled the smallest values of r for which the probability of correct selection (PCS) $\geqslant 0.95$ and 0.99 for several values of u and pairs of success probabilities, γ and η, for treatments A and B, respectively. Treatment A denotes the better treatment, so $\gamma > \eta$. Let ASN (average sample number) denote the expected number of patients in the RPW phase. Let ITN refer to the expected number of patients allocated to the inferior treatment. Values of ASN and the ITN are tabled by Cornell et al. (1986) for combinations of r, u, γ, and η for which PCS $\geqslant 0.95$ and 0.99. Indices of possible patient selection bias (PSB) are also given.

The calculation of ASN and ITN was based on the recursive calculation of probabilities denoted by Π_{ab}, where Π_{ab} is the probability of adding a balls of type A and b balls of type B to the urn as a function of η, γ, and u. Initially, $\Pi_{00} = 0$. Also, $\Pi_{rr} = 0$ since random allocation ceases once r balls of either type are added to the urn. Otherwise,

$$\begin{aligned}
\Pi_{ab} &= [P_{a-1,b}\gamma + (1-P_{a-1,b})(1-\eta)]\Pi_{a-1,b} + [P_{a,b-1}(1-\gamma) + (1-P_{a,b-1})\eta]\Pi_{a,b-1} \\
\Pi_{rb} &= [P_{r-1,b}\gamma + (1 - P_{r-1,b})(1 - \eta)]\Pi_{r-1,b} \qquad (1) \\
\Pi_{ar} &= [P_{a,r-1}(1 - \gamma) + (1 - P_{a,r-1})\eta]\Pi_{a,r-1}
\end{aligned}$$

for a, $b = 0, 1, \ldots, r - 1$, where $\Pi_{ab} = 0$ for either a or $b < 0$.

Equation (1) utilizes the probability, P_{ab}, of an allocation to treatment A, given that a balls of type A and b balls of type B have been added to the urn. This probability is given by

$$P_{ab} = \frac{u + a}{2u + a + b} \qquad (2)$$

This follows from each allocation being made randomly with replacement from an urn with $u + a$ balls of type A and $u + b$ balls of type B.

Since A denotes the better treatment and randomization stops after r balls of either type are added to the urn,

$$\text{PCS} = \sum_{b=0}^{r-1} \Pi_{rb} \tag{3}$$

$$\text{ITN} = \sum_{a=0}^{r-1} \sum_{b=0}^{r-1} \Pi_{ab}(1 - P_{ab}) \tag{4}$$

For the ECMO randomization phase, u was set to equal 1, the minimum such that either a control or treatment allocation was possible for each admission to the trial. The stopping rule, determined in advance, was to discontinue the randomization whenever 10 balls of one type were added to the conceptual urn. For $r = 10$, the tables in Cornell et al. (1986) show that PCS $\geqslant 0.95$ for all $\eta \leqslant 0.5$ and $\delta \geqslant 0.4$. These ranges of η and δ values were chosen to give an adequate PCS even if η were larger, or δ were smaller, than anticipated.

G. Statistical Analysis

The statistical analysis planned for the randomization phase consisted simply of selecting the treatment, A or B, which had r balls added to the urn. Then the identity of the selected treatment was ascertained. If it were ECMO, allocation to ECMO would continue using the same admission criteria. If it were standard therapy, additional allocations to standard therapy under the admission protocol for this study would be unnecessary, since standard therapy was known to yield a high mortality rate. If allocation to ECMO were continued, the planned method of analysis was confidence interval calculation, using all data on ECMO outcomes from both the randomization and continuation phases. Since the study was completed, Wei (1988) has presented a permutation method for testing the null hypothesis of no difference in treatment effect with a play-the-winner treatment allocation rule.

H. Results

When the ECMO trial was carried out, an r of 10 was attained after only 10 patients were treated, one of whom was randomized to conventional therapy and died, and nine of whom were randomized to ECMO and survived. Later Wei (1988) calculated a significance level of 0.051 for the RPW phase of the trial. At the time the trial was done, the RPW phase merely led to the selection of ECMO for further study without randomization.

Two additional patients were successfully treated with ECMO at the time of the publication by Bartlett et al. (1985). Later Cornell et al. (1986) reported that 19 successes without any failures had been obtained with ECMO. They calculated a lower one-sided 99% confidence limit for the probability of survival on ECMO (γ) of 0.785. Data from the treatment of ECMO patients at Michigan has been entered into a multicenter registry for which Toomasian et al. (1988) reported a survival rate of 81% for 715 cases. These rates are well above the survival rate observed for conventional therapy in the past and confirm that the choice of ECMO as the better treatment for survival was appropriate.

III. THE DESIGN OF AN RPW TRIAL FOR HYPOTHESIS TESTING

A. Objective

The use of the RPW design in the ECMO trial has been criticized primarily because it afforded little opportunity for the comparison of ECMO and standard treatment (Ware and Epstein, 1985; Paneth and Wallenstein, 1985; Begg, 1990). It relied heavily in its design and interpretation on evidence that the survival rate on conventional intensive therapy was low for neonates eligible for the trial and on the desire to minimize the ITN subject to a high probability of selection of the better treatment.

The ECMO trial did not lead to a test of hypothesis, but only to a decision to evaluate ECMO further without continued randomization to control therapy. Ware (1987) has pointed out that the PCS corresponds to power in a hypothesis-testing setting, so our RPW design has high power against specified differences δ, but does not necessarily provide protection against a type I error based on concurrent observation of both conventional and new treatments. In fact, under the null hypothesis that $\eta = \gamma$, the probability of the selection of the control treatment is 0.5, which equals α in the terminology of hypothesis testing.

Currently there is interest in developing an RPW design for comparing ECMO and standard therapy for the treatment of severe respiratory conditions in older infants. An adaptive design is of interest to avoid an unnecessarily large ITN. However, reduction in the ITN is no longer the primary concern because it is expected that the survival rate will be high in both the ECMO and standard therapy arms. The reason is that the protocol calls for switching any infant in the standard therapy arm to ECMO if sufficient deterioration takes place, so the comparison is between ECMO and a regimen that combines standard therapy with ECMO as rescue therapy.

The accrual of patients is expected to take a considerable period of time. Thus a reduction in the ASN is of primary interest. The use of an RPW design with a data-dependent stopping rule in addition to an adaptive randomization plan leads to the possibility of a reduction in sample size. The objective is to test the null hypothesis of equal treatment effects, instead of only treatment selection, with control over both the probability of a type I error and the power.

Ware (1989) describes a design with a data-dependent stopping rule but without adaptive allocation probabilities. His design calls for stopping randomized allocation once a prescribed number of deaths is observed either on conventional therapy or ECMO. This design was used for an experimental evaluation of ECMO at Harvard (O'Rourke et al., 1989) subsequent to the RPW clinical trial described by Bartlett et al. (1985).

Cornell et al. (1986) have suggested design modifications that enable the RPW design, with both adaptive randomization and a data-dependent stopping rule, to be used for hypothesis testing. These design features and their implementation are described here.

B. Decision Criteria

First a modified decision criteria is presented that requires $b \leqslant t < r$ when a reaches r in order for rejection of the null hypothesis that ECMO is not better than control therapy. The method of calculation of t is different from that suggested by Cornell et al. (1986), who used a formula for posterior probability.

Let η be the probability of successful treatment on control therapy. Let γ be the corresponding probability of success on ECMO. Under the null hypothesis, $\gamma = \eta$. Under the alternative hypothesis, $\gamma > \eta$. Note that these definitions are consistent with those given earlier in terms of the probability of success under the inferior and superior treatments. Similarly, a and b now will be used to refer to the numbers of ECMO and control balls added to the urn, respectively.

The design considered here provides for a modification in the decision criterion. Before the treatment selected for further study was the treatment for which r balls were added to the urn first. Now a critical value t, where $t < r$, is specified at the design stage. The null hypothesis (H_0) is rejected in favor of the alternative hypothesis (H_1) only if r is achieved for ECMO and the number of balls added to the urn for the control treatment at the time that the rth ball is added for ECMO, denoted by s, is such that $s < t$.

Note that the change in the decision rule leads to a modification in the stopping rule. If a $(t + 1)$st control ball is added to the urn, the null hypothesis can be retained without waiting to accumulate r balls of either type. So the stopping rule calls for stopping whenever r ECMO balls or $t + 1$ control balls are added, whichever occurs first.

The critical value t for any given r is the largest integer for which the probability of a type I error is less than or equal to a prespecified maximum α. This probability is calculated by modifying equation (3) for PCS in two ways:

the upper limit of summation is t instead of $r - 1$, and γ is set equal to η in the calculation of the Π_{ab} terms. Thus the actual α for given r is given by

$$\alpha = \sum_{b=0}^{t} \Pi_{0;rb} \tag{5}$$

where $\Pi_{0;rb}$ denotes Π_{rb} calculated under H_0 with $\gamma = \eta$. The probability P_{ab} is the probability of an allocation to ECMO in this hypothesis-testing setting.

As before, the integer assigned to the design parameter r is the minimum value for which the power is greater than a specified value. The formula used for power is the same as that for PCS given earlier, calculated with η and an alternative value of $\gamma > \eta$, except for one modification. The upper limit for the summation is t instead of $r - 1$, since the null hypothesis is rejected only if $s \leqslant t$. Thus the power, denoted by $1 - \beta$, is given by

$$1 - \beta = \sum_{b=0}^{t} \Pi_{1;rb} \tag{6}$$

where $\Pi_{1;rb}$ denotes Π_{rb} calculated under H_1 with $\gamma > \eta$.

Equation (5) gives the value of α for a one-sided test. For a given t, the sum in equation (5) should be doubled for a two-sided test. Another term, equal to $\Sigma_{a=0}^{t}\Pi_{1;ar}$, should be added to the sum in equation (6) to calculate $1 - \beta$ for a two-sided test. Moreover, a two-sided test also requires that the stopping rule be modified so that r balls of either type may be added provided that not more than t balls of both types are added. A one-sided test is appropriate for our ECMO example. Therefore, to avoid complexity, the rest of the formulas presented will be for one-sided tests only.

When $s \leqslant t$, equation (5) can also be used to calculate the empirical significance level, denoted by P, after a RPW trial is completed, by replacing t by s in the upper limit of summation. For $s = t + 1$, a formula to estimate P is

$$P = \sum_{b=0}^{t} \Pi_{0;rb} + \sum_{a=q}^{r-1} [P_{at}(1 - \gamma) + (1 - P_{at})\eta]\Pi_{0;at} \tag{7}$$

where q is the number of ECMO balls added to the urn before the $(t + 1)$st control ball is added.

C. Rate of Adaptation

In using an RPW trial for hypothesis testing, it is desirable to take u large so that initial allocation probabilities are not very sensitive to the early results of the experiment. However, this could increase the ITN inordinately and make the RPW design little different than one with equal allocation probabilities throughout.

To counter the specification of a large value of u, Cornell et al. (1986) suggest another design modification. They present a formula that accelerates the divergence of the allocation probabilities as the results in favor of one of the treatments becomes pronounced. They set

$$P_{ab} = \left(\frac{1}{2}\right)\left[1 + \operatorname{sign}(a-b)\left|\frac{a-b}{2u+a+b}\right|^{v}\right] \qquad 0 \leqslant v \leqslant 1 \tag{8}$$

where $\operatorname{sign}(a-b) = 0$ when $a = b$. When $v = 1$, equations (2) and (8) are equivalent and there is no acceleration. When $v = 0$, $P_{ab} = 0$ or 1 and maximum acceleration is attained.

D. Design Specification

Values of r and t can be calculated for specified maximum α and power. Values of η and γ must also be determined. Under the null hypothesis, this requires the specification of η with γ set equal to η. Under the alternative hypothesis, a minimum threshold value of γ is required. Design parameters u and v must also be chosen.

Once these specifications are made, $\Pi_{0;ab}$ and $\Pi_{1;ab}$ can be calculated recursively. The sums in equations (5) and (6) for α and power can be accumulated concurrently, as can those for ITN and ASN. Equation (4) for ITN is modified by replacing Π_{ab} with $\Pi_{1;ab}$ since it is important to minimize allocations to control therapy only when ECMO is better. The modified stopping rule is incorporated into the upper limit on the second sum, which is t instead of $r-1$. The resultant equation for ITN is

$$\mathrm{ITN} = \sum_{a=0}^{r-1} \sum_{b=0}^{t} \Pi_{1;ab}(1 - P_{ab}) \tag{9}$$

The equation for ASN is

$$\mathrm{ASN} = \sum_{b=0}^{t} \Pi_{1;rb}(r+b) + \sum_{a=0}^{r-1} [P_{at}(1-\gamma) + (1-P_{at})\eta]\Pi_{1;at}(a+t+1) \tag{10}$$

Note that equation (10) is also presented under H_1. The sample size never exceeds $r+t$ under H_0 or H_1.

In the calculation of design parameters, a trial value of r is selected and a corresponding value of t is determined which satisfies equation (5). Then equation (6) is used to see if r is large enough to meet the power requirement. If not, r is increased by one and the procedure is repeated. If the trial r is large enough, it is reduced by one to see if a smaller value could be used. The final (r, t) pair selected is the one that minimizes r subject to the restraints on α and power.

The recursive and iterative nature of the calculations lends itself to computer programming. We have prepared a BASIC program for this purpose.

E. ECMO Examples

In the setting of the original ECMO trial, with $\eta = 0.2$, $\gamma = 0.6$, $u = 0$ or 1, and $v = 1$ (no acceleration), tables in Cornell et al. (1986) display a minimum r value of 9 and an ASN = 17 for PCS $\geqslant 0.95$. The corresponding values of ITN for $u = 0$ and 1 are 4.7 and 5.2, respectively. Suppose that we require $\alpha \leqslant 0.05$ and $1 - \beta \geqslant 0.90$ for a one-sided test of hypothesis. The procedure described here, with $u = 0$, leads to a minimum value of r of 27 paired with a t of 18. The corresponding values of ASN and ITN are 39.6 and 13.5. Note that the limitation imposed on the probability of a type I error has led to larger values for r, ASN, and ITN despite the reduction in minimum power (PCS) from 0.95 to 0.90. Also note that ITN < ASN/2, unlike a design with equal allocation probabilities throughout.

For the experiment under consideration, a reasonable specification for η is 0.50. A threshold value for γ under the alternative hypothesis is 0.85. It is required that $\alpha \leqslant 0.05$ and $1 - \beta \geqslant 0.80$ for a one-sided test. For $u = 10$ and $v = 1$, $r = 27$, $t = 15$, ASN = 36.2, and ITN = 15.4. A value of u this large makes the initial allocation probabilities quite stable, but the expected sample size is too large to be feasible. Acceleration of the adaptation of the allocation probabilities, once the results favor one treatment over the other, may be achieved by taking $v = 0.5$. This reduces r, t, ASN, and ITN to 20, 10, 24.1, and 8.7, respectively. This illustrates the advantage of accelerated adaptation when combined with initial stability of the allocation probabilities.

IV. DISCUSSION

We have reviewed the design of an RPW clinical trial that led to the selection of ECMO for continued evaluation as an alternative to conventional intensive therapy. This was preceded by individual case studies and followed by the formation of an ECMO registry. These studies form a progression with the study design changing in response to accumulated information for both ethical and scientific reasons.

One important aspect of the RPW ECMO study has been the discussion generated on adaptive randomized clinical trials. Much of this is contained in published comments and rebuttals following the papers by Ware (1989), Begg (1990), and Royall (1991).

Criticisms of the RPW phase of the ECMO trial mainly concern the lack of concurrent information on the control treatment, the use of a treatment selection procedure without protection against making a type I error and the use of the randomized consent procedure. These criticisms would be valid in the absence of substantial historical information on the poor performance of the control treatment and without the great but unproven potential for better results with the new treatment, ECMO.

Although the survival rate with ECMO was high during both the randomization and the continuation phases of the initial clinical trial, the lack of concurrent testing with control patients led many scientists to doubt the findings. However, many physicians accepted the results and many clinical centers have established ECMO teams for the treatment of respiratory distress in newborn infants. Moreover, the findings of the initial study have been confirmed in a subsequent study at Harvard with a similar two-phase design.

The experience with the initial ECMO trial has led to the modifications presented here which make the RPW approach appropriate for experiments aimed at the comparison of two treatments with a test of hypothesis. These modifications provide for more allocations to the control treatment and protection against a type I error. They lead to larger experiments and more allocations to the inferior treatment than in the original RPW trial. A procedure for acceleration of the adaptation rate is suggested to lessen the impact of protection against rejection of control therapy in favor of a new experimental therapy. However, even with acceleration, a RPW procedure would not be preferred to a traditional experiment with equal allocation probabilities unless the potential exists for the new treatment to be much better than the control treatment.

REFERENCES

Bartlett, R. H., Roloff, D. W., Cornell, R. G., Andrews, A. F., Dillon, P. W., and Zwischenberger, J. B. (1985). Extracorporeal circulation in neonatal respiratory failure: a prospective randomized trial. *Pediatrics 76*: 479–487.

Begg, C. B. (1990). On inferences from Wei's biased coin design for clinical trials. *Biometrika 77*: 467–473.

Cornell, R. G. (1987). Play-the-winner in pediatrics. *Proceedings of the Biopharmaceutical Subsection of the American Statistical Association*, pp. 243–245.

Cornell, R. G., Landenberger, B. D., and Bartlett, R. H. (1986). Randomized play-the-winner clinical trials. *Commun. Stat. Theory Methods 15*: 159–178.

O'Rourke, P. P., Crone, R. K., Vacanti, J. P., Ware, J. H., Lillihei, C. K. W., Parad, R. B., and Epstein, M. F. (1969). Extracorporeal membrane oxygenation and conventional medical therapy in neonates with persistent pulmonary hypertension of the newborn: a prospective randomized study. *Pediatrics 84*: 957–963.

Paneth, N., and Wallenstein, S. (1985). ECMO and the play the winner rule. *Pediatrics 76*: 622–623.

Royall, R. (1991). Ethics and statistics in randomized trials. *Stat. Sci. 6*: 52–62.

Toomasian, J. M., Snedecor, S. M., Cornell, R. G., and Bartlett, R. H. (1988). National experience with extracorporeal membrane oxygenation for newborn respiratory failure: data from 715 cases. *ASAIO Trans. 34*: 140–147.

Ware, J. H. (1987). Evaluation of new technologies of potential great benefit. Presentation at the *Meeting of the Biometric Society and the American Statistical Association*, Dallas, March 22–25.

Ware, J. H. (1989). Investigating therapies of potentially great benefit: ECMO. *Stat. Sci. 4*: 298–306.

Ware, J. H., and Epstein, M. F. (1985). Extracorporeal circulation in neonatal respiratory failure: a prospective randomized study. *Pediatrics 76*: 850–851.

Wei, L. J. (1988). Exact two-sample permutation tests based on the randomized play-the-winner rule. *Biometrika 75*: 603–606.

Wei, L. J., and Durham, S. (1978). The randomized play-the-winner rule in medical trials. *J. Am. Stat. Assoc. 73*: 840–843.

Zelen, M. (1969). Play the winner rule and the controlled clinical trial. *J. Am. Stat. Assoc. 64*: 131–146.

Zelen, M. (1979). A new design for randomized clinical trials. *N. Engl. J. Med. 300*: 1242.

Index

Printed in the United States
by Baker & Taylor Publisher Services

Printed in the United States
by Baker & Taylor Publisher Services